UPPERS, DOWNERS, ALL AROUNDERS

Physical and Mental Effects of Psychoactive Drugs

Third Edition

Darryl S. Inaba, Pharm.D.

Director, Drug Detoxification, Rehabilitation, and
Aftercare Program of the Haight-Ashbury Free
Medical Clinics and Associate Clinical Professor of Pharmacology,
University of California Medical Center, San Francisco

William E. Cohen

Communications and Education Consultant,
Haight-Ashbury Detox Clinic

Michael E. Holstein, Ph.D.

Southern Oregon State College,
School of Social Science, Education, Health, and Physical Education

CNS Publications, Inc.™

Ashland, Oregon

CNS Publications, Inc. ™
Paul J. Steinbroner—Publisher
130 Third St.
P.O. Box 96
Ashland, OR 97520
Tel: (541) 488-2805   Fax: (541) 482-9252

Uppers, Downers, All Arounders
Third Edition
Second Printing

Book Design: By Design/Wendy LaChance
Illustrations: Impact Publications/David Ruppe
Cover Design: Lightbourne Images
Printing and Color Separations: Cedar Graphics, Cedar Rapids, Iowa
Editor: Carol A. Caruso
Photo Rights and Coordination: Paul J. Steinbroner

Special thanks to

Michael Aldrich, Ph.D., Curator, Fitz Hugh Ludlow Memorial Library, San Francisco, California

Carlton Blanton, Ph.D., Associate Professor and Advisor, Department of Health and Nutritional Science, Cal State University, Los Angeles, California

Dana C. DeWitt, Ph.D., Coordinator, Law Enforcement Program, Department of Justice Studies, Chadron State University, Chadron, Nebraska

Lou Hughes, Ph.D., Drug Prevention Consultant, Professor, Cal State University, Los Angeles, California

Jerry Lotterhos, M.S.W., Director, Substance Abuse Track, Department of Rehabilitation Studies, East Carolina University, Greenville, North Carolina

Peter Myers, Ph.D., Director, Addictions Studies Program, Essex County College, Newark, New Jersey

Rick Seymour, M.A., Director of Training and Education, Haight-Ashbury Free Clinic, San Francisco, California

David E. Smith, M.D., Founder, Haight-Ashbury Free Clinics, San Francisco, California

DISCLAIMER: Information in this book is in no way meant to replace professional medical advice or professional counseling and treatment.

ISBN 0-926544-25-X

*D*edicated to all those who provide drug abuse education, prevention, treatment, and aftercare. May you find continued fulfillment and joy in your work. The authors also acknowledge a debt of gratitude to those clients of the Haight-Ashbury Detox Clinic who so generously shared their stories of addiction and recovery so that others may learn from their experiences.

PREFACE

The information and quotations in this book are based on the experiences and clinical expertise of the 130 staff members of the Haight-Ashbury Detox Clinic in San Francisco, California and on the experiences of more than 85,000 clients who have been treated at the Clinic over the last 30 years.

The Haight-Ashbury Detox Clinic treatment program has one of the highest caseloads and best success rates in the country due in part to its success in drug education. They have found that objective nonjudgmental information about drugs and their effects is important in treatment and crucial in drug abuse prevention.

THE THIRD EDITION

The changes in the Third Edition of **Uppers, Downers, All Arounders** are based on the teaching experiences of the hundreds of professors and instructors, including the authors, who have used the previous editions in numerous teaching situations. We have endeavored to make the information presented in each chapter clear and accurate through chapter profiles, precise headings, chapter summaries, and expanded illustrations. In addition, the Third Edition presents the latest research on addiction, trends in drug use, and new concepts in the field of chemical dependency based on the practical experience in the Clinic and other treatment centers.

At the suggestion of many instructors using the Second Edition of Uppers, Downers, All Arounders, we have reorganized this Third Edition into 10 chapters instead of the previous 12 in order to make the book easier to use.

Highlights

Chapter 1: A more extensive survey of history with expanded illustrations; more precise classifications of psychoactive drugs.

Chapter 2: An integration of the various theories of addiction, including new research on the neurochemistry of addiction.

Chapter 3: Expanded coverage of meth-amphetamine and tobacco.

Chapter 4: The latest information on the heroin trade, prescription drug diversion, and smuggled sedatives, such as Rohypnol®.

Chapter 5: Expanded coverage on alcohol from neurochemical, health, and sociological perspectives.

Chapter 6: A greatly expanded marijuana section, including new insights from users as well as information on the latest research. GHB, MDMA, and other "rave" club drugs are examined.

Chapter 7: Called **Other Drugs and Other Addictions**, this chapter covers inhalants and sports drugs as well as new sections on compulsive gambling, eating disorders, and other addictive behaviors.

Chapter 8: Prevention is now the driving force of this chapter. It examines the reasons each age group uses drugs and then describes prevention techniques for that group.

Chapter 9: A greatly expanded comprehensive look at all phases of treatment based on addiction theory and the experience of the Haight-Ashbury Drug Detox Clinic.

Chapter 10: A more detailed examination of the connection between mental health and drug abuse; also covers the latest information on psychiatric medications.

Appendices: A greatly enhanced bibliography; a more extensive index for reference purposes; and detailed review questions which reinforce the information presented in each chapter.

Trademark symbol: In order to distinguish between trade (brand) and chemical (generic) names of prescription and over-the-counter drugs, we have included the symbol ® after all trade names.

CONTENTS

CHAPTER 9   365

TREATMENT

CHAPTER 10   417

MENTAL/EMOTIONAL HEALTH AND DRUGS

Mental Health and Drugs

Dual Diagnosis or the Mentally Ill Chemical Abuser (MICA)

Psychoactive Drugs:
History and Classification

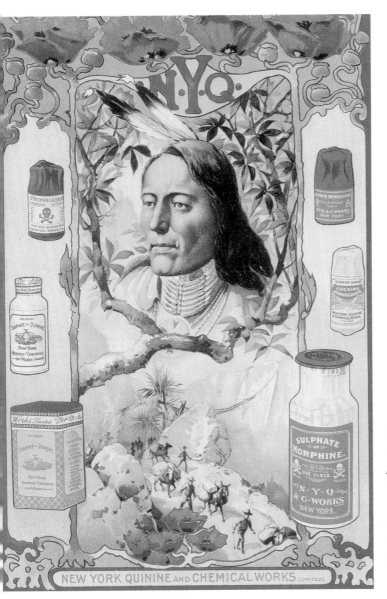

*T*he New York Quinine and Chemical Works (c. 1901) carried products that would treat multitudes of ill-nesses and moods.

(Collection Theodore Robinson, Richboro, P.A. Courtesy of Harry N. Abrams, Inc., New York)

HISTORY OF PSYCHOACTIVE DRUGS

- **Prehistory:** Mind-altering drugs have been used by humans since before recorded history.

- **Ancient Civilizations:** The earliest psychoactive drugs were alcohol, opium, marijuana, coca (cocaine), and psychedelic mushrooms.

- **Middle Ages:** Other psychedelic plants (e.g., khat, caffeine, henbane) were discovered. Ruling classes kept control of the supply.

- **Renaissance and Enlightenment:** Tobacco use, distilled alcoholic beverages, and opium smoking spread. Governments controlled much of the trade for economic gain.

- **Nineteenth Century:** New refinement techniques (e.g., synthesis of heroin from opium), new delivery methods (e.g., hypodermic needle), and new manufacturing and marketing techniques (e.g., cigarette-rolling machine and advertising) increased use, abuse, and addiction liability.

- **Twentieth Century:** Wider distribution channels, better refining techniques, and new synthetic drugs made legal and illegal use much more widespread. Government control and criminality increased.

- **Today and Tomorrow:** After a decline in the 1980s, use of illegal drugs in the '90s is increasing, especially marijuana, methamphetamines, MDMA, LSD, and heroin. Alcohol and tobacco remain the most dangerous drugs.

CLASSIFICATION OF PSYCHOACTIVE DRUGS

- **What Is a Psychoactive Drug?:** Psychoactive drugs can be identified by chemical name, trade name, or street name. This book classifies drugs by their general effects.

- **Major Drugs:**

  Uppers: Stimulants, such as cocaine, amphetamines, Ritalin®, caffeine (coffee, tea, colas), and nicotine (cigarettes, chewing tobacco), force the release of energy chemicals. The strongest stimulants (cocaine and amphetamines) produce intense euphoria or a "rush."

  Downers: Depressants include opioids (e.g., heroin, codeine), sedative-hypnotics (e.g., Xanax®, barbiturates), and alcohol. They depress circulatory, respiratory, and muscular systems. They can also sedate, lower inhibitions, and cause some euphoria.

  All Arounders: Psychedelics (e.g., marijuana, LSD, MDMA) can cause some stimulation, but mostly they alter sensory input and can cause illusions and hallucinations.

- **Other Drugs:**

  Inhalants: Organic solvents, volatile nitrites, and nitrous oxide (laughing gas).

  Anabolic Steroids and Other Sports Drugs: Drugs used to enhance performance in sports.

  Psychiatric Medications: Antidepressants, antipsychotics, and antianxiety drugs prescribed to rebalance brain chemistry.

1921

HARDING'S PEN SPEEDS DRIVE AGAINST DRUGS

President Signs Congress Re-solution to Join with Other Nations in Limiting Supply

Negotiations to Open at Once with Lands That Grow the Bases of Opium and Cocaine

1929

COOLIDGE SIGNS BILL FOR DOPE-CURE FARMS

NEW U.S. LAW WILL HELP END NARCOTIC EVIL, SAVE ADDICTS

JANUARY. 20, 1929
All Drug Slave" Convicts Will Be Sent to Farms First for Rehabilitation

Washington, Jan. 19 - President Coolidge today signed the Porter Bill, creating two Federal farms where narcotic drug addicts may be cured of their affliction.

1986

Reagan, Congress Call for Drug War

Washington
House and Senate leaders and President Reagan called for bipartisan cooperation against drugs yesterday while all sides continued to maneuver for the political spotlight on what is becoming a major issue of the 1986 Congressional Campaign.

The administration wants to spend a few hundred million dollars and some members of Congress are talking of a billion and a half or more.

Clinton Reveals New Drug Strategy

Plan increases enforcement on methamphetamine
1996

"Finally, the president ends his silence on the drug problem," said Senator Paul Coverdell, R-Ga. "For three long years, the president stood mute, as illegal drugs ravaged our schools. neighborhoods and

recycled proposals he has made before. It reiterated the call in his 1997 budget for $15.1 billion in federal drug spending, an increase of about 9 percent over the amount budgeted for this year. About two-

HISTORY OF PSYCHOACTIVE DRUGS

Drug use in contemporary life is by no means a new or unique phenomenon. For much of history, humans have searched for ways to alter their states of consciousness. Whether it has been to reduce pain, forget harsh surroundings, alter a mood, explore feelings, promote social interaction, escape boredom, treat a mental illness, stimulate creativity, or enhance the senses, some people have felt a desire to chemically change their perception of reality. Which drugs are to be used, how they are to be used, what constitutes abuse, and how abuse is prevented, treated, or punished have varied from culture to culture and within the same cultures during different periods of human history.

PREHISTORY

Many of the drugs available today are of recent discovery, refinement, or synthesis but most of them have antecedents in plants that have been around for millions of years. More than 4,000 plants yield psychoactive substances. About 60 have been in constant use throughout history, with Cannabis, opium, coca, tea, coffee, tobacco, and plants that yield alcohol predominating.

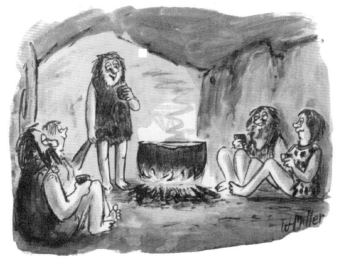

"Hey, what is this stuff? It makes everything I think seem profound."

Drawing by Miller; © 1978 The New Yorker Magazine, Inc.

Evidence exists that Neanderthals used medicinal plants 50,000 years ago. One hypothesis maintains that mind-altering or "psychoactive" drugs were used by prehistoric shaman healers throughout Eurasia and that the earliest Native Americans brought their interests in these drugs with them as they migrated from Asia to the Americas about 20,000 years ago.

There are many ways other than using drugs to radically change our perception of reality: through religious experiences, such as fasting, meditating, and praying; by going without sleep, food or drink; by chanting, dancing, working, loving, or creating music or art; by intense exercise or sports. But over the centuries, most cultures have also chosen psychoactive drugs as one of the routes (albeit a shortcut) to altered states of consciousness.

ANCIENT CIVILIZATIONS

Civilizations have also differed in the religious and social controls placed on drug use. In ancient times, geographic isolation kept the customs of different peoples localized. But migration, exploration, conquest, and trade made various psychoactive substances more widely available. The spread of Cannabis along ancient trade routes is one example. The more contact people had with other cultures, the more drugs and drug practices there were to choose from.

ALCOHOL

Alcohol has been with us since the beginning of civilization. Perhaps hunger, thirst, or curiosity made early humans eat or drink foods that had begun to ferment. Liking the taste and the psychoactive effects, they learned how to make some themselves. Many ancient cultures looked on alcohol, particularly wine, as a gift from their gods. In legends, Osiris gave alcohol to the Egyptians, as did Dionysus to the Greeks. In ancient Egypt, alcohol was given to workers building the great pyramids. The Jewish people have historically used wine as part of their religious celebrations.

An early documented attempt to regulate and control alcohol use dates back to the Babylonian Code of Hammurabi in

Make not	thyself helpless	in	drinking in the

beer shop. For will not the words of [thy] report repeated

slip out from { thy mouth } without { thy knowing } { that thou hast uttered them ? }

Falling down   thy limbs   will be broken, [and]

no one will   give thee { a hand [to help] thee up}   as for thy

companions in the   swilling of beer,   they will get up

and say, " Outside with   this   drunkard."

This hieroglyphic from 1500 B.C. advised moderation in drink as well as avoidance of other compulsive behaviors.
Translation from *Precepts of Ani*, World Health Organization.

2000 B.C. This code set forth standards of measurement for beer and wine, offered consumer protection guidelines, and outlined the responsibilities of alcohol servers.

"The vine bears three types of grapes: the first of pleasure, the next of intoxication, and the third of disgust."
Anacharsis, 600 B.C.

Heavy drinking was recognized as a problem by the Egyptians in 1500 B.C. when their hieroglyphics started to advise the moderate consumption of beer. As early as the fourth century B.C., Aristotle wrote that "women who drink wine excessively give birth to children who drink excessively of wine." By the first century B.C. in Rome, alcohol use was distinguished from alcohol abuse by the philosopher Seneca. By the fourth century A.D., heavy drinkers were led through town by a cord strung through their noses. Habitual offenders were tied with a nose cord in the public square and left for ridicule.

OPIUM

More than 6,000 years ago, the Sumerians, living in the area we now call Iran, cultivated the opium poppy. They named it, "the joy plant." The milky white fluid from the dried bulb was boiled to a sticky gum and chewed, burned and inhaled, or mixed with fermented liquids and drunk. It was used for both its medicinal properties of pain relief or diarrhea control and its mental properties of euphoria and

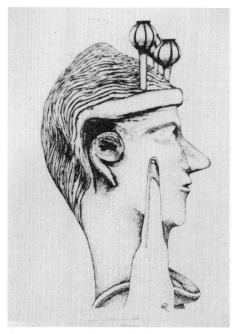

Sumerian crown decorated with incised opium poppies c. 3000 B.C.
Courtesy of the Fitz Hugh Ludlow Memorial Library

CANNABIS (marijuana)

According to legend, in 2737 B.C., the Chinese emperor Shen-Nung, in the first medical herbal encyclopedia called the *Pen-tsao,* wrote about the medicinal uses of Cannabis (marijuana) along with 364 other drugs he had tested on himself. Over the centuries, it was recommended for constipation, rheumatism, absent-mindedness, female disorders, malaria, beriberi, and for the treatment of wasting diseases. Other evidence shows that the Chinese were well aware of its stupefying and hallucinogenic properties. In the fifth century B.C., a Taoist priest reported that necromancers (channelers of dead spirits who foretell the future) used it in combination with ginseng root to "set forward time and reveal future events." In India, almost 1,500 years before the birth of Christ, the *Atharva-Veda* (sacred psalms) sang of Cannabis as one of five plants that give freedom from distress or anxiety.

About 500 B.C., the Scythians, whose territory ranged from the Danube to the Volga River in Eastern Europe, threw Cannabis on hot stones placed in small tents and inhaled the vapors. The Greek historian Herodotus wrote, "No Grecian vapor bath can surpass the Scythian tent. The Scythians, transported with the vapor, shout for joy." Most often, though, Cannabis was prized as a source of fiber and oil, for its edible seeds, and as a medicine. Archaeologists have found traces of its use 10,000 years ago in Asia.

PSYCHEDELIC MUSHROOMS

The Vedas of ancient India also sang of various other psychedelic drugs. Aryan tribes drank an extract of the *Amanita muscaria* mushroom, also called the fly agaric. In fact, "Soma," their name for the hallucinogen, was also the name of one of

sedation. Because it was a potent and, therefore, desirable substance, rulers and holy men often tried to limit its use to increase their control over society.

Opium was used in many ways. Ancient Egyptian medical texts referred to opium both as a cure for illness and as a poison. In Egypt, it was a remedy for crying babies. The substance, called "shepen," was described as opium mixed with fly-specks (or more probably opium poppy seeds). About 700 B.C. in *The Odyssey,* Homer spoke about another opium mixture called nepenthe, given by Helen of Troy to Telemachus "to lull all pain and bring forgetfulness of grief." Even Hippocrates, the Father of Medicine, wrote about poppy juice and its usefulness as a narcotic painkiller.

their most important gods. Over 100 holy hymns from the Rig-Veda are devoted to Soma. (The name "Soma" has been used to represent such diverse drugs as a mythical psychedelic in Aldus Huxley's novel *Brave New World* and a modern prescription muscle relaxant.) The intoxication, hallucinations, and delirium produced by psychedelic mushrooms have been employed over the centuries in religious ceremonies by native tribes from India and Siberia. A totally different species of mushroom was used in Aztec and Mayan cultures in pre-Columbian Mexico.

MIDDLE AGES

PSYCHEDELIC PLANTS

Other psychedelics used over the centuries include members of the nightshade family *Solanaceae* which contain the psychedelic chemicals atropine and scopolamine. Commonly abused plants in this family are belladonna, henbane, mandrake root, and jimson weed or thornapple. They were sometimes used by medicine men and women accused of witchcraft. Henbane had been referred to as early as 1500 B.C. It was used as a poison and a painkiller. It was also used to mimic insanity, produce hallucinations, and generate prophecies. Belladonna, known as "witch's berry" and "devil's herb," dilates pupils and inebriates the user. Mandrake, a root occasionally shaped like a human body, was used in ancient Greece as well as in medieval times. Its properties, similar to those of belladonna and henbane, cause disorientation and delirium.

PSYCHEDELIC MOLD (ergot)

Another psychedelic which has persisted through the ages is found in ergot, a

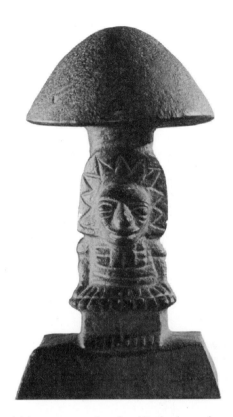

A Mayan stone god, sculpted in the shape of a mushroom (c. 500 A.D.), is one of many sculptures of the psychedelic Psilocybe mushroom. Some date back to 100 A.D.
Courtesy of the Archives Sandoz, Basel

brownish purple fungus that grows on rye or wheat plants and contains lysergic acid diethylamide, the natural form of the synthetic LSD. This drug, considered a poison until 1943 when its psychedelic nature was recognized, is referred to in ancient Greek literature. Over the centuries, there have been numerous outbreaks of ergot poisoning when whole towns, particularly in rye-consuming areas of Eastern Europe, seemed to go mad, occasionally with great loss of life. Hallucinations, sometimes permanent insanity, and gangrene were com-

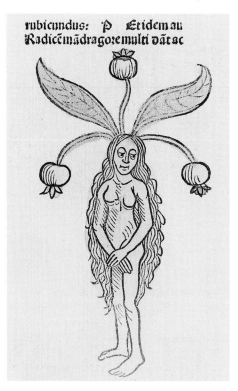

rubicundus: p Etidem au
Radicēmādragoremulti vātac

This representation of a mandrake root shows how its similarity to the human form might have been thought to increase the magic aura surrounding its use.

Courtesy of the National Library of Medicine, Bethesda

mon. One of the outbreaks gave the name "St. Anthony's Fire" to the affliction because victims developed a strange burning sensation in their extremities. Another outbreak is speculated to have been a stimulus for the Salem witchcraft trials in seventeenth-century America.

ALCOHOL

In the Middle Ages, European monasteries cultivated grapes to assure a supply of wine for their meals and for the Eucharistic sacrament. Since alcohol also killed bacteria and micro-organisms that lived in water, alcoholic beverages were often the only safe liquids to drink. As the hordes of invading barbarians, from the Goths to the Huns, swept through Europe, Europeans found solace in wine.

During the late Middle Ages, people learned how to increase the alcoholic content in beverages from 14% up to 50% by the process of distillation, making it easier to get drunk and aggravating the problems caused by heavy drinking.

ISLAMIC SUBSTITUTES FOR ALCOHOL

After the seventh century throughout the Arab Empire, opium was seen as an acceptable substitute for alcohol which was forbidden by the Koran. Opiates were taken to control pain and diminish grief. They were also used recreationally. Later, coffee, tobacco, and hashish were employed as substitutes for alcohol in order to alter consciousness.

Khat, a stimulant, was also permissible in Islamic cultures. It was used during long prayer ceremonies to help the people stay awake. Khat also seems to have paved the way for coffee among Islamic peoples. In 1238 A.D., the Arab physician Naguib Ad-Din distributed khat to soldiers to prevent hunger and fatigue. In the fourteenth century, another Arab king, Sabr Ad-Din, gave it freely to subjects he had recently conquered to placate them and quell their revolutionary tendencies.

COFFEE (caffeine)

The coffee plant, originally found in Ethiopia about 600 A.D., was intensely cultivated in Arabia where it was both popularized and persecuted. Called "the wine of Islam," it was to Arabia what tea had become to China since the third century B.C. At first, coffee was consumed by chewing the beans or by infusing the leaves in water. It was used for medicinal purposes until the fourteenth century. Then, during the later Middle Ages, coffee, like alcohol, was made even more potent once people learned how to roast and grind the beans, producing a cheaper and tastier version. It took 500 more years until caffeine, the active ingredient in coffee and tea, was finally identified.

COCA (cocaine)

Almost eight centuries ago in South America, the Incan Emperor Manco Capac controlled use of the coca leaf, the natural source of cocaine. Written accounts said, "The right to chew the coca leaf was prized far above the richest presents of silver and gold." All the nobility carried their precious supply of coca leaves in ornate bags strapped to their wrists. A plentiful supply of the drug, which was considered divine, was buried with the mummified nobility. The use of coca never reached Europe because of the difficulty in cultivating the plant outside South America.

PSYCHEDELIC FUNGI AND PLANTS

To the north of the Incan Empire, about the time Columbus arrived in the Americas, the Aztec, Huichol, Cora, and Tarahumare Indians of Mexico were digging up the peyote cactus (containing mescaline), "magic mushrooms" (containing psilocybin), and the ololiuqui vine (containing DMT-like psychedelic constituents). They celebrated the hallucinogenic effects of these plants in sacred ceremonies. However, the Spanish conquistadors and Christian clerics considered peyote and other hallucinogenic drugs to be Satanic instruments. In fact, a manual published in 1760 that contained a list of

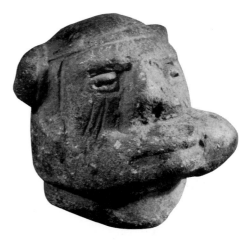

Colombian stone head depicting user's cheek stuffed with concada, coca leaf mixed with powdered lime.
Courtesy of the Fitz Hugh Ludlow Memorial Library

questions to ask potential converts included the question, "Have you practiced cannibalism or eaten peyote?"

RENAISSANCE AND ENLIGHTENMENT

Two general trends continued the spread of psychoactive substances. Beginning with Portuguese and Spanish exploration and colonization, Europeans encountered diverse cultures and new psychoactive substances, most notably coffee from Turkey and Arabia, tobacco from the New World, tea from China, and the kola nut from Africa. Similarly, European explorers, soldiers, merchants, traders, and missionaries carried their own culture's drugs and drug-using customs, especially beers, wines, and later distilled spirits, to the rest of the world. Greater secularization of life, urbanization, and spreading wealth increased contact with new drugs. These factors, combined with growing personal freedom, increased use.

COFFEE

Coffee drinking became widespread, first among wealthy classes, then as quantities increased and prices declined, among middle and lower classes. Coffee became a favorite drink to try to counteract alcohol abuse. In cities, it was drunk in coffee houses which became popular centers of intellectual, political, and literary discussion and news circulation. In both Turkey and England, coffee houses were closely watched by authorities as possible hotbeds of political dissent, sedition, and revolution. With the British conquest of India in the early eighteenth century, cheap tea became widely available in England and began to replace coffee as the favorite stimulant drink.

TOBACCO

In 1492 after sailing the ocean blue, Columbus noted that the American Indians smoked tobacco. They used it as part of their religious rituals and also as remedies for snake-bite, stomach and heart pains, skin diseases, and a variety of other ailments. (He also noted that the Caribbean natives snuffed cohoba, which is a potent psychedelic substance.) Soon the Spaniards were exporting tobacco to Europe where it was received enthusiastically not only for its mental effects but also for its supposed medicinal qualities (an

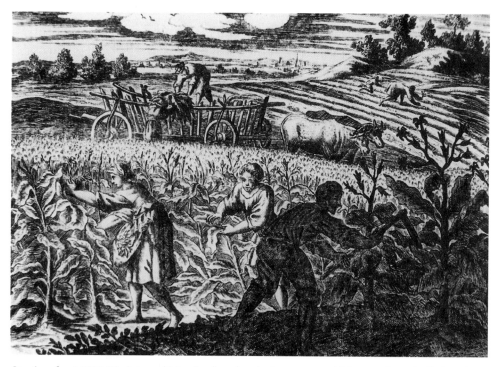

Starting about 1610, Virginia and Maryland produced tobacco crops which were planted, tilled, and picked by slave labor and which supported the Chesapeake Colonies for two centuries.
Courtesy of the National Library of Medicine, Bethesda

idea that lost favor after a few hundred years).

Seeds were brought from Brazil to France, where tobacco was eventually called "nicotiana" after Jean Nicot who described its medicinal properties. Portuguese sailors introduced tobacco to Japan where its cultivation began about 1605. Despite prohibition, prison sentences, and fines, its use spread. The Portuguese probably introduced tobacco to China as well where it was highly regarded as a medicine. It was carried throughout China by soldiers, then banned, then taxed. It was in vogue first at the Emperor's court, then among the people, and then actively propagated throughout Asia.

"The use of tobacco is growing greater and conquers men with a certain secret pleasure, so that those who have once become accustomed thereto can later hardly be restrained therefrom." Sir Francis Bacon, 1610

The dangers of fire, the congregation of smokers in tobacco houses or tobacco taverns where ideas and politics were discussed, and the abuse of tobacco by the clergy led to vigorous attacks by various authorities, including King James I of England.

"[Smoking is] a custome lothsome to the eye, hatefull to the Nose, harmefull to the braine, dangerous to the Lungs, and the blacke stinking fume thereof, neerest resembling the horrible Stigian smoke of the pit that is bottomless."

King James I, A Counter-Blaste to Tobacco, 1604

Pope Urban VIII forbade smoking under pain of excommunication. It was also forbidden in Turkey by sultans under pain of torture and death and banned by Czars Michael and Alexis in Russia under similar

penalties. But smuggling and widespread covert use by clergy, by commoners, and by people at court defeated all attempts at prohibition. Eventually, tobacco became a large source of revenue for many governments, especially for Spain and later for England. It also helped finance much of the U.S. Revolutionary War.

OPIUM

During the Renaissance in the fifteenth and sixteenth centuries, the use of opium in medicinal concoctions came back into favor when the works of the second-century physician Galen and the Moorish physician Avicenna became widely taught in medical education. Theriac, one of the opium preparations that came into favor again, was used in the Middle East and in Europe. It originally contained more than 70 ingredients in addition to opium, and Galen added over 30 more. Among other things, it was prescribed for poisoning, inflammation, and pestilence. Galen prepared it for several Roman Emperors. Since opium controls diarrhea, pain, headaches, and anxiety and produces a certain euphoria, its presence in theriac is thought to be the main reason for the popularity of the drug.

In 1524, Paracelsus (Theophrastus von Hohenheim) returned from Constantinople to Western Europe with the secret of laudanum, a tincture of opium in alcohol. It was employed as a panacea or cure-all medication and, for many, a simple way to soothe a crying child. It was readily available, inexpensive, and soon was widely used (and abused) in all strata of society. Laudanum, like both nepenthe and theriac before it, was found in most home remedy chests. Scrooge drank it in Charles Dickens' *A Christmas Carol*, and it is still in use today.

Benjamin Franklin, one of America's Founding Fathers, died addicted to opium which he was taking for gout. Samuel

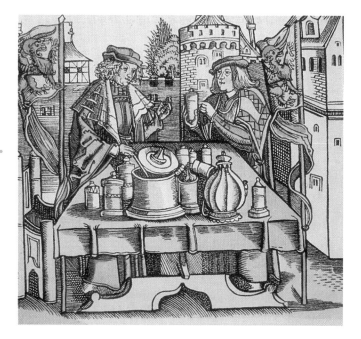

The preparation of theriac, the ancient cure-all, is depicted in this sixteenth century woodcut. From H. Brunschwig, Das Neu Distiller Buch, *Strassburg, 1537.*

Courtesy of the National Library of Medicine, Bethesda

Taylor Coleridge probably wrote his famous poem *"Kubla Khan"* while under the influence of opium.

> *Beware! Beware!*
> *His flashing eyes, his floating hair!*
> *Weave a circle round him thrice,*
> *And close your eyes with holy dread,*
> *For he on honey-dew hath fed,*
> *And drunk the milk of Paradise.*
> Samuel Taylor Coleridge, 1797

Coleridge was a miserable, guilt-ridden addict who drank laudanum daily to control the pain of chronic heart disease. In fact, alcohol, opium, and other drugs have been an occupational hazard for many writers and philosophers throughout the centuries.

DISTILLED LIQUORS (alcohol)

The availability of rum, gin, whiskey, and other ardent spirits in the eighteenth century also led to widespread drunkenness. Beer and wine had long been part of the European diet. Ancient beer, much thicker than modern beer, was a food, contributing B vitamins and other nutrients to European diets. But now, some people began to drink distilled spirits having virtually no nutritional content just to get drunk.

Gin, first made in Holland during the 1600s from fermented mixtures of grains flavored with juniper berries, became popular throughout Europe. When the English began producing their own, consumption, urban alcoholism, and the mortality rate skyrocketed. During "the London gin epidemic" from 1710 to 1750, the novelist Henry Fielding said that gin was the principal sustenance of more than 100,000 Londoners, and he predicted that "should the drinking of this poison be continued at its present height, during the next 20 years, there will be by that time very few of the common people left to drink it." It was estimated that one house in six in London was a gin house. Only stiff taxes and the

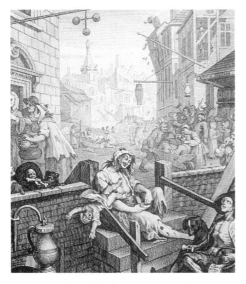

The gin epidemic devastated London from 1710 to 1750. Engraving by William Hogarth depicts "Gin Lane."
Courtesy of the National Library of Medicine, Bethesda

strict regulation of sales brought the epidemic under control.

During the latter half of the eighteenth century, rum was the chief medium of exchange in the slave trade and a mainstay of the economy of colonial America (as were tobacco and Cannabis or hemp), producing probably the highest level of alcohol consumption in American history. Around 1790, per capita consumption was three times what it is today. Similarly, white trappers and settlers trading whiskey ("firewater") to Native Americans for furs in the late eighteenth and early nineteenth centuries led to epidemics of alcoholism among both settlers and indigenous peoples.

CANNABIS (marijuana, hemp)

King George III of England sent a proclamation to America in 1761 to encourage the planting of hemp. His purpose was to establish an American textile and rope industry so the colonies could depend on a local supply. George Washington cultivated hemp at his Mount Vernon plantation, and he too encouraged its production as a domestic source of rope and sails for the fledgling navy of the United States. Until the Civil War, hemp was the nation's second largest crop behind cotton. But because hemp was dependent on slave labor, it was no longer profitable after the slaves were freed.

NINETEENTH CENTURY

NITROUS OXIDE

Inhaling a gas (as opposed to smoking a drug) became popular in the 1800s with the discovery of nitrous oxide or "laughing gas." Nitrous oxide was first used as an intoxicant and later found to be an anesthetic. Several other gases used for anesthesia were also developed during the century, namely chloroform and ether. Both men and women participated in "gas frolics" in the 1830s.

OPIUM

The production and distribution of drugs have often had economic motives. Since the Chinese did not want to buy anything that the English sold, the British government grew opium in India to trade for tea with China in order to balance their trade. The Chinese had banned opium use and imports because of the terrible costs of crime, corruption, and addiction, but the British insisted on their "right" of free trade. "The Wars for Free Trade," as the British called them, or the "Opium Wars" (1839–42, 1856–60) as the rest of the world called them, were fought to enforce the British right to sell opium to Chinese merchants who, in turn, sold it to the peasants, creating one of the world's worst drug

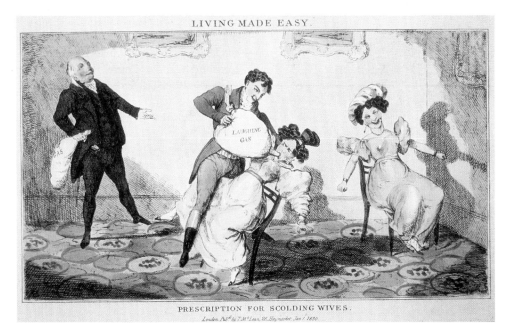

This 1830 print from England with its caption, "Living Made Easy," depicts a "gas frolic."
Courtesy of the National Library of Medicine, Bethesda

problems. Later in the century, the French as well as the English both owned a monopoly on the distribution of opium throughout their empires. The resulting addiction of many Chinese, the indignities of China's defeat, and the unequal treaties imposed by Western countries after the Opium Wars continue to complicate China's relations with the West even today.

About 1800, a German pharmacist, Frederick W. Serturner, developed morphine from opium. Morphine is much more powerful than opium and was incorrectly thought to have no negative side effects. By mid-century, morphine tablets were being dispensed and were widely used, as was injected morphine by the time of the Civil War. By 1868, both opium and morphine had become cheaper than drinking alcohol and use had spread so widely (especially among women) that Dr.

Horace B. Day, a nineteenth century physician, declared an opium epidemic in the United States. In his book, *The Opium Problem: Suggestions as to Remedies,* Dr. Day stated that 1 out of every 300 Americans was an opium addict, a proportion surprisingly close to the ratio of U.S. heroin addicts in 1996.

DRUG REFINEMENT

In the 1860s, soon after the hypodermic needle was developed, cocaine was isolated from the leaf of the coca bush. In 1874, heroin was refined from morphine at St. Mary's Hospital in London. In 1898, the German Bayer Company began marketing heroin as a remedy for coughs. Using drugs in their natural forms (chewing coca leaves or smoking opium) could cause addiction. But more potent versions of drugs and

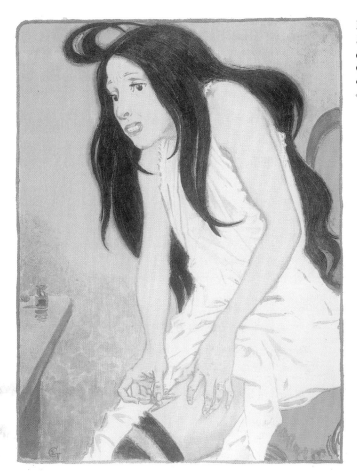

Morphinomania *by Eugene Samuel Grasset, 1897.*

Courtesy of the Ars Medica Collection. Philadelphia Museum of Art

more rapid delivery systems (snorting processed cocaine powder or shooting heroin into veins with hypodermic needles) accelerated the number of compulsive users.

TEMPERANCE AND PROHIBITION MOVEMENTS

The first temperance movement in the United States had been started about 1785 by Dr. Benjamin Rush, a noted physician and reformer who warned against overuse of alcohol but praised limited amounts for health reasons. In spite of the warnings, alcohol use continued to grow until it peaked in 1830 in the United States with per capita consumption of 7.1 gallons of pure alcohol versus 1.8 gallons today. In fact, at Andrew Jackson's inauguration in 1833, the new President's staff stopped serving alcohol because they were afraid drunken revelers would destroy the White House. But it wasn't until 1851 that Maine passed the first prohibition law. Within four years, one-third of the states had laws controlling the sale and use of alcohol, and consumption fell to one-third of pre-Prohibition and temperance levels. The Civil War stalled and in some cases reversed the prohibition movement, but after the war, the Women's Crusade, the Women's Christian Temper-

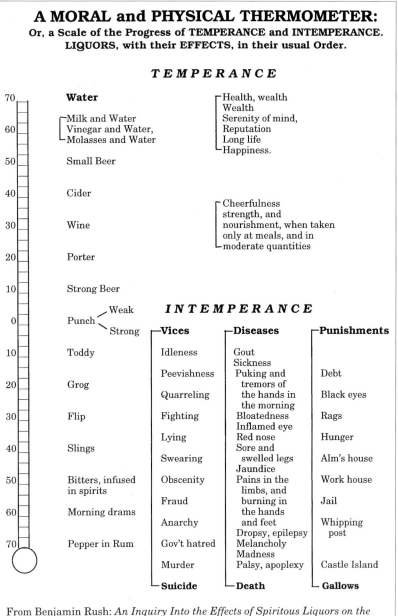

A MORAL and PHYSICAL THERMOMETER:

Or, a Scale of the Progress of TEMPERANCE and INTEMPERANCE.
LIQUORS, with their EFFECTS, in their usual Order.

T E M P E R A N C E

70	**Water**	⌐Health, wealth
		Wealth
	⌐Milk and Water	Serenity of mind,
60	Vinegar and Water,	Reputation
	└Molasses and Water	Long life
		└Happiness.
50	Small Beer	
40	Cider	
		⌐Cheerfulness
		strength, and
30	Wine	nourishment, when taken
		only at meals, and in
		└moderate quantities
20	Porter	
10	Strong Beer	

I N T E M P E R A N C E

	Liquor	⌐Vices	⌐Diseases	⌐Punishments
0	Punch ╱ Weak ╲ Strong			
10	Toddy	Idleness	Gout	
			Sickness	
		Peevishness	Puking and	Debt
20	Grog		tremors of	
		Quarreling	the hands in	Black eyes
			the morning	
30	Flip	Fighting	Bloatedness	Rags
			Inflamed eye	
		Lying	Red nose	Hunger
40	Slings		Sore and	
		Swearing	swelled legs	Alm's house
			Jaundice	
50	Bitters, infused in spirits	Obscenity	Pains in the limbs, and	Work house
		Fraud	burning in	Jail
60	Morning drams		the hands	
		Anarchy	and feet	Whipping
			Dropsy, epilepsy	post
70	Pepper in Rum	Gov't hatred	Melancholy	
			Madness	
		Murder	Palsy, apoplexy	Castle Island
		└Suicide	└Death	└Gallows

From Benjamin Rush: *An Inquiry Into the Effects of Spiritous Liquors on the Human body*, 1790

Published in 1785, the Moral Thermometer *by Dr. Benjamin Rush, an early temperance pioneer, allowed for the moderate and medicinal use of alcohol but warned that excess use would eventually lead to the stocks, insanity, death, jail, or the gallows. His booklet,* An Inquiry into the Effects of Ardent Spirits upon the Human Mind and Body, *was widely distributed in post-Revolutionary America.*

ance Union, and the Anti-Saloon League led the temperance movement, which later became the prohibition movement, into the twentieth century.

TOBACCO

By the middle of the century, both men and women used snuff and smoked pipes. In addition, men smoked cigars, chewed tobacco, and spat tobacco juice where and when they pleased. One of the changes that propelled tobacco to a grave health problem was the invention of the automatic cigarette-rolling machine in the late 1800s. Historically, only small amounts of tobacco had been used—a pinch of snuff, a leaf in the cheek, or a gram in a pipe. It wasn't until later in the century that automation, advertising, and a more plentiful supply of tobacco vastly expanded the use of cigarettes.

HEROIN AND COCAINE IN TONICS AND PATENT MEDICINES

Cocaine was very popular in America by 1885. In 1887, the Hay Fever Association declared cocaine to be its official remedy. It was offered for sale in drug stores, by mail order, and in catalogues. There were coca cigarettes and small cigars. Vin Mariani, a fine Bordeaux wine laced with coca leaf extract, became quite popular beginning in the 1890s, spurred on by the first celebrity endorsements from such luminaries as Thomas Alva Edison and President William McKinley. From its formulation in 1886 until 1903, Coca-Cola® contained, about 5 milligrams of cocaine or one-third to one-half of a "line." Today, the beverage contains a nonnarcotic coca flavoring and caffeine.

Over-the-counter medicines sold at the turn of the century had imaginative names, such as Mrs. Winslow's Soothing Syrup,

Roger's Cocaine Pile Remedy, Lloyd's Cocaine Toothache Drops, and McMunn's Elixir of Opium, all loaded with opium, heroin, cocaine, and usually alcohol. Needless to say, patent medicines were very popular in all strata of society and were used to cure any illness from lumbago to depression, much like nepenthe, theriac, and laudanum centuries before.

TWENTIETH CENTURY

TOBACCO

A variety of factors increased the use of cigarettes and decreased the cigar smoking and tobacco chewing that had marked the nineteenth century: public health campaigns against chewing tobacco and spitting; better cigarette paper and machinery for producing more cigarettes at a cheaper cost; development of a milder strain of tobacco which enabled smokers to inhale smoke deeper; and encouragement of women and children to learn to smoke.

The pioneer in the "mild" cigarette was the "Camel" brand produced by R.J. Reynolds. During the 1920s, this brand began to be actively marketed to women (as a symbol of female emancipation), to young people, and to those on diets. Inspired by the success of Prohibition, antismoking efforts redoubled. State laws were passed prohibiting cigarettes, but they were largely unenforceable and were repealed by the late 1920s. By the '30s, taxes on cigarettes provided a rich source of revenue for federal and state governments during the Depression and World War II. By the end of the war, demand for cigarettes sometimes exceeded supply, and smoking was considered socially acceptable.

By mid-century, smoking was entrenched in American society. It was a source of revenue for advertisers, retailers,

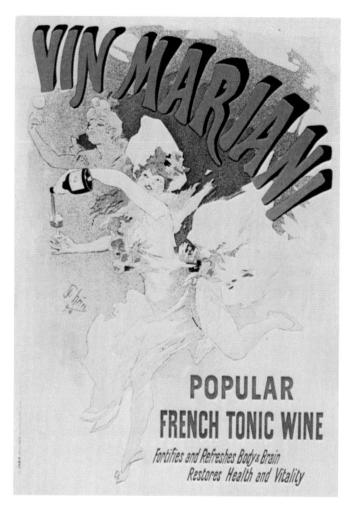

Ad for French tonic wine, made with coca leaf extract. It promised to help the user's digestion and disposition (c.1896 by Charles Levy).
Courtesy of the estate of Timothy C. Ploughman

tobacco farmers, the media, and government treasuries. Warnings of the health hazards of smoking were issued as early as 1945 by the Mayo Clinic. Warnings continued throughout the early 1950s from the American Cancer Society and various heart and physicians' associations. The tobacco industry ridiculed health concerns and responded to health warnings with slogans, such as "Old Golds: For a treat instead of a treatment," and with the formation of The Tobacco Institute, the chief political lobbying group of the industry. In 1964, the Surgeon General issued a report that con-cluded, "Cigarette smoking is a health hazard." Smoking generally decreased through the '60s, then began rising during the '70s, and then went into a long decline that continues into the present.

REGULATION

Heroin/cocaine kits were advertised in newspapers and sold in the best stores. Even though by the 1890s physicians understood the addictive and psychosis-inducing effects of cocaine, it took another two decades before regulation began. The

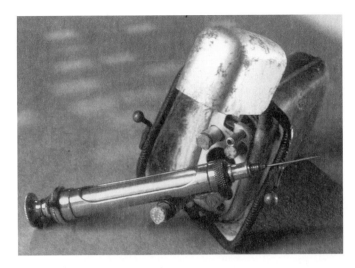

Drug kit on sale at Macy's (c. 1908) included vials of cocaine, heroin, and a reusable syringe.
Courtesy of the Fitz Hugh Ludlow Memorial Library

Pure Food and Drug Act (1906), the Opium Exclusion Act (1909), and the Harrison Narcotic Act (1914) eliminated the over-the-counter availability of opiates and cocaine. Unfortunately, the tight control of all supplies encouraged the development of an illicit drug trade.

ALCOHOL PROHIBITION

In 1918, it took 12 months to ratify the Eighteenth Amendment prohibiting the manufacture and sale of liquor. Thirteen years later it only took 10 months to repeal that same amendment. Americans hadn't changed their feelings about the benefits or liabilities of alcohol. They had simply found out that Prohibition created other devastating problems for America.

Unfortunately, by that time, a new coalition of smugglers, strong-arm thieves, Mafia members, corrupt politicians, and crooked police had developed a lucrative trade in the distribution and sale of illicit alcohol. With the return of alcohol to legal status, this coalition turned to other illicit drugs, like heroin and cocaine, which eventually gave rise to a multi-billion dollar business that continues to make illegal drugs the leading cause of crime and corruption in the world today.

With the end of Prohibition, alcoholism increased again, though it took 20 years for per capita drinking to reach pre-Prohibition levels. Higher levels of alcoholism were answered by the creation of an organization to help alcoholics recover. Alcoholics Anonymous (AA), a spiritual

PROHIBITION REPEAL IS RATIFIED AT 5:32 P. M.;
ROOSEVELT ASKS NATION TO BAR THE SALOON;
NEW YORK CELEBRATES WITH QUIET RESTRAINT

Headlines of the time seemed to be happy about the end of Prohibition.

State House Bootlegger Is Barred in Maryland	CITY TOASTS NEW ERA	The Repeal Proclamation	FINAL ACTION AT CAPITAL
Special to THE NEW YORK TIMES. ANNAPOLIS, Md., Dec. 5.—	Crowds Swamp Licensed	Special to THE NEW YORK TIMES. WASHINGTON, Dec. 5.—The text of the proclamation	President Proclaims the

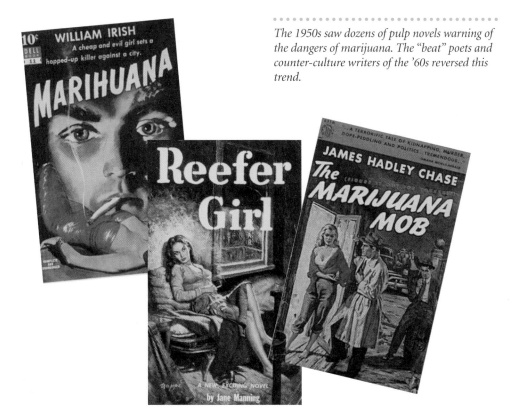

The 1950s saw dozens of pulp novels warning of the dangers of marijuana. The "beat" poets and counter-culture writers of the '60s reversed this trend.

program that teaches alcoholics 12 steps to recovery, was founded in 1934 by two alcoholics, Bill Wilson and Dr. Bob Smith. Over the years, AA and its offshoots, such as Narcotics Anonymous, have proved themselves to be the most successful drug treatment programs in history.

MARIJUANA (Cannabis)

In 1937, *Cannabis sativa* (marijuana) was banned despite its use in numerous medicines for over 5,000 years. Although sterilized hemp seeds could still be used for birdseed under the Marijuana Tax Act, the other economic uses of hemp for fiber, rope, paper, and oil were effectively prohibited except for a brief period during World War II when hemp fiber was needed by the military. Banning medicinal uses of mari-

juana was unusual since opiate-based medications, which are stronger than marijuana, were never banned, only controlled through prescription. One reason that marijuana was banned was an antimarijuana campaign by the Hearst newspapers. Publisher W. R. Hearst had his papers popularize the Spanish word "marijuana" to make the drug sound more foreign and menacing.

During the 1950s, marijuana use was confined mainly to jazz musicians and residents of urban ghettos. It was celebrated in the novels and poetry of the "Beat Generation" poets and writers, chiefly Allen Ginsberg, Jack Kerouac, and Gregory Corso. By the 1960s, a new generation began to defy prohibitions against marijuana use, in part because they discovered it was not the demonic drug portrayed in pulp fiction.

AMPHETAMINES

In an attempt to improve the physical performance of soldiers during World War II, American, British, German, and Japanese army doctors routinely prescribed amphetamines ("speed") to fight fatigue, heighten endurance, and "elevate the fighting spirit." Illicit amphetamine abuse also increased greatly during the 1940s and '50s among civilian truck drivers and workers engaged in monotonous factory jobs.

SEDATIVE-HYPNOTICS

Barbiturates, first used at the turn of the century, came into their own in the 1950s. The indiscriminate prescribing of these drugs, plus the development of Miltown® and other "milder" tranquilizers, created an era of prescription downer abuse during the '40s and '50s.

LSD

Dr. Timothy Leary encouraged the youth of the '60s to *"Turn on, tune in, and drop out."* The so-called guru of LSD advocated drug experimentation to "alter the mind." Psychedelics and stimulants such as LSD, marijuana, and "speed" were the most popular. Better communication, faster travel, a "do-your-own-thing" attitude, along with criminal organizations engaged in drug trafficking, helped spread the use of illicit psychoactive drugs. In the years to come, a flood of new psychedelic drugs like DOB, DMT, PCP, 2CB, CBR (nexus), and others, combined with the new experimental attitude of the times, made many believe in the slogan, "Better living through chemistry."

LEGAL AND MEDICAL RESPONSES

The increase in drug use was met with attempts to address the problem of abuse, addiction, and crime brought on by drugs. The methods tried were interdiction and stricter laws concerning use (**supply reduction**) and prevention and treatment (**demand reduction**).

As research findings were compiled, understanding of the process of addiction grew and treatment facilities expanded. Alcoholism and other addictions were slowly being defined and, to a certain extent, accepted as illnesses. The treatment of compulsive use became a medical as well as a social science. Some of the treatment protocols tried were therapeutic communities, treatment hospitals, free clinics, 12-step fellowships, and methadone maintenance.

METHADONE AND HEROIN

Developed during the 1960s in New York, methadone maintenance treatment programs substituted the legalized narcotic methadone for heroin. They spread throughout the country. Methadone maintenance programs attempted to bring the heroin addict population under control. The idea was that if addicted people didn't have to steal for their drug, crime would go down. It was an early example of a harm-reduction goal primarily benefiting society rather than a drug-free treatment goal benefiting the addict. Methadone maintenance continues today as the medical treatment model for opiate or opioid addiction.

In the 1970s, an unpopular war in Vietnam, along with a flood of opium from the Golden Triangle (Burma, Laos, and Thailand), encouraged the use of downers, such as heroin, Valium®, and the barbiturates. A new group of heroin addicts was created during the years of America's involvement in the war. Only a few Vietnam veterans continued their heroin use after the war. The bulk of this new wave of heroin abusers was composed of counter-culture and inner-city youth.

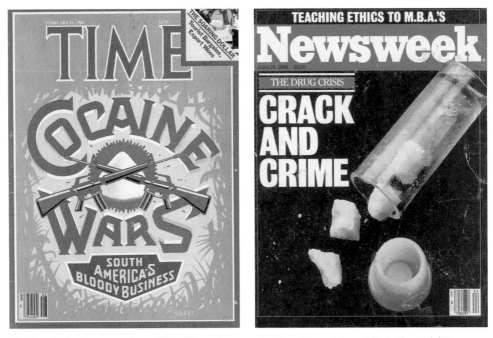

The hundreds of cover stories and headlines about cocaine that deluged the public in the mid–'80s gave the impression that everyone used cocaine. Surveys, however, indicated that only two or three percent of the adult population used the drug.

STIMULANTS (cocaine and amphetamines)

From the 1930s to the 1960s, cocaine use was limited primarily to the inner city, underworld, and jazz musicians. During the 1980s, a decade of stimulant abuse, a barrage of publicity surrounding cocaine use by athletes, musicians, and media stars promoted the drug. Cocaine became the fashionable drug. Restricted to the wealthy and elite at first, cocaine use became widespread as supplies increased and prices dropped.

Snorting, the traditional method for using cocaine, gave way to smokeable cocaine, known most commonly as "freebase," "crack," or "rock." The ensuing "crack epidemic" was partly fueled by the media's heavy-handed news coverage. But mostly, smokeable cocaine became popular because of the low cost of a "hit," the addictive properties of this form of cocaine, and its spread into both the suburbs and the inner city. At the beginning of the 1990s, "crack" was firmly entrenched in the drug culture.

In the late '80s, a new and more powerful smokeable amphetamine, called "ice," came onto the scene. Also called "L.A. glass" and "rose quartz," it was stronger and its effects lasted longer than regular methamphetamines. The initial center of "ice" abuse was Hawaii. By the beginning of the '90s, its use hadn't spread nearly as rapidly as had been feared, perhaps because of the greater severity of its toxic effects.

La. becomes only state where 18 is drinking age

1996

Load 'em up,
a's drinking
18 Friday

one 18-to-20 to buy or drink liquor, but it was legal to sell it to them. After 10 years of lobbying by organizations such as Mothers

1996

1996

Pot use by teenagers skyrockets

The Associated Press

WASHINGTON — Marijuana use by black males as young as 11 has tripled in four years. For white girls, it's more than doubled. And teens who carry guns or join gangs are more likely to use cocaine, a national survey says.

Against this bleak statistical backdrop, President Clinton said Thursday he will convene a White House conference in January to

Heroin Finds a New Market Along Cutting Edge of Style

By TRIP GABRIEL

LOS ANGELES, May 4 — The rising young fashion photographer was acting jumpy. He scratched the label off a beer bottle and skittered his fingers over the buttons of a cellular phone without ever dialing. For m

Fast-Lane Killer

A special report.

and early 80's, when cocaine was the cocktail of choice for the chic, before red down to the mass of urban sionals and, then, in its cheapd most destructive form, as to the poor. High-grade heroin an be smoked rather than inhas caught on, on both coasts, les whose habits often set — young people piloting the e in the film, rock and fashion es.

1996

Neighborhood meth lab surprised Medford cops

By PETER WONG
of the Mail Tribune

Wayne Fairchild says he suspected nothing about his neighbors. Lee and Brenda Poulton say they suspected something.

"They were the worst neighbors we ever had," Lee Poulton said.

But all of them said Saturday they were as surprised as the Medford police who came Friday to the house at 2411 Crater Lake Ave., not far from North Medford High School.

Police summoned the Jackson County Narcotic Enforcement Team, the Oregon State Police crime lab and the U.S. Drug Enforcement Administration. Cleanup took most of the day Saturday.

Sheriff's Lt. Ed Mayer, JACNET commander, said Saturday that methamphetamine labs usually turn up in rural areas, not in Medford neighborhoods.

"A neighbor was talking to me and said he came up from California to get away from these labs," an appalled Fairchild said. "Yet here it is, right down the street. I said Medford is getting really bad."

tive Steve Edson as he sat in a car parked in a vacant lot north of the house.

Rodney Michael Lubin, 34, was arrested Friday afternoon, and April Michelle Baker, 28, was arrested late Friday night. They were lodged as fugitives without bail Saturday at the Jackson County Jail.

In addition to stolen-property warrants from Washington state, they were held on two counts each of endangering the welfare of minors — neighbors say they have two children — and possession of methamphetamine. Lubin also was held on a charge of manufacturing the drug.

Wayne Fairchild is an older man whose home is two lots north of the site.

he let Lubin use his vacant

Aug. 1996

Teen Drug Use Doubled in 1992-95, Study Says

Rise attributed to marijuana

Reuters

Washington

Drug use among teenagers more than doubled from 1992 to 1995, a federal study said yesterday, prompting Republicans to blame the Clinton administration.

Much of the increase was due to big jumps in the percentage of 12- to 17-year-olds who said they had used marijuana in the past month. Some drug experts call marijuana, the most commonly used illic

it drug, a "gateway" to harder drugs such as cocaine.

In 1995, the rate of drug use during the past month by such teenagers rose to 10.9 percent, more than twice the 5.3 percent low point reached in 1992, according to the Health and Human Services Department's 1995 National Household Survey on Drug Abuse. The survey put the total number of 12- to 17-year-olds at 22.2 million.

In presenting the findings, Health Secretary Donna Shalala took pains to emphasize that youth attitudes toward marijuana began changing as early as 1990 during the administration of Republican President George Bush.

"What we are seeing is ... a multiyear trend that began before we came to Washington, before this administration came to Washington," this trend began, but it continues today," she said at a joint outdoor news conference at a local Boys and Girls Club meant to dramatize the dangers of drugs to youth.

Republican presidential candidate Bob Dole, campaigning in Louisville, Ky., called the report's findings "nothing short of a national tragedy" and said he would make the war on drugs the "priority No. 1 once again."

White House spokesman Mike McCurry said Clinton has focused much attention on the drug problem and would con

tinue to do so. "This is something the president talks about regularly and has identified as an area that he wants to work on personally," he said.

McCurry rejected Republican charges that Clinton's initial cuts in the office of drug policy had exacerbated the problem.

Although drug abuse began rising sharply in the early 1990s, it remains down from the 16.3 percent peak reached in 1979 among adolescents. That year, which was the peak for illicit drug use, rates were 38 percent for those aged 18 to 25, 20.8 percent for ages 26 to 34, and 2.9 percent for 35 and over.

In contrast, in 1995, the percentage of

adults reporting drug use in the past month were 14.2 percent for those 18 to 25; 8.3 percent for those 26 to 34, and 2.8 percent, the same as in 1979, for those age 35 and older, the survey showed.

McCurry said he believed the administration's plan to fight drugs was on the right track. "We think it's the right strategy to control use, to control imports," he said. "Above all, this has to be a bipartisan effort that all join into."

Jim Copple, president of the Community Anti-Drug Coalitions of America, said blame should be shared by Republicans and Democrats for cutting funds for drug control programs and losing interest in the issue.

UPPER-DOWNER CYCLE

Beginning in the mid-nineteenth century, the United States saw a curious popular cycle of alternating depressant and stimulant abuse. Renewed heavy use of alcohol and a generation of morphine (depressants) abusers produced by the Civil War were followed by the widespread use and abuse of the stimulant cocaine and energy tonics less than a generation later. The opium dens and opium-based tonics at the start of the twentieth century gave way to renewed cocaine use along with expanded cigarette smoking and coffee drinking in the "Roaring '20s." The end of Prohibition ushered in an era of alcoholic downer abuse symbolically coinciding with the Great Depression.

During World War II, amphetamines and cigarettes (stimulants) were dispensed to troops almost as freely as chipped beef on toast. The abuse of depressants like Miltown®, other tranquilizers, and alcohol ("three martini lunches") followed in the downer decade of the '50s. Along with psychedelics and marijuana (all arounders), illegal "speed" or "meth" and legal diet pills became fashionable in the 1960s, followed by the depressants heroin, Quaaludes®, and alcohol in the '70s. The '80s saw the spread of cocaine, particularly smokable "crack" cocaine, and a resurgence of methamphetamines.

The reasons for these cycles seem to have most to do with people's desire to experiment with psychoactive drugs, changing political climates, the exigencies of war, general economic conditions, and social amnesia about the damage done in previous generations by abuse of certain substances.

TODAY AND TOMORROW

COCAINE

From years of peak use in the early and mid-1980s, cocaine use has generally trended lower, the exact levels of use depending on the age group. Hard-core use hasn't dropped quite so dramatically and has spread more to the inner cities. By the mid-'90s, cocaine remained in use, whether by itself (snorted, smoked or injected), or in combination with other drugs. The *1995 U.S. Household Inventory Study* documents that at least 3.6 million Americans had used cocaine during 1995.

AMPHETAMINE

The mid–1990s have seen street chemists developing newer and more effective ways of manufacturing illicit methamphetamines sold as "crank," "crystal," "meth," and "speed." Some of the drugs are produced on stovetops, but most of the manufacture and wholesaling is done by Mexican gangs. They either manufacture the drugs in Mexico and smuggle them into the United States or they supply raw materials and personnel to set up labs in the United States, mostly in California. In addition, an increase in smoking as the route for methamphetamine has also promoted this resurgence of "speed" abuse.

PSYCHEDELICS AND "RAVE" CLUBS

There has also been an increase in the use of psychedelics, particularly LSD, MDMA, and high potency marijuana. LSD is sold in lower dosages than in the '60s and '70s and acts more like a stimulant than a psychedelic. A newer chemical variation, created in the 1990s and called LSD-49 or "illusion," produces more visual distortions, much like the stronger doses of LSD-25 sold in the '60s. It is one of the drugs used in "rave" clubs, a '90s version of the psychedelic rock clubs of the '60s. At these parties, sometimes held in legitimate clubs, sometimes in hastily rented warehouses, dancing, partying, and drug use are the

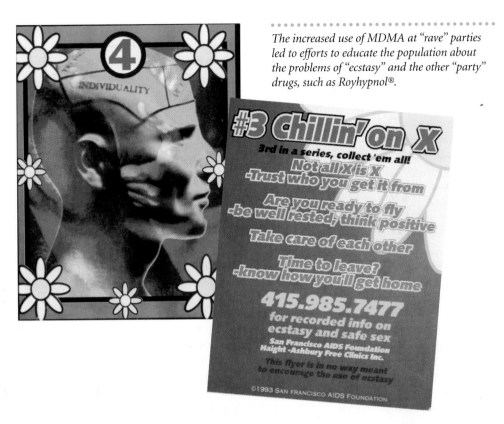

The increased use of MDMA at "rave" parties led to efforts to educate the population about the problems of "ecstasy" and the other "party" drugs, such as Royhypnol®.

rule of the day. MDMA, LSD, amphetamines, Rohypnol® (a sedative), GHB, alcohol, Ketamine® ("special k"), and "smart drinks", used individually or in combination with each other, are the most common substances taken at "raves."

MDMA, also known as "ecstasy," "X," "Adam," and "rave," is a stimulatory psychedelic. It has become more widely used in the '90s, much as MDA, a similar drug, was in the '60s. Users claim it is mellower than its chemical kin, amphetamines. MDMA users also claim that it promotes closeness and empathy, along with a loss of inhibitions.

INHALANTS

Another disturbing '90s trend is the use of spray-can solvents and their propellants as inhalants. Younger and younger students are inhaling ("huffing") anything from fabric stain protectors to ethyl chloride. Metallic paints and glue are even more common. Young people use inhalants alone or at "huffing parties." Up to 1,200 deaths from inhalant abuse are reported in the United States annually.

HEROIN

Heroin use continues to see a resurgence in the 1990s. Not only are there the traditional "China white" (from the Golden Triangle in Asia) and "Mexican brown" types of heroin, but also "Persian brown," "Mexican tar heroin," "Afghani," "Colombian," "African tar," and even an American domestic opium in limited quantities. Since the illegal heroin trade can be so lucrative, many of the Colombian drug lords have added it to their cocaine trade to diversify their business. Because of the money involved and the growing number of users, Chinese tongs (criminal societies) have tried to wrest control of the heroin trade in the United States from the Mafia. Indeed, for the first time, federal reports now list the Golden Triangle in Asia as the primary source of street heroin sold in the United States, instead of Turkey and Mexico. However, the Mexican gangs are fighting back and spreading into distribution of not only heroin but cocaine, marijuana, and methamphetamine as well.

MARIJUANA (Cannabis)

Marijuana is one of the drugs that has never been out of favor and is still popular in the 1990s. The biggest change in this drug is the increase in the availability of highly potent marijuana (up to 14 times as strong as varieties available in the '70s) and the increase in price which has gone up 10- to 30-fold since the early '70s. Just as the refinement of coca leaves into cocaine and opium into heroin led to greater abuse of the drugs, so have better cultivation techniques increased the compulsive liability of marijuana use. There is also an increase in the practice of mixing marijuana with other drugs like cocaine, amphetamine, and PCP. Some users even smoke marijuana "joints" which have been soaked in formaldehyde and embalming fluid for a bigger kick.

In recent years, there has been a drive to legalize marijuana for medical purposes. NORML (National Organization for the Reform of Marijuana Laws) and other groups have also pressed for legalization of marijuana, citing among other reasons, the use of hemp to make paper or other products. Opponents contend that legalization is a cover for use of marijuana as a eupho-

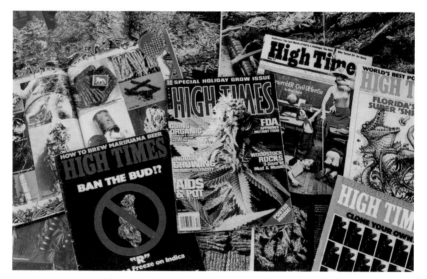

Marijuana continued its popularity as different brands proliferated. High Times, a counter-culture magazine that started in the early '70s, documented the hundreds of different kinds of "grass." The sinsemilla-growing method produces a higher THC concentration, which is bringing more marijuana users with bad experiences into emergency rooms and drug clinics in the '90s.

riant, that there is not enough sound medical evidence of the drug's usefulness in medical treatment, and that other drugs are medically more effective. The controversy is likely to continue well into the future.

ALCOHOL

The other drug that has never been out of favor is alcohol It is still widely used by every age group and in every country (except Muslim nations). It is used for a dozen different reasons from supplementing meals, reducing the risk of heart attacks, lowering inhibitions, being social, getting high, or becoming drunk. But, as in the past, used separately or in combination with other psychoactive drugs, alcohol kills over 130,000 persons a year in the United States, compared to only 8,000 killed by all other illicit psychoactive drugs combined. There were an estimated 10 to 12 million Americans suffering from alcoholism in 1996.

TOBACCO

From the peak smoking year of 1962, tobacco use in the U.S. has been gradually declining. This decline resulted in part from the U.S. Surgeon General's Report on the dangers of smoking in 1965, anti-smoking information campaigns, warnings printed on packaging and advertising, legislation prohibiting smoking on aircraft and in public places, an acceptance by the public of the dangers of smoking, legal suits against tobacco companies, and restrictions placed on tobacco advertising on radio and television. Between 1962 and 1995, per capita tobacco use declined by 30%.

Statistics in 1995 documented about 3,500 cigarette smokers who quit each day and 1,178 who die each day in the United States. The tobacco companies have responded by developing generic brands, cutting prices, developing foreign markets, as well as targeting females, minorities, and younger smokers. In certain urban areas, for example, Joe Camel is now more recognizable by children than Mickey Mouse.

CONCLUSION

Few histories can rival that of the continuous use and abuse of mind-altering substances by human beings over thousands of years of development and culture. Some historians have even suggested that the drive to alter states of consciousness is as essential to human nature as the drive to survive and procreate. Further, there is a theory that civilizations arose as a direct result of the desire to have a continued, uninterrupted access to substances which alter perceptions of the world. For example, agriculture in the Mesopotamian River valley in the Mideast may have evolved some 10,000 years ago to cultivate the opium poppy (which offered no food value) to provide a reliable supply of opium for medicinal, cultural, and ritualistic uses.

History provides us with valuable lessons about psychoactive substances like opium. Cultures quickly learned that most of these substances could create a drive or compulsion to continue using which was so powerful that it could supersede all other life instincts. Attempts to address this problem of the addictive potential of psychoactive substances are also well documented throughout the millennia, but most methods have failed. Technological, pharmacological, and communication advances in modern times have once again brought the abuse of psychoactive drugs to crisis proportions.

Partly, the problem of compulsion lies in the configuration of the human brain. We have evolved the neocortex which allows us to reason and to make more complex decisions than other creatures. Yet, because the action of drugs affects the neocortex in ways that disrupt reasoning and distort judgment, once addiction develops, compulsive use continues despite negative consequences experienced by the addict. It becomes very difficult to "reason" one's way out of addiction and to "will" abstinence. It is not surprising that addiction is now our society's major public health and social problem. Psychoactive drugs kill more humans every year than any other cause. Thus, it now seems that what may have stimulated the development of human civilization is now a major threat to its members.

Past history may also give us some clues to solving this modern crisis. In the fourth century B.C., Aristotle wrote that reason more than anything else makes humans distinctively human. Recognizing that all psychoactive drugs impair reason and judgment, we need to proceed with our clearest reasoning to find solutions to the crisis of substance abuse and addiction.

The basic reasons for wanting to change one's perception of reality and consciousness will probably stay the same in succeeding generations, and psychoactive drugs are one way that people will choose to try to bring about change. It is, therefore, crucial to understand psychoactive drugs because they will affect us directly (physically and mentally) or indirectly (economically and socially) for the rest of our lives.

CLASSIFICATION OF PSYCHOACTIVE DRUGS

WHAT IS A PSYCHOACTIVE DRUG?

- In ancient Egypt, the Pharaoh Ramses might have defined a psychoactive drug as the beer that kept his pyramid workers happy.
- In second-century Greece, the physician Galen would have defined it as theriac, an opium-based cure-all.
- About 1400 A.D., an Incan noble in Peru would have defined it as coca leaves, a gift from the gods.
- A pilot in World War II would have defined it as the amphetamine the medic gave him to stay awake on a night-bombing run and the cigarettes he smoked afterwards.
- In the 1990s, a college student might define a psychoactive drug as a joint of marijuana that will get her high.

- A law enforcement officer might define a psychoactive drug by its legal classification as a Schedule I, II, III, or IV substance whose illegal use and sale carry legal penalties.
- A counselor working at a drug treatment center might define a psychoactive drug as any substance whose compulsive use keeps the client from functioning in a normal manner.

Each culture, each generation, each profession, and particularly each user has a definition of what constitutes a psychoactive drug.

"I like nitrous oxide a lot better than the other two things, isobutyl or amyl nitrite. You shouldn't stand up or walk around when you do them." 26-year-old inhalant user ("huffer")

"I started drinking gin and tonic. And then after a while, about a month, I started

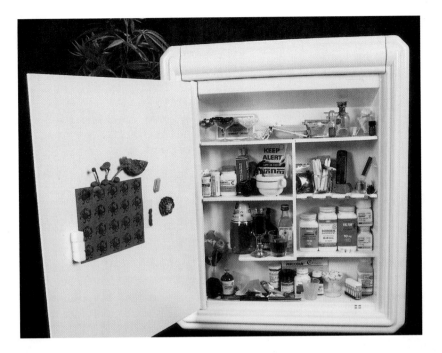

drinking gin over ice. And then I switched to brandy." *35-year-old recovering female alcoholic*

"Acid, in our heyday, was a lot stronger. One hit then was the equivalent of 5 or 6 hits today." *38-year-old LSD user*

"This doctor I went to started out giving me Nembutal®, Darvon®, a little Phenobarbital®, Valium®, and Compazine®. The drugstore delivered all at one time. My health insurance paid for them. I mean, luxury, right there." *35-year-old Valium® abuser*

"I'd been using 'China white' heroin, about 95% pure, for a year and a half. We ran out. I don't remember anything that happened for about four days. I do remember trying to drink alcohol to try to reduce the pain." *42-year-old heroin abuser*

"If the 'crack' is real pure, you get a real intense vibration, like waves of energy. Lots of times there's too much baking soda left in the rock, so it doesn't get you quite as high." *35-year-old "crack" cocaine smoker*

"A psychoactive drug is any substance that when injected into a rat gives rise to a scientific paper." *Darryl Inaba, Pharm.D., Director, Haight-Ashbury Clinic*

DEFINITIONS

Our definition of a psychoactive drug is any substance that directly alters the normal functioning of the central nervous system. In our modern society, there are any number of drugs that fit this definition. Today there are more psychoactive drugs to choose from than at any time in history. Modern transportation, a more open society, greater financial incentives for drug dealing, easy access to legal psychoactive drugs like tobacco, alcohol, caffeine, and prescription medications, new refinement techniques, along with the development of new drugs in sophisticated or street laboratories, have all come together to increase availability of these chemicals to all strata of society.

CHEMICAL, TRADE, AND STREET NAMES

The difficulty in studying, defining, and categorizing psychoactive drugs is that they have chemical names, trade names, and street names. For example, street names like "blunts," "illusion," "rave," "ice," "snot," "flip flop," "crack," "junk," "angel dust," "loads," "crank," "base," "window pane," "roofies," "chronic" (strong marijuana), "bammer" (weak marijuana), "Adam," "hubba," "rock," "horse," "ecstasy," and "U4Euh" continue to evolve almost daily among drug users. Each commonly used and abused substance may have 10 or more informal names. Just as confusing is the continued synthesis of new psychoactive drugs with chemical names such as methylenedioxyamphetamine and alpha-methyl-fentanyl. Trade names, such as Prozac®—instead of its chemical name fluoxetine, or Xanax®—instead of alprazolam, further confuse the issue of how to classify psychoactive drugs. Lawmakers have to be careful when outlawing a drug since they must describe its exact chemical formula. Customs officials have to examine imported herbal medicines carefully because some of them contain natural forms of restricted psychoactive substances.

CLASSIFICATION BY EFFECTS

A more practical way of classifying these substances is to distinguish them by their overall effects. Thus, the terms **Uppers** for stimulants, **Downers,** for depressants, and **All Arounders** for psychedelics have been chosen to describe the most commonly abused psychoactive drugs. Then there are so-called **"Other Drugs,"** such as inhalants, steroids, psychi-

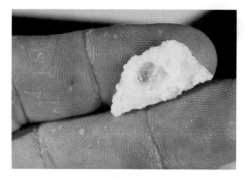

This piece of "crack" cocaine can be called "rock," "boulya," "hubba," or a dozen other street names.

atric medications, and a few more which don't fit one of these categories but which can be defined by their purpose, such as performance-enhancing sports drugs, antidepressants, or deleriants.

Caution: Since drug effects depend on amount, frequency, and duration of use as well as the makeup of the user and the setting in which the drug is used, reactions to psychoactive substances can vary radically from person to person and even from dose to dose. Our information about the action of drugs on the body should be used as a general guideline and not as an absolute guide.

MAJOR DRUGS

UPPERS (stimulants)

Uppers, central nervous system stimulants, include cocaine ("freebase," "crack"), amphetamines ("meth," "speed," "crank," "ice"), diet pills, Ritalin®, khat, lookalikes, nicotine, and caffeine.

Physical Effects

The usual effect of a small to moderate dose is over-stimulation of the nervous system, creating energized muscles, increased

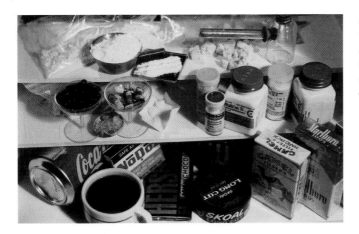

Several different types of uppers are available as illicit street drugs, prescription medications, or over-the-counter products.

heart rate, increased blood pressure, insomnia, and decreased appetite. Strong stimulants, like methamphetamines or cocaine, can also cause jitteriness, anger, aggressiveness, and dilated pupils. If large amounts are used or if the user is extra-sensitive, heart, blood vessel, and seizure problems can occur. Frequent use over a period of a few days will deplete the body's energy chemicals and exhaust the user. Although tobacco is a weak stimulant, its long-term health effects can be dangerous, causing such diseases as cancer, emphysema, and heart disease.

Mental/Emotional Effects

A small to moderate dose of the stronger stimulants can make someone feel more confident, outgoing, eager to perform, and excited. It can also cause a certain euphoria or rush, depending on the physiology of the user and the specific drug. Larger doses or prolonged use of the stronger stimulants can cause anxiety, paranoia, and mental confusion and can even mimic a psychosis.

DOWNERS (depressants)

Downers (central nervous system depressants) are divided into four main categories:

- **Opiates and Opioids:** Opium, heroin, codeine, Percodan®, methadone, morphine, Dilaudid®, Demerol®, Darvon®
- **Sedative-Hypnotics:** Benzodiazepines (Xanax®, Valium®, Halcion®, Rohypnol®), Doriden®, Miltown®, Soma®, barbiturates
- **Alcohol:** Beer, lite beer, wine, wine coolers, hard liquors, and mixed drinks
- **Others:** Antihistamines, skeletal muscle relaxants, lookalike sedatives, and bromides

Physical Effects

Small doses slow heart rate and respiration, relax muscles, decrease coordination, induce sleep, and dull the senses (e.g., diminish pain). Opiates and opioids can also cause constipation, nausea, and pinpoint pupils. Excessive drinking or sedative-hypnotic use can slur speech and cause digestive problems. Sedative-hypnotics and alcohol in large doses can cause dangerous respiratory depression. Large-dose use or prolonged use of any depressant can cause sexual dysfunction.

Mental/Emotional Effects

Initially, small doses (particularly with alcohol) seem to act like stimulants because

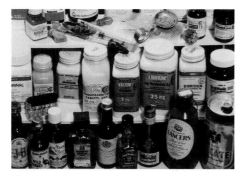

There are more depressants than any other category of psychoactive drugs, both legal and illegal. The most widely used depressant is alcohol.

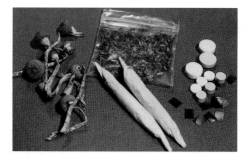

From dried psilocybin mushrooms to panes of LSD, from joints of marijuana to "ecstasy" pills, psychedelics come in a wide variety of shapes, sizes, and chemical compositions.

they lower inhibitions, but as more of the drug is taken, the overall depressant effect begins to dominate, relaxing and dulling the mind, diminishing anxiety, and controlling some neuroses. Certain downers can also induce euphoria, or a sense of well-being. Long-term use of any depressant can cause physical dependence.

ALL AROUNDERS (psychedelics)

All arounders or psychedelics are substances which can distort perceptions and induce illusions, delusions, or hallucinations: LSD, PCP, psilocybin mushrooms, peyote (mescaline), MDA, MDMA ("ecstasy"), marijuana, 2CB, methylpemoline ("U4Euh"), ayahuasca, and DMT.

Physical Effects

Most hallucinogenic plants, particularly cacti and some mushrooms, cause nausea and dizziness. Marijuana increases appetite and makes the eyes bloodshot. LSD raises the blood pressure and causes sweating. MDMA and even LSD act like stimulants. Generally, except for PCP which acts as an anesthetic, the physical effects are not as dominant as the mental effects.

Mental/Emotional Effects

Most often, psychedelics overload or distort messages to and from the brain stem, the sensory switchboard for the mind, so that many physical stimuli, particularly visual ones, are intensified or distorted. Imaginary messages (hallucinations) can also be created by the brain.

OTHER DRUGS

In this category, there are three main groups which can stimulate, depress, or confuse the user: inhalants, anabolic steroids and other sports drugs, and psychiatric medications.

INHALANTS

Inhalants are gaseous or liquid substances which are inhaled and absorbed through the lungs. They include organic solvents, such as glue, gasoline, metallic paints, and household sprays; volatile nitrites, such as amyl or butyl nitrate (also called "poppers"); and nitrous oxide (laughing gas).

Physical Effects

Most often, there is central nervous system depression. Dizziness, slurred speech, unsteady gait, and drowsiness are seen early on. Some inhalants lower the blood pressure, causing the user to faint or lose balance. The solvents can be quite toxic to lung, brain, liver, and kidney tissues.

Mental/Emotional Effects

With small amounts, impulsiveness, excitement, and irritability are common. Eventually, delirium with confusion, some hallucinations, drowsiness, and stupor can occur.

ANABOLIC STEROIDS AND OTHER SPORTS DRUGS

Performance-enhancing drugs, such as anabolic-androgenic steroids, are the most common. Others include stimulants (e.g., amphetamines); therapeutic drugs, such as pain killers; human growth hormones; HCG; caffeine; beta-blockers; and even diuretics.

Physical Effects

Anabolic steroids increase muscle mass and strength. Prolonged use can cause acne, high blood pressure, shrunken testes, and masculinization in women.

Mental/Emotional Effects

Anabolic steroids often cause a stimulant-like high, increased confidence, and increased aggression. Prolonged large-dose use can be accompanied by outbursts of anger, known as "rhoid rage."

PSYCHIATRIC MEDICATIONS

These medications are used by psychiatrists and others in an expanding field known as psychopharmacology to try to rebalance brain chemistry that causes mental problems, drug addiction, and other compulsive disorders. The most common are antidepressants (e.g., imipramine, Prozac®), antipsychotics (e.g., Thorazine®, Haldol®), antianxiety drugs (e.g., Xanax®, BuSpar®), and panic disorder drugs (e.g., beta-blockers). These drugs are being prescribed more and more frequently.

Physical Effects

Psychiatric medications are accompanied by a wide variety of physical side effects, particularly on the heart and skeletal-muscle systems, but their mental and emotional effects are the most important.

Mental/Emotional Effects

Antidepressants counteract depression by manipulating brain chemicals that elevate mood. Antipsychotics lower dopamine and control schizophrenic mood swings

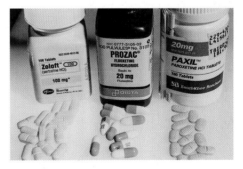

In the last few years, the number of available psychiatric drugs has increased. The most popular have been the new selective serotonin reuptake inhibitors and antidepressants, such as Prozac®, Zoloft®, and Paxil®.

and hallucinations. Antianxiety drugs also manipulate brain chemicals in ways that calm a person.

There are a number of other drugs, such as those which affect sexual perfor-mance, those which can aid in treatment, and even herbal medications, which have psychoactive effects. These will also be dis-cussed in later chapters.

CHAPTER   SUMMARY

HISTORY OF PSYCHOACTIVE DRUGS

Prehistory

1. More than 4,000 plants yield psychoactive substances. Their use dates back 50,000 years or more.

2. Psychoactive drugs have been used throughout history as a shortcut to an altered con-sciousness.

Ancient Civilizations

3. Drugs and their uses gradually spread as contacts among different cultures increased.

4. Alcohol, opium, Cannabis, and psychedelic mushrooms were the earliest psychoactive drugs employed by various civilizations.

5. Four uses of opium throughout history have been to stop pain, control diarrhea, lessen anxiety, and induce euphoria.

6. Two of the psychoactive drugs available in ancient Egypt were alcohol (as a reward for pyramid builders) and opium (as a medicine and a remedy for crying babies).

7. Two of the drugs used in ancient India were Cannabis (as a medicine and vision-induc-ing drug) and *amanita muscaria* mushrooms (called "Soma" and used for visions and sacred ceremonies).

Middle Ages

8. During the Middle Ages, distillation increased the alcoholic content of beverages in Europe. In Arab countries, tobacco, hashish, and especially coffee were employed as sub-stitutes for alcohol, which was forbidden by the *Koran.*

9. *Psilocybin* mushrooms and coca leaves were used in the Americas in pre-Columbian times.

10. Regulation of psychoactive drugs was one way political and religious leaders kept con-trol of their people.

11. Six psychedelic plants that have been employed in religious, magic, or social ceremonies throughout history are psychedelic mushrooms, belladonna, henbane, peyote, mari-juana, and coca leaves.

Renaissance and Enlightenment

12. European explorers brought back various drugs to Europe and carried European drugs, principally alcohol, to other peoples they encountered.

13. Tobacco was introduced to Europe and the Americas in the 1500s. Tobacco and hemp helped support many colonies and helped finance the American revolution.

14. Opium was used as a "cure-all" throughout history. Theriac, made from opium and many other ingredients, was used for almost 2,000 years. Laudanum, made from opium and alcohol, was available for over 400 years.

15. Consumption of distilled liquors like rum, gin, and whiskey increased alcohol abuse, sometimes to epidemic proportions.

Nineteenth Century

16. In the nineteenth century, nitrous oxide (laughing gas) was used as an anesthetic and intoxicant. Other anesthetics developed were chloroform and ether.

17. The invention of the hypodermic needle and the extraction of the active ingredients from opium and coca leaves encouraged abuse of drugs, especially morphine and heroin.

18. The China-Britain Opium Wars were fought for economic reasons: one was the right of the British to sell opium to China in order to improve the British balance of trade.

19. Opium and morphine were used as pain killers and in patent medicines in the United States during the Civil War and overseas in other wars (e.g., Crimean War). Use led to abuse and a new addict population.

20. The temperance movement, begun in the previous century in the United States, led to state prohibition laws.

21. The invention of the cigarette-rolling machine vastly expanded cigarette smoking.

22. Patent medicines at the turn of the century frequently contained opium, cocaine, and alcohol as their active ingredients.

Twentieth Century

23. Cigarettes gradually replaced cigars and chewing tobacco as the most popular method of nicotine consumption. Use increased through the first half of the century and then began to decline following public health campaigns.

24. In 1914, the Harrison Narcotic Act was passed to control opiates and cocaine. Marijuana was banned in 1937.

25. The alcohol Prohibition Amendment lasted from 1920 to 1933. It helped create the multi-billion dollar illegal drug business. The widespread abuse of alcohol encouraged the creation of Alcoholics Anonymous in 1934, the most successful drug treatment program in history.

26. Psychedelics, like LSD, PCP, MDA, and marijuana, became popular in the 1960s. MDA and PCP were also used.

27. An upper-downer cycle has been occurring in the United States: the downer alcohol in the 1930s; stimulants like amphetamines in the '40s; sedative-downers like Miltown® in the '50s; amphetamine uppers in the '60s; heroin and Valium® downers in the '70s; cocaine (including "crack") and amphetamine (including "ice") uppers in the '80s; and heroin or sedative-downers in the '90s.

Today and Tomorrow

28. In the 1990s, LSD and MDMA are making a comeback. Marijuana use has remained fairly constant, although its potency has greatly increased. Alcohol remains the number one drug problem in most of the world. Newer drugs like Rohypnol®, GHB, and Herbal Nexus® or 2CV are reminiscent of psychedelic drug patterns seen in the '60s.

CLASSIFICATION OF PSYCHOACTIVE DRUGS

What Is a Psychoactive Drug?

29. The major classes of psychoactive drugs are uppers (stimulants), downers (depressants), and all arounders (psychedelics).

Major Drugs

30. Uppers include cocaine, amphetamines, diet pills, plant stimulants, caffeine, and tobacco. Major effects are increased energy, feelings of confidence, and raised heart rate and blood pressure. Euphoria occurs initially with stronger stimulants. Overuse can cause jitteriness, anger, depletion of energy, and paranoia.

31. Downers include opiates (e.g., heroin, codeine), sedative hypnotics (e.g., benzodiazepines, barbiturates), and alcohol (beer, wine, distilled liquor). These drugs depress circulatory, respiratory, and muscular systems. The stronger opiates and sedative-hypnotics can initially cause euphoria. Prolonged use can cause health problems and dependence.

32. All arounders include marijuana, LSD, MDMA, PCP, psilocybin mushrooms, and peyote. Major mental effects are illusions, hallucinations, and confused sensations. Physically, many psychedelics cause stimulation, but marijuana usually causes relaxation.

Other Drugs

33. Other psychoactive drugs include inhalants, which are depressants but also cause dizziness and delirium accompanied by confusion; steroids and other sports drugs, which are used to enhance performance, such as muscle growth or relief from pain; and psychiatric drugs, which help rebalance brain chemistry disrupted by mental illness (e.g., antidepressants, antipsychotics, and antianxiety drugs).

Heredity, Environment, Psychoactive Drugs

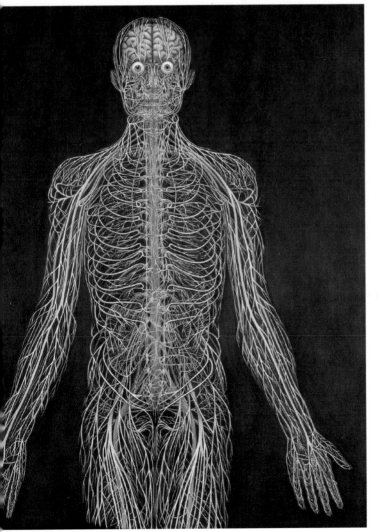

T he central and peripheral nervous systems communicate with the outside world and with each other to help human beings survive. Psychoactive drugs affect this com-munication.

The Nervous System by Alex Grey. Reprinted by permission, from Sacred Mirrors—The Visionary Art of Alex Grey, Inner Traditions International.

HOW PSYCHOACTIVE DRUGS AFFECT US

- **How Drugs Get to the Brain:** No matter how a drug is put in the body, it travels through the blood until it reaches the central nervous system (the brain and spinal cord).

- **The Brain:** Desire for psychoactive drugs mostly resides in the old brain which can override the reasoning of the new brain.

- **Neuroanatomy:** Psychoactive drugs affect the chemistry of the brain, especially neurotransmitters (which transmit messages throughout the body).

- **Neurotransmitters:** Psychoactive drugs mimic or modify the effects of neurotransmitters. These manipulated neurotransmitters cause most of the effects on the mind and body.

- **Physiological Responses to Drugs:** In addition to direct effects, phenomena such as tolerance, tissue dependence, withdrawal, and metabolism determine a user's reaction to psychoactive drugs.

FROM EXPERIMENTATION TO ADDICTION

- **Desired Effects Versus Side Effects:** People use psychoactive drugs to get high, to self-medicate, to oblige family or friends, and for many other reasons. All drugs also have undesired effects (side effects) especially when the drug is used to excess.

- **Levels of Use:** The amount, frequency, and duration of drug use help indicate level of use from abstinence, experimentation, and social use, up to habituation, abuse, and addiction.

- **Theories of Addiction:** Theories of addiction emphasize heredity, environment, psychoactive drugs, or a combination of those factors as the basis for compulsive use.

- **Heredity, Environment, Psychoactive Drugs:** Three major factors determine at what level a person might use psychoactive drugs.

  Heredity: Family history can indicate a susceptibility to compulsive drug use.

  Environment: The pressures of growing up, forged by the friendliness or hostility of the home, school, community, or society, mold people's personalities and can make them more susceptible (or less susceptible) to compulsive drug use or addiction.

  Psychoactive Drugs: Drugs can activate a genetic/environmental susceptibility. More important, psychoactive drugs themselves can change brain chemistry and lead to even more compulsive use.

- **Alcoholic Mice and Sober Mice:** A classic experiment with mice strongly suggests the interrelationship between heredity, environment, psychoactive drugs, and level of use.

- **Compulsion Curve:** The way heredity, environment, and drug use combine to increase susceptibility to compulsion and addiction in human beings can be visualized with compulsion curves.

Compulsions Tracked in Images of Brain

Psychiatrists able to see circuitry that is involved

By Daniel Goleman

The approach is adding a new level of detail to psychiatry's understanding of what goes wrong in the brains of patients when symptoms as diverse as posttraumatic stress, obsessions, phobias and delusions have them in their grip.

tures of psychiatric symptoms they will eventually be able to use imaging methods to bring greater precision to diagnosis and treatment. "One day, brain imaging may help s▢▢▢ ▢▢▢ which patients would ben▢▢▢▢▢▢▢▢▢▢▢▢▢▢ ment," said

would be in a "neutral" state.

But as symptoms wax and wane, the images rendered of patients' brains can change drastically. "Simply asking patients to lie quietly fails to control for whether ▢▢▢ daydreaming,

Early Violence Leaves Its Mark on the Brain

By DANIEL GOLEMAN

With rates of violence among teenagers rising precipitously, the argument over the causes of violent behavior has never been more charged.

The research on golden ham took advantage of that species of living singly, and being fi protective of their nesting te — or, in this case, laboratory

In the wild, adolescent ha ordinarily go off on their o establish a solitary nest. Bu

Scientists Pinpoint Brain Irregularities In Drug Addicts

Researchers seek treatments to alter chemical imbalances.

By DANIEL GOLEMAN

A radically new approach to fighting drug abuse is emerging from discoveries of brain irregularities that make certain people much quicker to become addicted than others, and much harder to cure.

For several years, scientists have suspected that at least some drug addicts suffer imbalances in brain chemistry that make them vulnerable to depression, anxiety or intense restlessness. For such people, addiction becomes a kind of self-medication in which drugs correct the chemical imbalance and bring a sort of relief.

Now researchers are beginning to identify the particular imbalances associated with addictions to particular ugs like cocaine, heroin or alcohol.

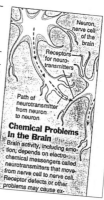

Neuron, nerve cell of the brain

Receptors for neurotransmitters

Path of neurotransmitter from neuron to neuron.

Chemical Problems In the Brain

Brain activity, including emotion, depends on electro▢▢ chemical messengers called neurotransmitters that move from nerve cell to nerve cell. Receptor defects or other problems may cause ex-

Nurture, Not Nature, Boosts IQ, Studies Show

But training must start in infancy

can be improved with techniques ranging from random play to purposeful training.

HOW PSYCHOACTIVE DRUGS AFFECT US

"I don't think that a drug is evil in and of itself, but just as drugs can be used to help heal a person, they can result in destroying a life as they did to me. So it really depends on the individual—what and how he chooses, and how wisely he uses or chooses not to use medications and drugs."
28-year-old recovering sedative-hypnotic abuser

To understand psychoactive drugs, it is valuable to first examine how these substances affect brain chemistry and then to look at the factors, particularly heredity, environment, and other special qualities of the psychoactive drugs, that determine how a person will use those drugs.

HOW DRUGS GET TO THE BRAIN

The methods that people use to put a psychoactive drug in their bodies, the route the drug takes to the brain, the speed of that trip, and the affinity of that drug for nerve cells and neurotransmitters all help determine the effects generated by the substances as well as their abuse potential.

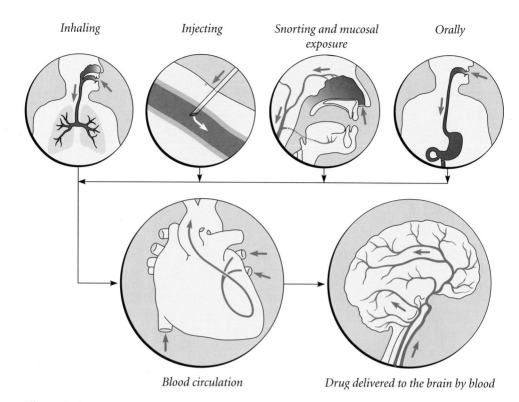

Inhaling *Injecting* *Snorting and mucosal exposure* *Orally*

Blood circulation *Drug delivered to the brain by blood*

Figure 2-1 •
Whether inhaled, injected, snorted, eaten, drunk, or put in contact with the skin (not shown here), the drug enters the bloodstream and is then pumped to the brain. It continues to circulate until it is eliminated from the body.

ROUTES OF ADMINISTRATION

There are five common ways that drugs may enter the body (Fig. 2–1). They are arranged in the order of the speed with which they will reach the brain and begin to have an effect (the shortest to the longest).

Inhaling

When a person smokes a marijuana joint, inhales freebase cocaine, or "huffs" airplane glue, the vaporized drug enters the lungs and is rapidly absorbed through the tiny blood vessels lining the air sacs of the bronchi. From the lungs, the drug-laden blood is pumped back to the heart and then directly to the brain and rest of the body, thus acting more quickly than any other method of use (7 to 10 seconds before the drug reaches the brain and its effects are felt).

Injecting

Substances such as heroin, cocaine, and "speed" can be injected directly into the body with a needle. Drugs may be injected into the bloodstream intravenously (IV or "slamming"), into a muscle mass (intramuscular, IM, or "muscling"), or under the skin (subcutaneous or "skin popping"). Injection is a quick and potent way to absorb a drug (15 to 30 seconds in a vein compared to 3 to 5 minutes in a muscle or under the skin for effects to begin). It is also the most dangerous method because it bypasses most of the body's natural defenses, thereby exposing the user to many health problems, such as hepatitis, abscesses, septicemia, or HIV infection.

Snorting and Mucosal Exposure

Certain drugs, such as cocaine and heroin, can be snorted into the nose and absorbed by the tiny blood vessels enmeshed in the mucous membranes lining the nasal passages. The effects are usually more intense and occur more quickly than with the oral route. A similar method involves placing a drug, such as crushed coca leaves (mixed with ash) or tobacco snuff, under the tongue or on the gums where it is absorbed through mucous membranes (3 to 5 minutes for effects to begin).

Orally

When someone swallows a codeine or Valium® tablet, the drug passes through the esophagus and stomach to the small intestine where it is absorbed into the tiny blood vessels (capillaries) lining the walls. Drugs taken by this route have to pass through mouth enzymes and stomach acids before they can get to the brain, so the effects are delayed (20 to 30 minutes for effects to begin). Some drugs are absorbed on the way to the small intestines. Alcohol (beer, wine, and distilled liquor) is partially absorbed by the stomach and can therefore reach the brain quicker (10 to 15 minutes for effects to begin). The majority of the alcohol is still absorbed by the small intestines.

Contact

Liquid LSD can be dropped into the eye where it is rapidly absorbed by ocular capillaries then propelled by the heart to the brain (3 to 5 minutes for effects to begin). Drugs can be applied to the skin through saturated adhesive patches which release measured quantities of the drug over a long period of time for up to 7 days (1 to 2 days for effects to begin). In hospices for terminally ill patients, morphine suppositories are used for patients too weak for an injection or an oral dose of a painkiller (10 to 15 minutes for effects to begin).

DRUG CIRCULATION

No matter how a drug enters the body, it eventually ends up in the bloodstream (Fig. 2–2). Drug molecules then circulate and travel to and through every organ, fluid, and tissue in the body where they will either be ignored, absorbed, or transformed. In the bloodstream, the drug may be carried inside the blood cells, in the plasma outside the cells, or it might hitch a ride on protein molecules.

The distribution of a drug within the body depends on the characteristics of the drug as well as on blood volume. The lighter the person, the less blood volume there is, so a small child of 12 might only have three to four quarts of blood to dilute the drug instead of the six to eight quarts in an adult circulatory system.

The effect of a drug on a specific organ or tissue is also dependent on the number of blood vessels reaching that site. For example, veins and arteries saturate the heart muscles, and since all drugs pass through these vessels, a drug such as cocaine can have a direct effect on heart function. Bones and muscles have fewer blood vessels, so most drugs will have less effect at these sites.

Figure 2-2 •

This drawing shows only a fraction of the blood vessels of the human body. Miles of capillaries deliver blood to the tissues including the nerve cells of the central nervous system.

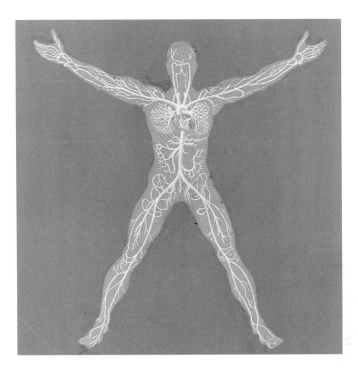

Most important, within only 10 to 15 seconds after entering the bloodstream, the drug will reach the gateway to the central nervous system, the blood-brain barrier. On the other side of the barrier, the drug will have its greatest effects.

The Blood-Brain Barrier

The drug-laden blood flows through the internal carotid arteries toward the central nervous system, also called the CNS (the brain and spinal cord). The walls of the capillaries surrounding the nerve cells, which make up the CNS, consist of tightly sealed cells so that only certain substances can penetrate and affect the CNS. Normally, substances such as toxins, viruses, and bacteria can't cross this barrier. One class of drugs which can infiltrate this blood-brain barrier (Fig. 2–3) is psychoactive drugs (stimulants, depressants, psychedelics, inhalants). Psychotropic drugs, such as antipsychotics or antidepressants, also cross this barrier as do most steroids and some muscle relaxants.

One reason why many psychoactive drugs, including cocaine, nicotine, alcohol, and marijuana, cross this barrier is that they are fat soluble, so they get to the nerve cells of the brain quickly. This occurs because the brain and blood-brain barrier, being essentially fatty, keep watery substances out and let fatty substances in. For example, morphine is partly fat soluble, so it takes 20 to 30 seconds to effectively cross the barrier. Users who are anxious for quicker effects prefer heroin because it crosses this barrier much faster. "Crack" cocaine is more fat soluble than cocaine hy-

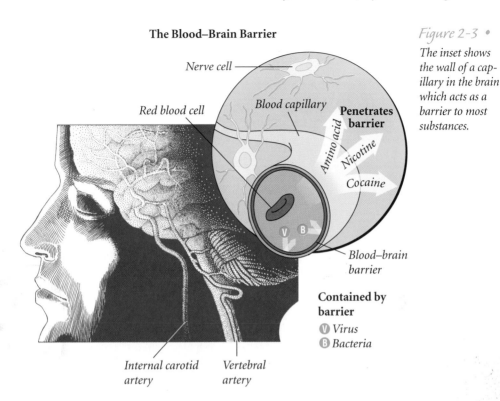

The Blood–Brain Barrier

Nerve cell

Red blood cell

Blood capillary

Amino acid

Penetrates barrier

Nicotine

Cocaine

Blood–brain barrier

Contained by barrier

Ⓥ Virus

Ⓑ Bacteria

Figure 2-3 •

The inset shows the wall of a capillary in the brain which acts as a barrier to most substances.

drochloride, so it too crosses the barrier more quickly and gives the user a faster, and often more intense, reaction.

Note, also, that since the brain is the most protected organ of the body, drugs which can penetrate its highly protective barrier possess the ability to penetrate and affect most other organs and tissues in the body.

THE NERVOUS SYSTEM

Since the principal target of psychoactive drugs is the central nervous system, it is important to understand how this network of 100 billion nerve cells and 100 trillion connections functions. The central nervous system is half of the complete nervous system. The other half is the peripheral nervous system which is further divided into the autonomic and the somatic systems (Fig. 2–4).

Peripheral Nervous System

The **autonomic nervous system**, which consists of the sympathetic division and the parasympathetic divisions, controls involuntary functions such as circulation, digestion, respiration, and reproduction. It automatically helps us breathe, sweat, pump blood, and so forth, to preserve a stable internal environment.

The **somatic nervous system** transmits sensory messages from the environment to the central nervous system and then transmits instructions back to muscles, organs, and other tissues, allowing us to respond appropriately.

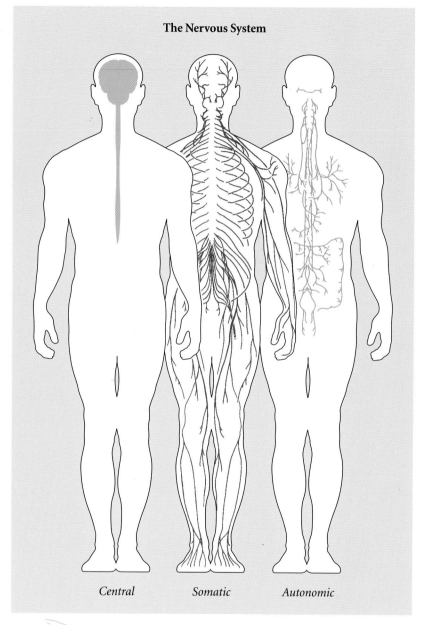

Figure 2-4 •

The three parts of the complete nervous system.

Central Nervous System (brain and spinal chord)

The central nervous system, especially the brain, acts as a combination switchboard and computer, receiving messages from the peripheral and autonomic nervous systems, analyzing those messages, and then sending a response to the appropriate system of the body: muscular, skeletal, circulatory, nervous, respiratory, digestive, excretory, endocrine, and reproductive. It also enables us to reason and make judgments.

A psychoactive drug, being a powerful external agent, can alter information sent to our brain from our environment; it can disrupt messages sent back to the various parts of the body; and it can disrupt our ability to think, reason, and interpret sensory input. A psychoactive drug not only affects the nervous system, it can affect other systems of the body as well. It can affect them directly while passing through the organ or tissue and it can affect them indirectly by manipulating nerve cell chemistry in the brain which then sends messages back to that organ.

THE BRAIN

The brain can be anatomically divided into its component parts (e.g., cerebellum, amygdala), or it can be divided by function (e.g., speech areas, breathing areas). For the purposes of understanding how psychoactive drugs work and what causes addiction, we have found it valuable to look at the brain in an evolutionary sense.

OLD BRAIN–NEW BRAIN

The brain can be divided into the old brain and the new brain. The **old brain**, also called the primitive brain, consists of the brain stem, cerebellum, and the mesocortex or midbrain. The old brain exists in all animals from a fish to a human being (Fig. 2-5). The two main functions of the old brain are:

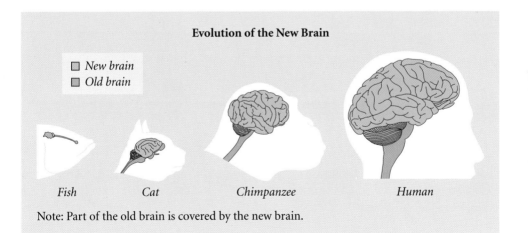

Evolution of the New Brain

☐ *New brain*
☐ *Old brain*

Fish   *Cat*   *Chimpanzee*   *Human*

Note: Part of the old brain is covered by the new brain.

Figure 2-5 •

On the evolutionary scale, from a fish, to a cat, to a chimpanzee, and finally to a human being, the new brain has grown in proportion to the old brain. Though the new brain is much larger, the old brain tends to override it, particularly in times of stress.

- to regulate physiologic functions of the body (e.g., respiration, heartbeat, body temperature);

- to experience basic emotions and cravings (e.g., anger, fear, hunger, thirst, sex, pleasure).

The emotions experienced by the old brain occur in response to internal changes in the body or external influences in the environment. For example, if a man has not had enough liquid, the old brain feels the body's thirst and creates a craving for water. If a deer hears a twig snap in the woods, the old brain feels fear and creates a desire to escape from that danger.

The **new brain**, also called the neocortex (cerebrum and cerebral cortex), processes information that comes in through our senses or from the old brain. So, if a human being is thirsty and craves water, the new brain can figure out the nearest source of water and how to get there. If there is danger, the new brain might figure out a smarter way of avoiding that danger instead of just running away. The new brain allows us to speak, reason, and create. Over millions of years, the new brain has grown over the old brain until, in humans, it had to fold in on itself to make room for all the billions of new cells. The higher up on the evolutionary ladder, the larger the new brain. The new brain works with the old brain, trying to make sense of the feelings and emotions coming from its more primitive half.

One would think that since the old brain is so much smaller, the new brain rules, but that's not the case. The old brain is the senior partner. It was there first and the new brain is the latecomer. Whenever the two brains are challenged by a crisis, such as fear or anger, there's an automatic tendency to revert to old brain function. And since the desire to use a psychoactive drug (craving) often resides in the old brain, the desire for the pleasure, pain relief, and excitement that drugs promise can be very powerful. That craving can override the new brain's rational arguments which say, "too expensive," "bad side effects," or "there's a midterm exam in the morning, so no partying tonight."

"The impact of that drug, the impact of that sensation and how it immobilized me and made me incapable of dealing with the simplest realities of walking to the bus, of going into my office, of getting on the phone, and of picking up my children was so frightening to me that I did not want to repeat it. I was, however, very compelled to repeat the use of methamphetamine which I did for years." Recovering methamphetamine abuser

If a person is to live a balanced life, there has to be good communication between the old brain and new brain. Communication can be disrupted by psychoactive drugs (it can also be disrupted by a hostile environment or mental illnesses).

THE REWARD/PLEASURE CENTER

The area of the old brain that is affected by many psychoactive drugs and is responsible for much of drug craving is called the reward/pleasure center. This center, which is really several structures in the old brain (Fig. 2–6), is one of the main reasons that people use drugs and eventually accelerate their use of drugs. The reward/pleasure center, which exists in all mammals, is a survival mechanism which gives us a surge of pleasure when we've satisfied some need of our body, such as thirst, hunger, or sex. This area of the brain was first pinpointed in 1954 by American biologist Dr. James Olds. What Dr. Olds and others have hypothesized, and to a large extent proven, is

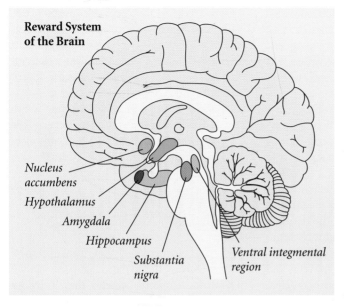

Reward System of the Brain

Nucleus accumbens

Hypothalamus

Amygdala

Hippocampus

Substantia nigra

Ventral integmental region

Figure 2-6 •

The reward/pleasure center is really a combination of several structures in the old brain that are activated when the person fulfills some emotion or feeling that has arisen, such as hunger, thirst, or sexual desire.

Courtesy of Kenneth Blum, John Cull, Eric Braverman, and David Comings

that the reward/pleasure center in the brain is a powerful motivator. Experimentally, when a rat had its nucleus acumbens (part of the reward/pleasure center) connected to an electrical switch and was allowed to stimulate that part of its brain, it kept pressing the switch to keep stimulating this center. In fact, it was so powerful a reinforcer, the rat would press the switch 5,000 times an hour. It wouldn't eat, it wouldn't sleep, it would just keep pushing the switch. Dr. Olds and other researchers found that many psychoactive drugs also stimulate this same reward/pleasure center. When they had the rat push a lever which gave it a shot of cocaine, the rat would push that lever in much the same way it pushed the lever for the electrical stimulation of the reward/ pleasure center, only this time, it was drug-induced stimulation.

The reward/pleasure centers in the old brain are tightly intertwined with the physiologic regulatory centers of the body as well as reaching out to the new brain. When drugs are used for intoxication or

pleasure, especially stimulants and depressants, they also affect physiologic functions, such as heart rate and respiration. They affect the way the old brain experiences emotions and the way the new brain reacts to those emotions. Psychedelics seem to have a greater affect on the new brain although they will affect physiologic functions in the old brain. Most drugs also affect memory in one way or another because memory involves both the new and old brains' activity.

NEUROANATOMY

NERVE CELLS

Understanding the precise way messages are transmitted by the nervous system is crucial to understanding how psychoactive drugs affect a user's physical, emotional, and mental functioning. For example, if a dentist pulls a lower left molar, the damaged mandibular nerve endings

(Fig. 2-7) send minute electrical pain signals towards the brain with a frequency of up to 1,000 pulses a second and at speeds up to 200 miles per hour. The message is routed from one neuron to the next until it reaches its target in the brain. At that point, the brain consults millions of other nerve cells, decides either consciously or unconsciously on a response, then reacts by sending the appropriate signals back to that part of the body that needs to react. The brain might tell the patient's neck muscles to move the head away from the drill, it might instruct the jaw to bite the dentist's finger, or it might tell the vocal muscles to ask the dentist to prescribe a painkiller.

The building blocks of the nervous system, the nerve cells, are called neurons (Fig. 2-8). They have four essential parts: **dendrites** which receive signals from other nerve cells; the **cell body** (**soma**) which nourishes the organism and keeps it alive; the **axon** which carries the message from the dendrites and cell body to the **terminals** which then relay the message to the dendrites of the next nerve cell.

The length of a neuron is determined by the length of the axon which varies from a fraction of a millimeter between brain cells, to a foot between the tooth and brain, to several feet between the spinal cord and toe. Terminals of one nerve cell do not touch dendrites of the adjoining nerve cell because a microscopic gap (called a **synaptic gap**) exists between them.

The message jumps this synaptic gap, from the presynaptic terminal to the postsynaptic dendrite, not as an electrical signal but as microscopic bits of messenger neurochemicals stored in vesicles of the nerve cell. This biochemical signal is then converted back to an electrical signal where it travels to the next synapse where it's converted to a neurochemical signal. It is similar to a relay race where one runner passes the baton (message) to the next runner who carries it on until it's passed to another runner and so on. This transmission process across the gap between nerve cells is called a synapse. Electrical and chemical signals alternate until the message reaches the appropriate section of the brain. (There are some synaptic gaps that are one-tenth the width of normal synapses. At these junctures, the signal, or synapse, is transmitted only electrically. Our focus is on the synapses that need neurochemicals to jump the gap.)

NEUROTRANSMITTERS

The biochemicals that transmit messages across the synaptic gap are called neurotransmitters because they transmit signals from one neuron to another. This chapter focuses on neurotransmitters because they are the parts of the central nervous system most affected by psychoactive drugs.

Some of the names of these neurotransmitters are dopamine, endorphin, enkephalin, serotonin, norepinephrine, GABA, substance "P," acetylcholine, anandamide, glycine, histamine, nitric oxide, and at least 50 more. Although each nerve cell usually produces only one type of neurotransmitter, a single neuron might ultimately cause the release of several types of neurotransmitters at different synapses. A pain message will release substance "P" at one synapse and enkephalin at another. In addition, the release of one neurotransmitter usually has a cascade effect where, for example, the release of serotonin will trigger the release of enkephalin which then triggers dopamine which will result in a feeling of well-being in the brain's emotional center.

Signal transmission works by sending the electrical message which forces the release of neurotransmitters from tiny holding sacs (vesicles) and sends them across the synaptic gap (magnified 10,000 times

Figure 2-7 •

View of the nerves that would transmit a message of pain from a left molar to the brain. A painkiller, such as Darvon®, might disrupt the pain message.

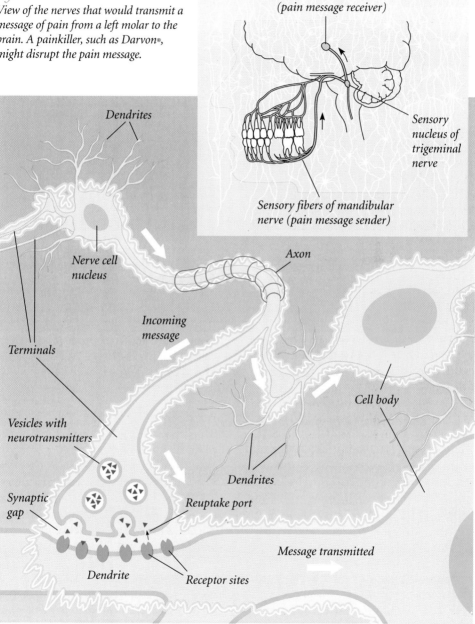

Posteromedial ventral nucleus (pain message receiver)

Sensory nucleus of trigeminal nerve

Sensory fibers of mandibular nerve (pain message sender)

Dendrites

Nerve cell nucleus

Axon

Incoming message

Terminals

Cell body

Vesicles with neurotransmitters

Dendrites

Synaptic gap

Reuptake port

Dendrite

Receptor sites

Message transmitted

Figure 2-8 •

Greatly magnified view of the junction of two nerve cells (neurons). The message that travels along this network must chemically jump the gap to continue its journey to the brain and eventually back to muscles and organs throughout the body.

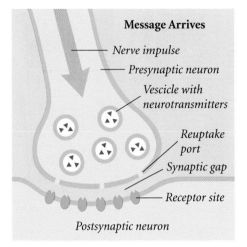

Message Arrives

Nerve impulse

Presynaptic neuron

Vescicle with
neurotransmitters

Reuptake
port

Synaptic gap

Receptor site

Postsynaptic neuron

Figure 2-9 •

*This is a simplified version of the synapse be-
tween nerve cells. The electrical message (nerve
impulse) arrives at the junction of two nerve
cells, the synaptic gap.*

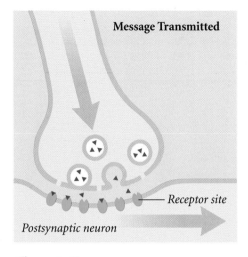

Message Transmitted

Receptor site

Postsynaptic neuron

Figure 2-10 •

*The electrical message is retriggered in the post-
synaptic neuron by neurotransmitters slotting
into specialized receptors.*

in Fig. 2-9). On the other side of the gap,
the neurotransmitters will slot into precise
and complex receptor sites, retriggering,
inhibiting, or modifying the electrical message (Fig. 2-10). Each receptor site is specific for a certain neurotransmitter. For example, a serotonin receptor will not
accommodate dopamine. When enough
neurotransmitters slot into receptor sites to
trigger a synapse, the receptor sites then release the neurotransmitters which are reabsorbed by the sending nerve cell terminals
and returned to the holding sacs (vesicles).
Some of the neurotransmitters don't make
it back and are metabolized by enzymes
outside the nerve cells.

AGONIST AND
ANTAGONIST

Psychoactive drugs are used because
they disrupt the process of message transmission in several different ways and produce desired (or undesired) reactions.

Generally, drugs that produce signals are
called agonists and drugs that block signals
are called antagonists.

- Drugs can chemically imitate part of a
  neurotransmitter and fool the receptor
  site into accepting it, thus creating a
  false message (agonist) or blocking a
  real one (antagonist).

- Drugs can prevent neurotransmitters
  from being reabsorbed into the sending
  neuron, thereby causing more intense
  effects of that neurochemical (agonist).

- Drugs can force the release of neurotransmitters which will, in turn, inhibit
  or force the release of another neurotransmitter.

- Drugs can cause the release of excess
  neurotransmitters to produce an exaggerated effect.

- Drugs can signal the neuron to slow
  down its production and release of
  neurotransmitters.

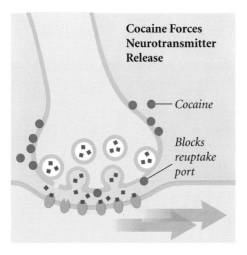

Cocaine Forces Neurotransmitter Release

Cocaine

Blocks reuptake port

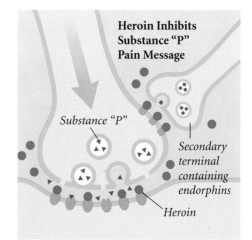

Heroin Inhibits Substance "P" Pain Message

Substance "P"

Secondary terminal containing endorphins

Heroin

Figure 2-11 •
Cocaine forces the release of extra neurotransmitters and blocks their reabsorption, thus increasing the frequency and therefore the intensity of the electrical signal in the postsynaptic neuron.

Figure 2-12 •
Heroin inhibits the release of substance "P" and also helps block most of the neurotransmitters that do get through. So, the electrical signal is greatly weakened each time it crosses a substance "P" synapse.

- Drugs can cause a combination of all these interactions.

A drug will sometimes disrupt communication in more than one of the above ways, for example, acting as an agonist at low doses and an antagonist at high doses. Sometimes the disruption of neurotransmitters is useful (blocking pain messages), sometimes desirable (releasing stimulatory chemicals), and sometimes it is extremely dangerous (blocking inhibitory neurotransmitters that control violent behavior). For example, a stimulant, such as cocaine, will force the release of norepinephrine (a stimulatory chemical) and dopamine (a pleasure-inducing chemical) from the vesicles and then prevent them from being reabsorbed. The net result is that there are then more of both those neurotransmitters available to exaggerate existing messages and stimulate new ones (Fig. 2-11).

A depressant, such as heroin, will mimic enkephalins and slot into opioid (enkephalin) receptors, thus inhibiting the release of substance "P," a pain-transmitting neurotransmitter, causing the pain signal to weaken. This is the reason that heroin and opioids lessen pain. It also slots into substance "P" receptor sites on the receiving neurons without causing pain and acts like an antagonist, further blocking pain transmission. Finally, it also attaches itself to certain receptor sites in the reward/pleasure center, inducing a euphoric sensation. This too is a desired effect. It also attaches itself to the breathing center, thereby depressing respiration. This is a dangerous effect (Fig. 2-12).

An all arounder, such as LSD, will release some stimulatory neurotransmitters, but mostly it will alter messages from the external environment, particularly visual and auditory images. It can distort, magnify, and even interchange visual and auditory images. Other psychedelics create images which don't exist at all in the external world. These imaginary images are called hallucinations.

NATURALLY OCCURRING SUBSTANCES

Although the first neurotransmitters were discovered in the 1920s (acetylcholine) and 1930s (norepinephrine), it was the discovery in the mid–1970s of endorphins and enkaphlins, neurotransmitters that produce the same effects as opioid drugs, that finally gave an understanding of how psychoactive drugs work in the body. For the first time, reaction and addiction to psychoactive drugs could be described in terms of specific, naturally occurring chemical and biologic processes.

Once the existence of endorphins and enkephalins was confirmed, the search for other natural neurochemicals which mimic other psychoactive drugs began in earnest. Over the next 20 years, researchers were able to correlate dozens of psychoactive drugs with the neurotransmitters they affect (Table 2-1).

Besides more than 60 known substances such as neurotransmitters and neuromodulators, it is estimated that eventually, several hundred brain chemicals will be identified.

One implication of the research implies that virtually any psychoactive drug works because it mimics or disrupts naturally occurring chemicals in the body that have specific receptor sites. It means that **psychoactive drugs cannot create sensations or feelings that don't have a natural counterpart.** It also implies that human beings can naturally create virtually all of the sensations and feelings they try to get through drugs, although many of them are not as intense as those received through highly concentrated drugs. Here are some examples.

- A genuine scare will force the release of adrenaline which will mimic part of an amphetamine rush.

- Prolonged running produces a runner's high through the release of endorphins and enkephalins, similar to a modified heroin rush.

- Sleep or sensory deprivation can produce true hallucinations through the

TABLE 2–1 PSYCHOACTIVE DRUG/NEUROTRANSMITTER RELATIONSHIPS

Drug	Neurotransmitters Directly Affected
Alcohol	GABA (gama amine butyric acid), met-enkephalin, serotonin
Benzodiazepines	GABA, glycine
Marijuana	Anandamide, acetylcholine
Heroin	Endorphin, enkephalin, dopamine
LSD	Acetylcholine, dopamine, serotonin
Nicotine	Adrenaline, endorphin, acetylcholine
Cocaine and amphetamines	Adrenaline, noradrenaline, serotonin, dopamine, acetylcholine
MDA, MDMA	Serotonin, dopamine, adrenaline, noradrenaline
PCP	Dopamine, acetylcholine, alpha-endopsychosin

same neurotransmitters affected by peyote.

- Relaxation and stress reduction exercises can calm restlessness through glycine and GABA modulation, similar to the effects of benzodiazepines, such as Xanax®.

- Shock can depress respiration and body functions in a similar fashion as a heroin overdose.

A big difference between natural sensations and drug-induced sensations is that drugs have side effects, particularly if used to excess, and the natural methods of producing the desired effects usually have no side effects. In addition, the more a drug is used, the weaker the effects become and the harder it becomes to reproduce the desired sensations. With natural sensations, the opposite is true. The desired effects become easier to reproduce over time.

Neurotransmitter research seems to indicate that some people are drawn to certain drugs because they have an imbalance in one or more neurotransmitter and they discovered through experimentation that a specific drug or drugs would help correct that imbalance. For example, people who are born with low endorphin/enkephalin levels or who have damaged their ability to make these chemicals, have a propensity for opioid and alcohol use because those drugs mimic the deficient neurotransmitters and make them feel normal, satisfied, and in control.

PHYSIOLOGICAL RESPONSES TO DRUGS

It is the way in which psychoactive drugs interact with neurotransmitters, nerve cells, and other tissues, such as liver, heart, and lung tissues, which helps determine how drugs affect people and why it is difficult to control their levels of use. Factors such as tolerance, tissue dependence, psychic dependence, withdrawal, and drug metabolism affect the way a person reacts to drugs.

TOLERANCE

"When I first started, I remember having a huge reaction to a small amount of 'speed.' Inside of a year, I could shoot a spoon of it easily, which is a pretty fair amount, and it finally got to a point where I couldn't even sleep unless I'd done some."
Recovering methamphetamine user

The body regards any drug it takes as a toxin. Various organs, especially the liver and kidneys, try to eliminate the chemical before it does too much damage. But if the use continues over a period of time, the body is forced to change and adapt to tolerate the continued input of foreign substances. The net result is that the user has to take larger and larger amounts to achieve the same effect (Fig. 2–13). For example, the body adapts to an upper, such as amphetamine, in order to minimize the stimulant's effect on various systems including pulse and heart rate, so the drug appears to weaken with each succeeding dose if it's used frequently. More has to be taken just to achieve the same effect. One amphetamine tablet on the 1st day of use will energize a user and trigger a euphoria that will take as many as 20 pills to reach on the 100th day of use.

Some degree of tolerance develops with all psychoactive drugs. One dose of LSD on the 1st day, 3 on the 7th day, and 9 on the 30th day might be needed to give the same psychedelic effect if the drug were taken daily. A glass of whiskey at the beginning of one's drinking career might give the same

Figure 2-13 •
This graph shows the gradually increasing amounts of amphetamine needed to produce stimulation or euphoria over time.

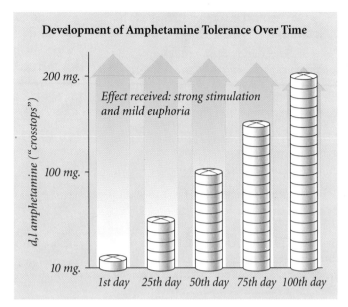

Development of Amphetamine Tolerance Over Time

Effect received: strong stimulation and mild euphoria

d,l amphetamine ("crosstops")

200 mg.

100 mg.

10 mg.

1st day   25th day   50th day   75th day   100th day

buzz as 5 drinks on New Year's Eve 4 years later.

The development of tolerance varies widely depending mostly on the qualities of the drug itself but it also depends on the amount, frequency, and duration of use, the chemistry of the user, and the psychological state of mind of the user. There are seven different kinds of tolerance.

Kinds of Tolerance

Dispositional Tolerance. The body speeds up the breakdown (metabolism) of the drug in order to eliminate it. This is particularly the case with barbiturates and alcohol. An example of this biological adaptation can be seen with alcohol. It increases the amount of cytocells and mitochondria in the liver that are available to neutralize the drug therefore more has to be drunk to reach the same level of intoxication.

Pharmacodynamic Tolerance. Nerve cells become less sensitive to the effects of the drug and even produce an antidote or antagonist to the drug. With opioids, the brain will generate more opioid receptor sites and produce its own antagonist, cholecystokinin.

Behavioral Tolerance. The brain learns to compensate for the effects of the drug by using parts of the brain not affected. A drunk man can make himself appear sober when confronted by police but might be staggering again a few minutes later.

Reverse Tolerance. Initially, one becomes less sensitive to the drug but as it destroys certain tissues and/or as one grows older, the trend is suddenly reversed and the user becomes less able to handle even moderate amounts. This is particularly true in alcoholics when, as the liver is destroyed, it loses the ability to metabolize the drug. An alcoholic with cirrhosis of the liver can stay drunk all day long on a pint of wine because the raw alcohol is passing through the body, time and again, unchanged.

"At first, I could drink a lot, for about eight or nine years. They'd say I finished 10 or more highballs in the bar, but I'd never get falling-down drunk. I'd be pretty high but never passed out. Now, especially since my liver is only slightly smaller than a Volkswagen and not doing its job, if I drink over about 4 drinks, I can't walk one of those white lines a cop makes you walk if he thinks you're DUI."

43-year-old alcohol user

Acute Tolerance (tachyphylaxis). In these cases, the body begins to adapt almost instantly to the toxic effects of the drug. With tobacco, for example, tolerance and adaptation begin to develop with the first puff. People who try suicide with barbiturates can develop an acute tolerance and survive the attempt and be awake and alert even with twice the lethal dose in their system even if they've never taken barbiturates before.

Select Tolerance. If increased quantities of a drug are taken to overcome this tolerance and to achieve a certain high, it's easy to forget or not even be aware that tolerance to the physical side effects also continues to escalate but not at the same rate. The dose needed to achieve an emotional high comes closer and closer to the lethal physical dose of that drug (Fig. 2-14).

"As many pills as I had, I would take. I didn't really care about overdose which I did many times." *Former barbiturate user*

Thus, people develop different rates of tolerance to different effects of the same drug. Codeine kills pain but causes nausea on the first day it is taken. Within a week, it still kills pain but no longer causes nausea.

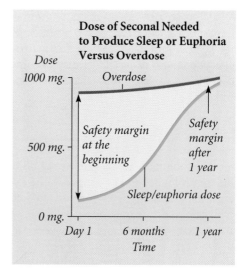

Dose of Seconal Needed to Produce Sleep or Euphoria Versus Overdose

Figure 2-14 •

With many drugs, tolerance to mental effects develops at a different rate than tolerance to physical effects.

Inverse Tolerance (kindling). The person becomes more sensitive to the effects of the drug as the brain chemistry changes. A marijuana or cocaine user, after months of getting a minimal effect from the drug, will all of a sudden get an intense reaction.

"At first I couldn't understand what people got out of methamphetamine. I'd shoot some and it gave me a little lift but that was it. Then one time I got a 1/4 gram, all for myself, and did it all in one shot and the effect was unlike anything I'd ever had before, like liquid fire. My brain was all of a sudden trained to recognize the effects. Then after that, when I'd use a smaller amount, I would experience those same effects though never quite as intense."

Recovering cocaine abuser

A cocaine or methamphetamine addict develops a greater risk of heart attack or stroke after prolonged use due to the toxic effects of those drugs. Thus they become more sensitive to the toxic effects over continued use.

TISSUE DEPENDENCE

The biological adaptation of the body due to prolonged use of drugs is quite extensive, particularly with downers. In fact, with certain drugs, the body can change so much that the tissues and organs come to depend on the drug just to stay normal. If the body doesn't have the drug, its biological adaptations can cause a series of side effects. For example, the increased numbers of cytocells and mitochondria in the liver of an alcoholic depend on repeated use of alcohol to maintain their existence. When alcohol is discontinued, their numbers return to normal levels. Enzymatic changes in the liver of a heroin addict trigger the need for regular doses of heroin to maintain the new chemical balance.

"I would start to feel very abnormal after two or three hours and it was like trying to maintain until I could begin to feel normal. And that was the only kind of normal that I knew, Darvon®-induced normality."
Recovering Darvon® user

In the past, a drug was called addicting only if an obvious tissue dependence developed but with breakthroughs in modern neurochemical research, more subtle changes in body chemistry can be measured. In addition, psychological dependence has been recognized in recent years as an important factor in the development of addictive behavior. Researchers, such as Dr. Anna Rose Childress at Veterans Hospital in Philadelphia, have shown that psychological dependence actually produces many physical effects, meaning that defining drug dependence as strictly physical or strictly mental is not accurate.

PSYCHIC DEPENDENCE AND THE REWARD/REINFORCING ACTION OF DRUGS

Psychic dependence and the positive reward/reinforcing action of drugs result from the direct influence of drugs on brain chemistry. Drugs cause an altered state of consciousness and distorted perceptions pleasurable to the user. These reinforce the continued use of the drug. Psychic dependence can therefore result from the continued misuse of drugs to deal with life's problems or from their continued use to compensate for inherited deficiencies in brain reward hormones.

Drugs also have the innate ability to guide and virtually hypnotize the user into continual use (called the **positive, reward/reinforcing action of drugs**). In the animal experiments in which rats were trained to press a lever which would feed them heroin or other drugs intravenously, they would continue to press the lever even before physical dependence had developed, showing that a psychoactive drug, in and of itself, can reinforce the desire to use.

"I have a choice about the first snort of cocaine I take. I have no choice about the second." Recovering cocaine user

WITHDRAWAL

When the user stops taking a drug that creates tolerance and tissue dependence, the body is left with an altered chemistry. There might be an overabundance of enzymes, receptor sites, or neurotransmitters. Without the drug to support this altered chemistry, the body, all of a sudden, tries to restore its balance. All the things the body was kept from doing while taking the drug, it does to excess while in withdrawal. For example, consider how the desired effects of heroin are quickly transformed into unpleasant withdrawal symptoms once a long-time user stops taking the drug (Table 2-2).

In fact, with many compulsive users, the fear of withdrawal is one reason they keep using. They don't want to go through the aches, pains, insomnia, vomiting, cramps, and occasional convulsions that accompany withdrawal.

"The rush I would get from shooting up again was, all of a sudden my body wouldn't be sick anymore from withdrawal. That was the high."

32-year-old recovering heroin user

Because the withdrawal as well as the fear of withdrawal can be so severe, many treatment programs use mild drugs to temper these symptoms. Withdrawal from opiates, alcohol, many sedatives, and even nicotine seems to be triggered by an area of the brain stem known as the locus cereleus. Drugs like Catapres®, Vasopressin®, and Baclofen®, which act on this part of the brain, block out the withdrawal symptoms of these drugs. There are three distinct types of withdrawal symptoms: nonpurposive, purposive, and protracted.

Kinds of Withdrawal

Nonpurposive Withdrawal. Nonpurposive withdrawal consists of objective physical signs that are directly observable upon cessation of drug use by an addict. These include seizures, sweating, goose bumps, vomiting, diarrhea, and tremors which are a direct result of the tissue dependence that has developed.

TABLE 2–2   OPIOID EFFECTS VERSUS WITHDRAWAL SYMPTOMS
(Withdrawal effects are often opposite of the drug's direct effects)

Effects	Withdrawal Symptoms
Numbness	becomes pain
Euphoria	becomes anxiety
Dryness of mouth	becomes sweating, runny nose
Constipation	becomes diarrhea
Slow pulse	becomes rapid pulse
Low blood pressure	becomes high blood pressure
Shallow breathing	becomes coughing
Pinpoint pupils	become dilated pupils
Sluggishness	becomes severe hyper-reflexes and muscle cramps

"When I ran out, it was severe. I mean, body convulsions, long memory lapses, cramps that were just enough to—you couldn't stand them. And, it lasted for about five days; the actual convulsions, the cramps, and the pain and stuff. And then, it took another couple of weeks before I ever felt anywhere near normal."
Recovering heroin user

Purposive Withdrawal. Purposive withdrawal results from either addict manipulation (hence "purposive" or "with purpose") or from a psychic conversion reaction from the expectation of the withdrawal process. Psychic conversion is an emotional expectation of physical effects which have no biological explanation. Since a common behavior of most addicts is manipulative behavior in an effort to secure more drugs, sympathy, or money, they may claim to have withdrawal symptoms that are very diverse and difficult to verify, e.g., *"My nerves are in an uproar. You've got to give me something, Doc!"* Physicians and pharmacists have to be very aware of these kinds of manipulations.

"It takes a doctor 30 minutes to say no, but it only takes him 5 minutes to say yes. We used to share doctors that we could scam. We called them 'croakers.'"
Recovering heroin user

Within the past few decades, the portrayal of drug addiction by the media, books, movies, and television has resulted in another kind of purposive withdrawal. When they run out of drugs, younger, addiction-naive drug users expect to suffer withdrawal symptoms similar to those portrayed in the media. This expectation results in a neurotic condition whereby they experience a wide range of reactions even though tissue dependence has not truly developed. Treatment personnel need to avoid overreacting to these symptoms.

Protracted Withdrawal (environmental triggers and cues). A major danger to maintaining recovery and preventing a drug overdose during relapse is protracted withdrawal. This is a flashback or recurrence of the addiction withdrawal symptoms and triggering of a heavy craving for the drug long after an addict has been detoxified. The cause of this reaction (similar to a posttraumatic stress phenomenon) often happens when some sensory input (odor, sight, noise) stimulates the memories experienced during drug use or withdrawal and evokes a reexperiencing of those symptoms and desire for the drug by the addict. For instance, the odor of burnt matches or burning metal (smells that occur when cooking heroin) several months after detoxification, may cause a heroin addict to suffer some withdrawal symptoms. Any white powder may cause craving in a cocaine addict; a blue pill may do it to a Valium® addict; and a barbeque can cause a recovering alcoholic to crave a drink.

"I had just got a disability check and that check was like a trigger for me. It just sent me into a state of nervousness or anxiety and I didn't know what to do. Today, I may not even walk on the same block that I used to walk on because I know if I'm feeling shaky, there could be a possibility that I'll run into somebody I want to use with, so I have to stay away from those areas."
Recovering "crack" cocaine user

Protracted withdrawal often causes users to try their drug again, generally leading to a full relapse. Unfortunately, these slips are associated with a greater chance of drug overdose since users are prone to use the same dose they were using when they quit. They often forget or ignore the fact that their last dose was probably a very high one that they could handle because tolerance had developed. They don't remember that abstinence allowed their bodies to return to a less tolerant state.

"We cleaned up because we didn't have any connections when we moved. We had about 15 clonidine pills to help us through and I was drinking. Then we shared one bag, one $20 dollar bag of cut, and both of us were on the floor."
33-year-old husband and wife heroin users

METABOLISM

Metabolism is defined as the body's mechanism for processing, using, inactivating, and eventually eliminating foreign substances such as drugs. As a drug exerts its influence upon the body, it is gradually neutralized, usually by the liver (Fig. 2–15). It can also be metabolized by the blood, the lymph fluid, or most any body tissue that recognizes the drug as a foreign substance. Drugs can also be inactivated by diverting them to body fat or proteins which hold the substances to prevent them from acting on body organs.

The liver, in particular, has the ability to break down or alter the chemical structure of drugs, making them less active or inert. The kidneys, on the other hand, filter the metabolites, water, and other waste from the blood and excrete the resulting urine through the ureter, bladder, and urethra. Drugs can also be excreted out of the body by the lungs, in sweat, or in feces.

Metabolic processes generally decrease (but occasionally increase) the effects of psychoactive drugs. For instance, the liver's enzymes help convert alcohol to water, oxygen, and carbon dioxide which are then excreted from the body through the kidneys, sweat glands, and lungs. Valium®, though, is transformed by the liver's enzymes into three or four compounds which are more active than the original drug.

If a drug is eliminated slowly, as with Valium®, it can affect the body for hours, even days. If it is eliminated quickly, as with smokable cocaine or nitrous oxide, the major actions might last just a few minutes, though other subtle side effects last for days, weeks, or even longer. Following are some other factors which affect the metabolism of drugs.

- *Age:* After the age of 30 and with each subsequent year, the body produces fewer and fewer liver enzymes capable of metabolizing certain drugs, thus the older the person, the greater the effect. This is especially true with drugs like Valium® and other benzodiazepines.

- *Race:* Different ethnic groups have different levels of enzymes. Over 50% of Asians break down alcohol more slowly than do Caucasians. They suffer more side effects, such as redness of the face, than many other ethnic groups.

- *Heredity:* Individuals pass certain traits to their offspring that affect the metabolism of drugs. They can have a low level of enzymes that metabolize the drug; they can have more body fat which will store certain drugs like Valium® or marijuana; or they can have a high metabolic rate which will usually eliminate drugs more quickly from the body.

- *Sex:* Males and females have different body chemistries and different body water volumes. Drugs such as alcohol and barbiturates generally have greater effects in women than in men.

- *Health:* Certain medical conditions affect metabolism. Alcohol in a drinker

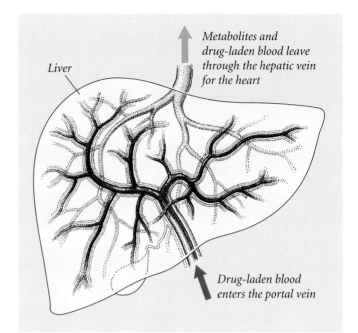

Figure 2-15 •
The liver deactivates a portion of the drug with each pass through the circulatory system.

Liver

Metabolites and drug-laden blood leave through the hepatic vein for the heart

Drug-laden blood enters the portal vein

with severe liver damage (hepatitis, cirrhosis) causes more problems than in a drinker with a healthy liver.

• **Emotional State:** The emotional state of the drug user also has a major influence on the drug's effects. LSD in someone with paranoia can be very dangerous because it can further disrupt the chemical imbalance of the brain and increase the paranoia.

• **Other Drugs:** The presence of two or more drugs can keep the body so busy metabolizing one that metabolism of the second drug is delayed. For example, the presence of alcohol keeps the liver so busy that a Xanax® or Seconal® will remain in the body two or three times longer than normal. Other drug interactions also cause increased or decreased effects and toxicity.

• **Other Factors:** In addition, factors such as the weight of the user, the level of tolerance, and even the weather can affect metabolism of a psychoactive drug.

• **Exaggerated Reaction:** In some cases, the reaction to a drug will be out of proportion to the amount taken. Perhaps the user has an allergy to the drug in much the same way a person can go into shock from a single bee sting. For example, a person who lacks the enzyme which metabolizes cocaine can die from exposure to just a tiny amount.

"When I took cocaine this one time, there was a heavy beating, tachycardia, a sense of not being able to get my breath. There was also the sensation of everything moving very quickly and intensely." Recovering cocaine user

FROM EXPERIMENTATION TO ADDICTION

DESIRED EFFECTS VERSUS SIDE EFFECTS

"Let's not kid ourselves. People initially do get something from drugs. They don't say, 'Well, I want to feel miserable so I think I'll swallow this.' They don't think, 'I'm gonna make myself cough by smoking a joint until my eyes become bloodshot.' They don't plan to get hepatitis or AIDS from a shared needle. They get something out of the drug, something desirable enough to throw caution to the wind."
Darryl S. Inaba, Director, Haight-Ashbury Detox Clinic

DESIRED EFFECTS

People take psychoactive drugs for the mental, emotional, and even physical effects they induce. In some cases, they are specific about the effect they want, and in other cases they are more abstract about their desires.

Curiosity and Availability

"I would be doing a lot better in school if I didn't get stoned. But marijuana is always around and everybody was doing it so I said, 'Why not?'" 16-year-old marijuana smoker

To Get High

"It's kind of like life without a coherent thought. It's kind of like an escape. It's like when you go to sleep, you kind of forget about things in your sleep. It's like everything's dreamlike and there's no restraints on anything." 17-year-old heroin user

Self-Medication

"I was very hyperactive, you know. Just always getting into trouble doing this, getting hurt, falling off of things, getting in fights, getting in arguments. And the more I smoked as the years went on, the mellower I got. I stopped getting into trouble."
23-year-old marijuana user

Confidence

"I felt I wasn't a whole person without it. I needed the drug to become myself, especially dealing with my peers. I was more of an introvert when I was off the drug. When I had the drug, I'd be really outgoing."
17-year-old "crack" cocaine user

Energy

"Very high energy, as though I could walk for miles. I would clean my apartment; use Brillo® on the floor; just lots of energy. It also made me feel very euphoric."
33-year-old amphetamine user

Pain Relief

"I'm always in pain. I have bad shoulders, arthritis, and all these things, so it was my excuse cause I knew this stuff would get me high, so I would take it. I would say, 'Oh, I'm just killing my pain.'" 26-year old opioid user

Anxiety Control

"It relieved certain anxieties. It alleviated depression which I had. Lots of depression.

You tell the doctor, 'I'm depressed.' 'Okay, take some Valium®.' Now they try to give you antidepressant medications prescribed by the doctor. I'll take the Valium®."
44-year-old Valium® user

To Oblige Friends (internal and external peer pressure)

"If your friends are all getting stoned, then you don't want to just sit there. Okay, you know, they're all going to be like having supposedly even more fun because they're stoned. You know, and then they make you look stupid because you feel stupid if you're not." 15-year-old marijuana smoker

Social Confidence

"Somebody walks in the room and what do you do, you offer them a drink. It's cordial. That's how you break the ice. You ask, 'Would you like a drink?' And I frankly don't know anyone who says no. I like to drink. Drink is good. It makes me happy. It makes everybody else I know happy. It's a social event." 42-year-old alcohol user

Boredom Relief

"They tell you you're going to school to get an education so you can get a good job, okay? They told me how to get a job, so that's eight hours a day. I knew how to sleep, that's eight hours a day. I had another eight hours a day that I didn't know how to fill and I used marijuana to fill those eight hours. Period."

35-year-old recovering marijuana user

Altered Consciousness

"I was really into the literature of the time —The Politics of Ecstasy, or something like that, by Timothy Leary, High Priest of the LSD movement. It was more like an adventure, looking for things in it. I think people doing it at the time were trying to find out what it was like to have some sort of spiritual experience."
48-year-old LSD user

To Deal with Isolation or Life Problems

"When I got addicted to the cocaine it was because I was being battered and I used that to hide. When I left the cocaine, I used the drinking to hide. When I left the drinking, the cigarettes kicked in. When I left the cigarettes, I began to overeat. It was like I had to fill up that hole with something."
28-year-old recovering compulsive overeater

Competitive Edge

"I was 125 pounds. Not big enough for the team. I started taking steroids I got from a weightlifter friend so I could bulk up. I also started eating like a hungry hog."
19-year-old steroid user

Oblivion

"I broke down after about six months over in Vietnam and I was in charge of a gun crew. I didn't respond to my duty of opening up an M-60 and some people's lives were lost in my outfit. And I'm responsible. They

flew me out to the States, and I immediately jumped into alcohol and heroin."
46-year-old Vietnam veteran

SIDE EFFECTS

If drugs did only what people wanted them to and they weren't used to excess, they wouldn't be much of a problem. But drugs not only generate desired emotional and physical effects, they also trigger side effects that can be mild, moderate, dangerous, or fatal. This competition between the emotional/physical effects that users want and those they don't want is one of the main problems with using psychoactive drugs. For example, a psychoactive drug such as codeine (an opioid-downer) can be prescribed by a physician to relieve pain, to suppress a cough, or to treat a bad case of diarrhea. It also acts as a sedative, gives a feeling of well-being, and induces numbness and relaxation. Thus, people who self-prescribe codeine just for the feeling of well-being or numbness will have slower reaction time and often become constipated. With moderate use, they can also be subject to nausea, pinpoint pupils, dry skin, and slowed respiration. And, if users keep using in order to recapture that feeling of well-being over a long period of time, they can instead become lethargic, lose sexual desire, and even become compulsive users of the drug.

Users try to learn how to take enough of a drug to get the desired emotional and physical effects without too many side effects that might disrupt their lives. They also try to keep drug use from accelerating to the point where craving for the drug overwhelms common sense. And if drug use continues to accelerate, toxic effects begin to overwhelm the desired effects.

Other complications of drug use include legal problems, relationship problems, financial problems, emotional problems, health problems, control problems, and work problems. The more compulsively a person uses, the more severe the various complications.

LEVELS OF USE

It is important to judge the level at which a person uses drugs, and thereby have a benchmark by which to judge whether drug use is accelerating or becoming problematic in others or in ourselves. To judge a person's level of use, it is necessary to first know the **amount, frequency**, and **duration** of psychoactive drug use. These three factors by themselves are not enough to judge the level of use. The second key factor is to know the impact the use has on an individual's life. For example, a man might drink a six-pack of lager beer (amount) twice a week (frequency) and keep it up for 12 years (duration) without developing any problems. Another man might only drink on Fridays but doesn't stop until he passes out. The second man might have more problems regarding health, the law, or money than the first man who drinks every evening but functions well on the job and works at his relationships.

The categories we've chosen to help people judge the level of use are abstinence, experimentation, social use, habituation, drug abuse, and addiction. The levels of use are presented as distinct categories although the transition from experimentation to habituation or habituation to addiction does not happen in distinct phases. Rather, it is a continuous process that can ebb and flow depending on whether the person is using, how much is being used, and what effect the use is having. Unfortunately, with most psychoactive drugs, a point is passed where it becomes harder and harder for people to choose the level at which they want to continue to use. That point can vary radically from person to person.

ABSTINENCE

Abstinence means people do not use a psychoactive substance except accidentally, for example, when they drink some alcohol-laced punch, take prescribed medication that has a psychoactive component they don't know about, or are in an unventilated room with smokers. The important fact to remember about abstinence is that even if people have a very strong hereditary and environmental susceptibility to use drugs compulsively, they will never have a problem if they never begin to use. If they never use, there is no possibility of developing drug craving. They might, however, have a problem with other compulsive behaviors, such as gambling, eating, TV watching, or obsessive sexual behavior. In addition, exposure to family drug use often affects people's behavior and life even if they remain abstinent from drugs. Adult children of addicts often have difficulty in maintaining relationships or work.

"I didn't like the way my father fought with mother when he drank, so I never drank a drop, not a drop, until I was 27. Then, it was like a light got turned on, and I tried to make up for lost time." 37-year-old drinker

EXPERIMENTATION

With experimentation, people become curious about the effects of a drug or are influenced by relatives, friends, advertising, or other media and take some when it becomes available to satisfy that curiosity. With experimentation, drug use is limited to only a few exposures. No patterns of use

develop and there are only limited negative consequences in the person's life except if

- large amounts are used at one time leading to accident, injury or illness (e.g., drinking binge);
- the person has an exaggerated reaction to a small amount (e.g., cocaine allergy);
- a preexisting physical or mental condition is aggravated (e.g., schizophrenia);
- the user is pregnant;
- legal troubles arise (e.g., drug test, possession arrest);
- a high genetic and/or environmental susceptibility to compulsive use triggers abuse;
- a history of addictive behavior with other psychoactive drugs leads to a relapse.

"I remember the first time a friend of mine gave me this little yellow 'popper,' and he said, 'Here's a present for you,' and I said, 'Oh, what's this?' and he said, 'Well, it's amyl nitrite, you know, and you snap it, and hold it up to your nose, and inhale it.' And so I said, 'Okay.'" Inhalant user

SOCIAL/RECREATIONAL

Whether it's a legal six-pack at a party, an illegal joint with a friend, or a couple of lines of cocaine at home, with social/recreational use, the person does seek out a drug and does want to experience a certain effect but there is no established pattern. Drug use is irregular, infrequent, and has a relatively small impact on the person's life except if it triggers exaggerated reactions, preexisting mental and physical conditions, an existing addiction, genetic/environmental susceptibility, or legal troubles.

"There's a lot of times you don't get stoned alone. You get stoned with your friends. If you come to school, you say to your friends, 'Hey Johnny, let's get stoned.' Everybody does it." Marijuana smoker

HABITUATION

With habituation, there is a definite pattern of use: the TGIF high, the 5 cups of coffee every day, the 1/2 gram of cocaine every weekend, the 2 packs of cigarettes while studying. No matter what happens that day or that week, the person will use that drug. As long as it doesn't affect that person's life in a really negative way, it could be called habituation. This level of use clearly demonstrates that one has lost some control of use of the drug. Regardless of how frequently or infrequently a drug is used, a definite pattern of use indicates that the craving for the drug is now starting to control the user.

"You would say that I was a habitual user, but I don't really think that's the case. So, it is a habit. I like a drink. And the question, you know, the question is could I go a day without having a drink? I think so, but I've never had a reason to try."
42-year-old habitual drinker

DRUG ABUSE

Our definition of drug abuse is **the continued use of a drug despite negative consequences**. It's the use of cocaine in spite of high blood pressure; the use of LSD though there's a history of mental instability; the alcoholic with diabetes; the two-pack-a-day smoker with emphysema; or the user with a series of arrests for possession. No matter how often a person uses a drug, if negative consequences are developed in relationships, social life, finances, legal status, health, work, school, or emotional well-being and drug use continues on a regular basis, then that behavior could be classified as drug abuse.

"I had an EEG and a CAT scan, and I was told that I had lowered my seizure threshold by doing so many stimulants. The reason I actually stopped was because I discovered heroin and I liked it better. I would probably have continued using 'speed' even with the seizures." 36-year-old "speed" user

ADDICTION

The step between abuse and addiction has to do with compulsion. If users

- spend most of their time either using, getting, or thinking about the drug;
- continue to use in spite of negative life and health consequences, mental or physical;
- often deny there's a problem, or claim that they can stop anytime they want;
- and, after withdrawal, still have a strong tendency to relapse and start using again, then that can be classified as addiction.

The users have lost control of their use of drugs and those substances have become the most important things in their lives.

"I guess about a year or so down the line I stopped caring about my appearance. I just didn't keep myself up anymore. I didn't keep my children up anymore. I started running out of food because I was spending money on the drugs." 24-year-old recovering "crack" user

THEORIES OF ADDICTION (addictionology)

In the past two decades, a tremendous amount of research and many theories have been generated to help understand the process of drug addiction. These theories govern the way drug abuse prevention is provided and the way addicts are treated. Traditionally, there have been three major schools of thought about addiction. One emphasized the effects of heredity (**Addictive Disease Model**), another the effects of environment and behavior (**Behavioral/ Environmental Model**), and the third, the physiological effects of psychoactive drugs (**Academic Model**).

ADDICTIVE DISEASE MODEL

This model maintains that the disease of addiction is a chronic, progressive, relapsing, incurable, and potentially fatal condition that is mostly a consequence of genetic irregularities in neurotransmitters, enzymes, and brain tissues which may be activated by the particular drugs that are abused. It also maintains that addiction is set into motion by experimentation with the drug by a susceptible host in an environment that is conducive to drug misuse. The susceptible user quickly experiences a compulsion to use, a loss of control, and a determination to continue the use despite negative physical, emotional, or life consequences.

Several studies of twins, along with other human and animal studies, strongly support the addictive disease theory that heredity and not environment is the stronger influence on uncontrolled, compulsive drug use. Other studies, however, cite environment as the stronger influence.

These hereditary differences in levels of neurotransmitters, receptor sites, enzymes, hormones, and other biochemicals cause addicts to react differently from nonaddicts to the same drug or life experience. Addictive disease, under this definition, is characterized by

- impulsive drug abuse marked by intoxication throughout the day and an overwhelming need to continue use;

- loss of control over the use of a drug with an inability to reduce intake or stop use;

- repeated attempts to control use with periods of temporary abstinence interrupted by relapse into compulsive, continual drug use;

- continuation of abuse despite the progressive development of serious physical, mental, or social disorders aggravated by the use of the substance;

- episodes or complications which result from intoxication, such as an arrest, heart attack, an alcoholic blackout, opiate overdose, loss of job, breakup of a relationship, or any other disabling or impairing condition.

BEHAVIORAL/ENVIRONMENTAL MODEL

This theory emphasizes the overriding importance of environmental and developmental influences in leading a user to develop addictive behavior. As seen in animal and human studies, environmental factors can change brain chemistry as surely as drug use or heredity. Many sociological and psychological studies suggest that physical/emotional stress, such as abuse, anger, peer pressure, and other environmental factors, cause people to seek, use, and sustain their continued dependence on drugs. For example, chronic stress can decrease brain levels of met-enkephalin (a neurotransmitter) in mice, making normal alcohol-avoiding mice more susceptible to alcohol use.

This model emphasizes the six levels of drug use: abstinence, experimentation, social/recreational use, habituation, abuse, addiction.

ACADEMIC MODEL

In this model, addiction occurs when the body adapts to the toxic effects of drugs at the biochemical and cellular level. The principle is that given sufficient quantities of drugs for an appropriate duration of time, changes in body/brain cells will occur which will lead to addiction.

Four physiological changes characterize this process:

- *tolerance:* resistance to the drug's effects increase, necessitating larger and larger doses;
- *tissue dependence:* actual changes in body cells occur because of excessive use, so the body needs the drug to stay in balance;
- *withdrawal syndrome:* physical signs and symptoms of tissue dependence appear when drug use is stopped;
- *psychic dependence:* the effects of the drug are desired by the user and these reinforce the desire to keep using.

· Currently, it is the belief of many researchers in the field of addictionology that the reasons for addiction are a combination of the three factors of heredity, environment, and psychoactive drugs. Because individuals' personalities, physiologies, and life styles vary, so each person's resistance or susceptibility to excessive drug use is different. It is necessary, therefore, to study the determining factors more closely in order to understand why one person might never use, another might use sparingly, a third will use for a lifetime and never have prob-

lems, and someone else will accelerate from experimentation to addiction in a few months. Expanded research has now linked these factors to other compulsive behaviors, like gambling, overeating, and uncontrolled sexual behavior. Thus, a recent definition of addiction describes it as a multivariable, genetic, compulsivity disease activated by environmental influences.

HEREDITY, ENVIRONMENT, PSYCHOACTIVE DRUGS

"Using is a kind of overlay of many different things. If you really want to drink, want to get drunk, and you want the high, that probably means that where you are when you're sober isn't as good as it could be."
22-year-old college student

To better understand current concepts of addiction and how heredity, environment, and psychoactive drugs interact with each other to cause abuse and addiction, it is necessary to study those factors in greater detail.

HEREDITY

In the past decade, there has been increased understanding of the way alcoholism and other compulsive behaviors can be passed on from generation to generation. Recent studies of animals, identical twins, neurological signs, body enzymes, and comprehensive reviews of alcoholics' or addicts' family histories, all provide strong evidence that alcoholism and compulsive drug use are, in part, an inherited condition.

For years, scientists have known that many traits are passed on through generations by genes: features such as such as eye and hair color, nose shape, bone structure, and most important for this chapter, the initial structure and chemistry of the nervous system. In recent years, scientists have expanded that list of genetically influenced traits to include more complex physical reactions and diseases such as juvenile diabetes, some forms of Alzheimer's disease, schizophrenia, some forms of depression, and even a tendency to certain cancers. Most surprisingly, many behaviors seem to have an inheritable component whether it's simply a brain chemistry that results in an exaggerated reaction to alcohol and other psychoactive drugs or a personality that gets a charge from taking risks.

Twin and Retrospective Studies

One set of proofs that a tendency to addiction has an inheritable component is twin studies that have been done in several countries over several decades. Dr. Donald Goodwin of Washington University School of Medicine in St. Louis looked at identical twins who were adopted into separate foster families shortly after birth. These studies strongly support genetics and heredity as the determining factor in alcohol use. Regardless of the foster parent family environment, adopted children developed alcohol abuse or abstinence patterns similar to their biologic parents' use of alcohol.

Other evidence of genetic alcoholism comes from reviewing the biologic family records of those alcoholics in various treatment programs across the United States. The statistics showed that if one biological parent was alcoholic, a male child was about 34% more likely to be an alcoholic than the male child of nonalcoholics. If both biological parents were alcoholic, the child was about 400% more likely to be alcoholic. If both parents and a grandparent were alcoholic, that child was about 900%

more likely to develop alcoholism. About 28 million Americans have at least one alcoholic parent.

Prior to 1990, most genetic studies on alcoholism focused on men simply because there were more men in treatment than women and because of biologic variables in women which made research more difficult. Recent studies of adopted, female identical twins has verified that women are at risk to genetic alcoholism similar to that seen in previous male twin studies.

Alcoholism-Associated Gene

Another breakthrough in this line of inquiry came in 1990 when a specific gene associated with alcoholism was discovered by Ernest Nobel and Kenneth Blum, researchers at the University of Texas. Many researchers believe this gene helps indicate a person's susceptibility to compulsive drinking. In some studies, this DRD_2A_1 Allele gene was found in greater than 70% of severe alcoholics in treatment but less than 30% in people who were assessed to be social drinkers or abstainers. What the presence of this gene and probably other yet to be discovered ones mean is that when people with these hereditary associations do use alcohol, they have a much higher chance of becoming alcoholics than drinkers in the general population. However, if they never drink, problems with alcohol can never occur.

"My grandmother told me, 'Our family can't drink. The only exercise your granddad got was bending his elbow. Your uncle died of cirrhosis of the liver. Your aunt died of a combination of alcohol and her sleeping pills. Your dad had four martinis every day of his business life, and that was just at lunch." 31 year-old recovering alcoholic

Kenneth Blum believes this gene (and others) also indicates a tendency to a number of compulsive behaviors, not just drinking. He refers to it as a compulsivity gene, not just an alcoholic gene.

In practical terms, what genetic associations mean is that people who are susceptible to developing alcoholism (or other compulsive drug use) begin drinking or using other drugs at a much quicker rate than people without that susceptibility. Though many susceptible people receive an intense reaction from alcohol with their first drinking experience, they also seem to need larger amounts of alcohol than others to get drunk, but when they reach that drunken state, it is much more intense and causes greater dysfunction. Many have blackouts, starting with the first few times they use, where they don't remember what happened to them while drunk.

"My first drunk was a blackout, and I was a weekend drinker until I was about 17 but I was considered an alcoholic by my friends by the age of 18. Drinking was what freed me up. See, for me, a few sips of booze and the whole world completely changes—completely changes the way it looks and the way I feel about it and how I feel about myself, whereas that doesn't happen to most people."
32-year-old recovering alcoholic

This exaggerated reaction to alcohol, the need for large amounts, and the greater dysfunction also happen with other drugs.

ENVIRONMENT

The environmental influences that help determine the level at which a person uses drugs can be positive or negative and as varied as stress, love, violence, sexual abuse, nutrition, living conditions, family relationships, health care, neighborhood safety, school quality, and television messages. The pressures and influences of environment, particularly home environment, actually shape, mold, and connect the nerve cells, tissues, and neurochemistry a person is born with, thereby helping to determine whether and how that person will use psychoactive drugs.

Environment and Brain Development

Environmental influences have the greatest impact on the development of the brain. Though we are born with all the nerve cells we will ever have, about 100 billion in the brain alone, environment influences the 100 trillion connections that develop between nerve cells (Fig. 2–16). In this way, environment molds the brain's architecture and neurochemistry, thus altering the way the brain reacts to outside influences. The growth and alteration are especially widespread in the first 10 years of life. The process of making new connections and altering brain chemistry continues thereafter, but at an increasingly slower rate. Early environmental influences (ages 0–10) seem to have the greatest influence on a person's development.

Through subtle chemical, structural, and biological changes, the brain keeps track of all that happens to a person in his or her lifetime. The stronger the environmental influences and the more often they are repeated, the more indelible the imprinting on the brain. For example, if a person uses a certain phone number again and again, the person memorizes it because the area of the brain responsible for numbers has physiologically written that information in the brain. Because a traumatic experience, such as an accident or war experience, is so intense, it can leave lasting impressions immediately.

Neurons Make Connections

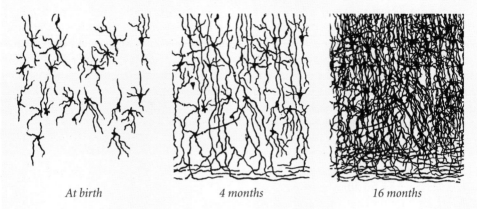

| At birth | 4 months | 16 months |

Figure 2-16 •

This representation of brain cells of a newborn is seen on the left. Notice that there are relatively few connections between cells. By the time it is born, the baby's brain will have all its 100 billion nerve cells. The influences of environment and learning will create new connections and patterns. By the age of 10, the number of interconnections between nerve cells will be about 100 trillion.

Children who are subject to excess emotional pain while growing up in a chaotic household remember that pain and may try different ways to deal with the hurt. They can try to understand why it happened, learn how to deal with it, find people to help them, and accept what happened or they can run away, become hyperactive, make jokes, use alcohol or other substances, anything to temper the pain or discomfort. If that stress continues long enough, the counter-behavior that the child learns also becomes ingrained in the brain. The brain remembers that counter-behavior just as it remembered the stress and pain. Once connections are made and chemistry altered in response to environmental challenges, particularly at a young age, they are very difficult to change (but not impossible).

One strong proof of environmental influences on drug abuse is found when one examines the social and family histories of addicts in treatment. They demonstrate an extraordinarily high level of experienced child abuse, incest, domestic violence, and rejection.

"Drinking really made the world all right. And without alcohol, I had to feel all these feelings that were unbearable in my childhood. I drank till I was 29 which is when I got sober, and even today it's extremely hard. Today, I still fight a lot of those same feelings of inadequacy, the feelings that my feelings aren't right, that I don't have the right to get angry, that I don't have the right to feel lonely." 32-year-old recovering alcoholic

Environment can make a person more liable to use and abuse psychoactive substances if stress is common in the home, if drinking or other drug use is common in the home, if different ways of reacting to stress or anger aren't learned and self-medication becomes the only solution, or if there are mental health problems triggered by the home environment.

People can also become more susceptible to use if society tells them in word and deed that drinking, smoking, and using drugs to solve all problems are a normal part of life. Massive advertising campaigns for tobacco or alcohol make people more likely to use. Belonging to a social, business or peer group where excessive drinking or drug use is considered normal increases use. Living in a community where access to legal and illegal drugs is easy increases use.

"I think it's gotten more of that social, habitual thing. It's like my parents have a glass of wine after they come home from work to relax and unwind. I'm the same way, just with marijuana. It's just kind of a regular thing that I do instead of alcohol or anything else."
17-year-old marijuana smoker

And if, in addition to these environmental stressors and influences, people have a hereditary susceptibility to use, the chances that they will slide into compulsive use (if they start drinking or taking drugs) greatly increase.

PSYCHOACTIVE DRUGS

The hereditary and environmental influences mean nothing in terms of alcoholism or addiction unless the person actually uses drugs, so the final factor that determines the level at which a person might use drugs is the psychoactive drugs themselves. Drugs can affect not only susceptible individuals but also those with no predisposing factors. This occurs because, by definition, psychoactive drugs are substances which affect the functioning of the central nervous system. Excessive, fre-

quent, or prolonged use of alcohol or other drugs inevitably modifies many of the same nerve cells and neurochemistry that are affected by heredity and environment, thus influencing not only the person's reaction to those substances when they are used but also the level at which they are used.

"It actually took me a long time to get strung out on crystal 'meth.' I first started using 'dexies' [Dexadrine®] in college to help me cram for exams. Several years later, I began using 'coke' and 'speed' to party with but never every day. Somehow, things began to change, slowly. I would get more and more depressed when I wasn't high. Then I started using the 'meth' every day just to keep awake."
45-year-old methamphetamine addict

The development of tolerance, tissue dependence, withdrawal, and psychic dependence are signs that the drugs themselves are causing physical and chemical changes in the body that tend to raise the level of use.

ALCOHOLIC MICE AND SOBER MICE

To better understand the close connection between heredity, environment, psychoactive drugs and drug abuse, it might be helpful to examine a series of classical animal studies done over the past 40 years by Drs. Gerald McLaren, T.K. Li, Horace Lo, and other researchers.

The basic experiment is as follows: years ago, two genetic strains of mice (Fig. 2-17) were discovered which helped researchers understand alcoholism. One of the strains of mice loved alcohol. When

Figure 2-17 •

Two strains of mice have been bred to help test theories of addiction.

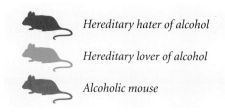

Hereditary hater of alcohol

Hereditary lover of alcohol

Alcoholic mouse

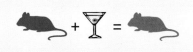

A Alcohol-hating mouse is force fed large quantities of alcohol.

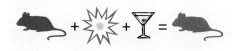

B Alcohol-hating mouse is subjected to stress and alcohol is made available

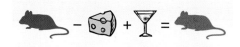

C Alcohol-hating mouse is nutritionally deprived and alcohol is made available.

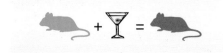

D Alcohol is made available to alcohol-loving mouse.

given the choice between water and even 70% concentrations of alcohol, these mice went for the alcohol, every time. If all they had was water, then they would grudgingly drink water. The other strain of mice hated alcohol. Given the same choice, even with concentrations as low as 2% alcohol, the mice always chose the pure water.

In the experiment, the researchers first took a group of the alcohol-hating mice and injected them with high levels of alcohol, the equivalent of what adult human beings would drink if they were heavy drinkers. Within a few weeks, these once sober mice came to prefer alcohol. In fact, if not stopped, they would drink themselves to death (Fig. 2-17A).

The researchers then took another group of the alcohol-hating mice and subjected them to stress by putting them in very small, constrictive tubes for intermittent periods of time. Within a few weeks, this group of sober mice also came to prefer higher and higher concentrations of alcohol to pure water. In essence, sober mice had been turned into alcoholic mice, first through stress (**environment**) and then through excessive use of alcohol (**psychoactive drugs**) (Fig. 2-17B).

Further, researcher Dr. Jorge Madronis, a nutritionist, took another group of alcohol-hating mice and restricted their diet of vitamin B and some essential proteins. This also resulted in increasing alcohol use after several months (**nutrition**) (Fig. 2-17C).

The mice whose **heredity** made them prefer alcohol from birth drank themselves to death, once they were given access to alcohol. Even when they were subjected to electrical shocks aimed at preventing them from drinking the alcohol (aversive therapy), they continued to drink, even until the shocks came close to being fatal (Fig. 2-17D). (Note that if they were never given alcohol, they could not become alcoholic mice even though they had the highest susceptibility to compulsive drinking.)

What was most interesting was that when the forced drinking, stress induction, and nutritional restriction were stopped, the originally sober, alcohol-hating mice did not return to their normal nondrinking habits. They had been transformed into alcohol-loving mice. And if given the chance to drink, they would be alcoholic mice.

When the brains of the four groups of mice were examined (the hereditary alcoholic mice, the stress-induced alcoholic mice, the drug-induced alcoholic mice, and the nutritionally restricted alcoholic mice), all had approximately the same (alcohol-loving) brain chemistry even though they started with different neurochemical balances. Most of the changes occurred in the old brain. This research suggests that whether the neurochemical disruption is caused by heredity, environment, psychoactive drugs, nutritional deficiency, or a combination of several of the factors, they can all lead to the same type of serious addiction.

COMPULSION CURVE

Human beings, of course, are different than mice. We are more complex: our brains are more intricate and our social patterns are much more complex. We have the power of reason, we have more control of our environment, we have self-awareness, and yet, research, especially over the last 10 years, shows that the basic drug-craving mechanisms, which reside mostly in the old brain, are similar to those of most other mammals. The difference is that in humans, it usually takes a combina-

tion of heredity, environment, and psychoactive drug use to increase compulsive use. In addition, the environmental factors are much more complex than with simpler animals, the new brain has the ability to override the old brain, and human beings have the capacity to change.

To help understand the interrelationship of heredity, environment, and the use of psychoactive drugs in human beings, we have developed a graphic representation of the ways that a user might advance from experimentation to addiction.

HEREDITARY SUSCEPTIBILITY

First, it's important to remember that all people are born with an inherited susceptibility to avoid, use, or abuse drugs. Some are more susceptible than others. That susceptibility is reflected by the brain's structure and neurochemical composition. The determining inherited factor might be that the person is born with a lack of dopamine, a satiation/reward neurotransmitter. The lack of this chemical makes that person more likely to use psychoactive drugs or engage in behaviors that increase the activity of that chemical and make him or her feel better (Fig. 2-18).

ENVIRONMENTAL FACTORS

If an individual is then subjected to stress (or other environmental factors like nutritional restriction) and the personality changes, the brain chemistry is altered and that individual can become more susceptible to the effects of the drug if he or she uses. (Note that people do not have to use to increase their susceptibility.) So as environmental stressors move a person up on the curve, the distance to habituation, abuse, and addiction shrinks (Fig. 2-19).

Figure 2-18 •
Initial susceptibility is
inherited.

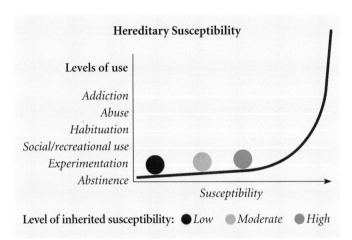

Figure 2-18 •
Initial susceptibility is
inherited.

Figure 2-19 •
Susceptibility increases due to
environment.

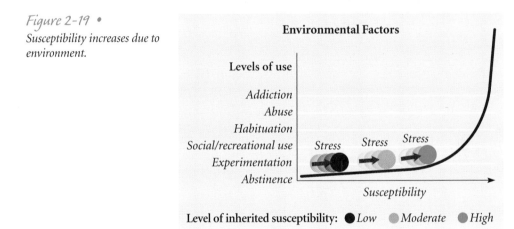

DRUG USE

If individuals then use psychoactive drugs, they are pushed further along the curve (Fig. 2-20). The stronger (more addictive) the drug, and the greater the amount, frequency, and duration of use, the closer to habituation, abuse, and addiction they will come. Those with a low inherited/environmental susceptibility to drugs would have to use a lot of drugs over a long period of time, or strong drugs over a shorter period, to push themselves along.

The drugs that push the hardest and the quickest towards addiction, are, in order from fastest to slowest

smoking tobacco;

smoking "crack" cocaine;

smoking or injecting heroin;

injecting methamphetamines;

snorting cocaine;

ingesting amphetamines;

ingesting sedative hypnotics;

drinking alcohol;

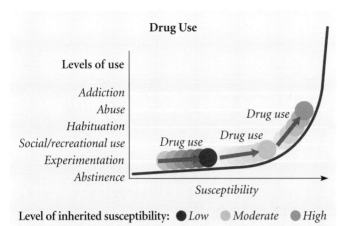

Figure 2-20 •
Susceptibility increases due to drug use.

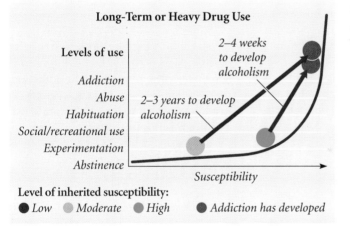

Figure 2-21 •
Addiction develops at different rates.

smoking marijuana;
ingesting or drinking caffeine;
ingesting PCP, MDMA, LSD;
ingesting peyote.

LONG-TERM OR HEAVY DRUG USE

It might take those with low susceptibility 10 years of drinking to become alcoholics or it might never occur. It might take them 2 years of occasional injecting to be-come a heroin addict or 6 months of smoking to get to a pack of cigarettes a day. People in the middle of the scale, with moderate inherited susceptibility, might need just 2 or 3 years of use to slip into alcohol abuse or addiction, or 6 months of heroin use to graduate to a $200-a-day habit, or 3 months of smoking to be a chain smoker. People with a high susceptibility might slip into compulsive, heavy drinking after just a couple of weeks of bingeing because their bodies are primed for compulsive use (Fig. 2-21). The highly

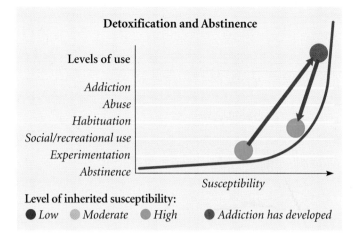

Figure 2-22 •
Susceptibility doesn't return to normal after detox and abstinence.

Detoxification and Abstinence

Levels of use

Addiction
Abuse
Habituation
Social/recreational use
Experimentation
Abstinence

Susceptibility

Level of inherited susceptibility:
● *Low*   ● *Moderate*   ● *High*   ● *Addiction has developed*

susceptible heroin user could be compulsive after a month of injecting and the high-risk smoker would be chain smoking within a couple of weeks.

The slope of the compulsion curve is very gradual at the low susceptibility end but dramatically steeper at the high susceptibility end. This visualizes the progressive and accelerating nature of addiction.

ABSTENTION

What happens if people stop taking the drug? Do they return to their starting point? Does their susceptibility go down? The answers are unclear. Current evidence and the experience with 85,000 clients at the Haight-Ashbury Detox Clinic suggest that there will be some rebound in the balance of the disrupted neurotransmitters, but those who have moved to addiction will have less of a rebound, particularly those with high inherited susceptibility (Fig. 2-22). Other evidence suggests that neurotransmitter levels in those with short-term, noninherited abuse or addiction rebound closer to normal levels once they stop using, but they are still at a higher susceptibility level than when they started to use.

RELAPSE

Since susceptibility doesn't return to normal, particularly in those with a strong hereditary component to their addiction, users are more at risk for a quicker return to addiction the next time they start to use. The brain is imprinted with memories of the drug-using habits and sensations experienced during use and abuse so drug craving increases. For example, if it took a person three years to develop Xanax® addiction and then that person abstains from use for a while, it might only take one month to relapse back into abuse or addiction. If it took four weeks to become addicted to cigarettes, it might take just one cigarette now to relapse (Fig. 2-23). Regardless of how one gets to the addictive end of the curve, the great majority of treatment professionals and recovering addicts agree that once there, it is virtually impossible to return to controlled experimental, social, or habitual patterns of use. Recovery from addiction is extremely difficult to accomplish without abstinence from all psychoactive drugs and assisted by treatment, counseling, education, support, and active participation in fellowships

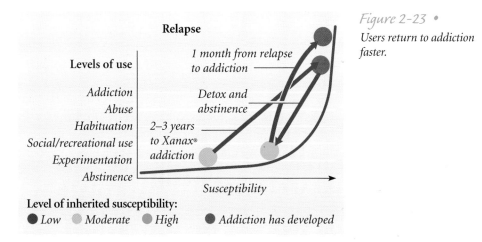

Figure 2-23 •
Users return to addiction faster.

(e.g., Alcoholics Anonymous or Rational Recovery).

CONCLUSIONS

The interrelations of heredity, environment, and psychoactive drugs emphasize that any study of addiction should focus on the totality of people's lives: their personality, relationships, how they live, and their family history. In succeeding chapters, this book will not only study stimulants, depressants, psychedelics, inhalants, and other drugs, but also look at compulsive behaviors such as compulsive overeating and gambling whose causes are similar to those that lead to drug use, abuse, or addiction.

C H A P T E R   S U M M A R Y

HOW PSYCHOACTIVE DRUGS AFFECT US

How Drugs Get to the Brain

1. Drugs can enter the body in five ways. In order of the speed with which they begin to exert their effects, they are: inhaling (including smoking), injecting, snorting (or under the tongue), eating or drinking, and contact (suppository, skin patches).

2. Drugs travel in the bloodstream to reach the central nervous system (CNS = brain and spinal cord) where they will have the greatest effect. They must cross the blood-brain barrier to reach the nerve cells of the brain.

3. Psychoactive drugs affect the rest of the body either directly or by acting on the nerves of the central nervous system.

4. The nervous system with 100 billion nerve cells and 100 trillion connections consists of the central nervous system (brain and spinal cord), the autonomic nervous system which controls physiologic functions, and the peripheral nervous system which connects the senses and organs to the autonomic and central nervous systems.

The Brain

5. The old brain controls physiologic functions, emotions, and feelings while the new brain controls reasoning, language, creativity, and other higher order functions.

6. Depressants and stimulants work mostly on the old brain, psychedelics work more on the new brain.

7. Drug craving seems to reside mostly in the old brain.

Neuroanatomy

8. A nerve cell consists of dendrites, cell body, axon, and terminals.

9. Messages travel from nerve cell to nerve cell as electrical signals. However, between most nerve cells there is a synaptic gap. Messages cross this gap as chemical signals called neurotransmitters and are then converted back to electrical signals. This message transmission process that occurs at the synaptic gap is called a synapse.

Neurotransmitters

10. Neurotransmitters are the biochemicals (e.g., dopamine, GABA, serotonin, norepinephrine, and endorphin) most affected by psychoactive drugs.

11. Psychoactive drugs increase, mimic, block, or otherwise disrupt the release of these chemicals. In turn, the neurotransmitters intensify signals (agonist) or inhibit signals (antagonist).

12. All psychoactive drugs mimic or disrupt naturally occurring neurotransmitters by slotting into existing receptor sites.

Physiological Responses to Drugs

13. When a person takes certain drugs over a period of time, the body becomes used to their effects so more is needed to achieve the same high. The user develops a tolerance to the drug.

14. The tolerance to the physical and psychological effects can develop at different rates.

15. The body tries to adapt to the increased quantities of drugs by changing its chemical balance and chemical composition of organs such as the liver.

16. The pleasurable effects of drugs reinforce the desire to continue to use the drug. The direct influence of drugs has the innate ability to keep someone using.

17. When a user stops taking a drug after tissue dependence has developed (mostly with opiates, alcohol, and sedative-hypnotics), the body experiences many of the unpleasant sensations and physical changes it was kept from feeling while taking the drug. This backlash is known as withdrawal.

18. Protracted withdrawal, which is a delayed psychic and physiological remembrance of drug experiences, is one of the main reasons for relapse.

19. The liver is the principal organ for neutralizing drugs. The kidneys are the principal organs for filtering drugs from the blood and excreting them in the urine.

20. A variety of factors, such as age, race, health, and sex, help determine how fast a drug is metabolized.

FROM EXPERIMENTATION TO ADDICTION

Desired Effects Versus Side Effects

21. People take drugs for a variety of reasons including getting high, self-medicating, building confidence, increasing energy, satisfying curiosity, obliging friends (peer pressure), and avoiding problems.

22. The major problem with psychoactive drugs is that some people who take them focus on the desired mental and emotional effects and ignore the potentially damaging physical and mental side effects that can occur.

Levels of Use

23. The level of use is judged first by the amount, frequency, and duration of use, then by the effect use has on the individual's life.

24. The six levels of use are abstinence, experimentation, social/recreational use, habituation, abuse, and addiction.

25. The hallmark of drug abuse is continued use despite adverse consequences.

26. The hallmarks of addiction are loss of control and compulsion to use.

Theories of Addiction

27. The addictive disease model says addiction is a chronic, progressive, relapsing, incurable, and potentially fatal condition that is mostly a consequence of genetic irregularities.

28. The behavioral/environmental model says that certain influences of one's environment, including stress, abuse, anger, and peer pressure, can induce addiction.

29. The academic model says that it's the use of drugs that causes the body to adapt through physiologic mechanisms such as tolerance, tissue dependence, withdrawal, and psychic dependence.

Heredity, Environment, Psychoactive Drugs

30. Heredity gives people their starting point in life. They begin with a certain susceptibility to use or not use drugs. This susceptibility is reflected in a certain neurochemical or neurostructural imbalance.

31. Environment, especially stress, then molds that basic architecture of the nervous system, further increasing or decreasing susceptibility to compulsive drug use.

32. Drug use itself triggers that existing hereditary/environmental susceptibility, and through tolerance and other physiological mechanisms, further pushes a user towards compulsive use.

Alcoholic Mice and Sober Mice

33. Animal experiments indicate that compulsive use can be reached through heredity, stress, nutritional restriction, or ingestion of large amounts of alcohol or other drugs.

Compulsion Curve

34. In humans, it is the combination of heredity, environment, and/or drug use that can push a person out of experimentation and social/recreational use towards habituation, abuse, and addiction.

Uppers

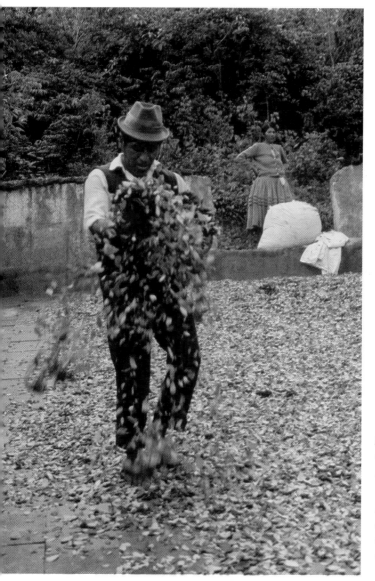

T his Bolivian farm worker is sorting coca leaves. It takes 250 kilos of leaves to make 1 kilo of cocaine.
Reprinted by permission, Alain Labrousse, Observatoire Geopolitique Des Drogues.

- **General Classification:** Uppers vary from very strong stimulants, such as cocaine and amphetamines, to weak ones, like caffeine and nicotine. However, nicotine causes the most severe long-term health problems.

- **General Effects:** Stimulants force the release of the body's own energy chemicals and stimulate the reward/pleasure center. They also constrict blood vessels, speed the heart, and raise blood pressure. Prolonged use of the stronger stimulants depletes energy resources, induces paranoia, and triggers intense craving.

- **Cocaine:** Ingested, injected, snorted, or smoked, cocaine causes the most rapid stimulation and subsequent comedown of all the stimulants.

- **Smokable Cocaine:** Smokable cocaine, also known as freebase cocaine and "crack" cocaine, has most of the same effects as snorting or injecting cocaine. Smoking "crack" or freebase is the most rapid and intense method of use.

- **Amphetamines:** Longer lasting and cheaper than cocaine, these synthetic stimulants have seen a rapid growth in the 1990s.

- **Amphetamine Congeners:** Ritalin® is used to treat hyperactive children whereas diet pills are used to control weight gain.

- **Lookalikes and Over-the-Counter Stimulants:** Legal mild stimulants can have additive effects. Some are falsely advertised as amphetamines or cocaine.

- **Other Plant Stimulants:** Other mild stimulants, like khat, ibogaine, betel nuts, and ephedra, are used worldwide in addition to coffee or other stronger stimulants.

- **Caffeine:** Coffee, tea, chocolate, and soft drinks contain caffeine and can be mildly addicting. Many over-the-counter medications also contain caffeine.

- **Nicotine (tobacco):** Nicotine is the stimulating and addicting component of tobacco. Hundreds of other by-products and additives, like tar and nitrosomines, can cause cancer and respiratory or cardiovascular problems.

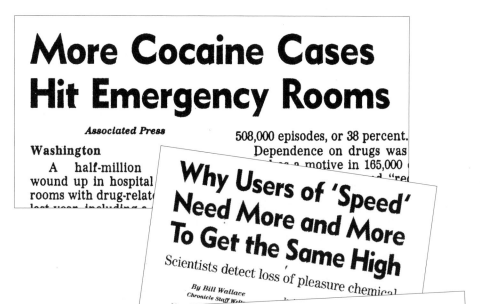

More Cocaine Cases Hit Emergency Rooms

Associated Press

Washington

A half-million wound up in hospital rooms with drug-relat...

508,000 episodes, or 38 percent. Dependence on drugs was ... motive in 165,000 ...

Why Users of 'Speed' Need More and More To Get the Same High

Scientists detect loss of pleasure chemical

By Bill Wallace
Chronicle Staff Wr...

Teenagers Not Kicking Cigarette Habit

Associated Press

Atlanta

A study shows young people are smoking as much as they did a decade ago despite efforts to warn them away from cigarettes, a federal health spokesman said yesterday.

"We have made no progress in

Smoking and Health in the Centers for Disease Control and Prevention.

The CDC released two surveys on smoking on the eve of the American Cancer Society's "Great American Smokeout."

One, by the University of Michigan, showed that 19 percent of

high school seniors has been fairly stable since 1984, when it was 18.7 percent.

The other survey, conducted by the CDC, showed that cigarette consumption among people over 18 is decreasing.

The CDC drew no direct con-

GENERAL CLASSIFICATION

From powerful stimulants, including methamphetamines and "crack" cocaine, to milder ones, such as caffeinated soft drinks and cigarettes, uppers are a regular part of life for many Americans. In the United States in 1995, according to the National Institute of Drug Abuse (NIDA) and other sources, almost 1.6 million Americans used amphetamines ("speed," "meth," "crank") for nonmedical reasons; over 3.6 million

used cocaine at least occasionally; 61 million smoked cigarettes; more than 100 million drank coffee; and almost as many took an over-the-counter medication containing caffeine.

Stimulants are found naturally in many plants, such as the coca bush (cocaine), the tobacco plant (nicotine), the khat tree (cathinone), the ephedra bush (ephedrine), and the coffee plant (caffeine). Other stimulants are synthesized in laboratories, for example, amphetamines, diet pills, Ritalin®, methcathinone, and lookalikes.

TABLE 3–1   UPPERS (stimulants)

Drug Name	Some Trade Names	Street Name
COCAINE (from coca leaf)		
Cocaine HCL (hydrochloride)	None	Coke, blow, toot, snow, flake, girl, lady, nose candy, big C, la dama blanca
Freebase cocaine	None	Crack, base, rock, basay, boulya, pasta, hubba, basuco, pestillos
AMPHETAMINES: (synthetic– "crank," "speed," "meth," "ice")		
d,1 amphetamine	Benzedrine®, Obetrol®, Biphetamine®	Crosstops, whites, speed, black beauties, bennies, cartwheels, pep pills
Dextroamphetamine	Dexedrine®, Eskatrol®	Dexies, Christmas trees, beans
Methamphetamine	Methadrine®, Desoxyn®	Crank, meth, crystal, peanut butter speed
Dextromethamphetamine base	None	Ice, glass, batu, shabu, yellow rock
Levo amphetamine	Vick's Inhaler®	
Freebase methamphetamine	None	Snot
AMPHETAMINE CONGERS (Ritalin®, diet pills)		
Methylphenidate	Ritalin®	Pellets
Phendimetrazine	Preludin®	Pink hearts
Pemoline	Cylert®	Popcorn coke
Phentermine HCL	Fastin®, Adipex®,	Robin's eggs, black and whites
Phentermine resin	Phenazine®, Bontril®, Plegine®, Trimtabs®, Melfiat®, Pendiet®, Statobex®, Ionamin®	
Fenfluramine	Pondimin®	
Dexfenfluramine	Redux®	
Diethylpropion	Tenuate®, Tepanil®	
LOOKALIKES AND OVER-THE-COUNTER STIMULANTS		
Can contain: caffeine, ephedrine, phenylephrine, phenylpropanolamine, pseudoephedrine	Lookalikes: Super Toot®, Super Caine® OTCs: Dexatrim®, Acutrim®, Benadryl®	Legal speed, robin's eggs, black beauties
Herbal caffeine, ephedra	Herbal Ecstasy®, Herbal Nexus®	

TABLE 3–1 (continued)

Drug Name	Some Trade Names	Street Name
OTHER PLANT STIMULANTS		
Khat (cathinone, cathine) (methcathinone is the synthetic version)		Qat, chat, Abyssinian tea (Cat, goob)
Betal nut (arecoline)		
Yohimbe (yohimbine)		
Ephedra		Ma Huang, marwath
CAFFEINE		
Coffee	Colombian, French espresso	Java, Joe, mud, roast, legal speed
Tea	Lipton®, Stash®	Cha
Colas (from cola nut)	Coca Cola®, Pepsi®,	Coke
Chocolate (cocoa beans)	Hershey®, Nestles®	
Over-the-counter stimulants	No Doz®, Alert®, Vivarin®	
NICOTINE (TOBACCO)		
Cigarettes, cigars	Marlboro®, Kents®	Cancer stick, smoke, butts, toke, coffin nails
Pipe tobacco	Sir Walter Raleigh®	
Snuff	Copenhagen®	Dip
Chewing tobacco	Day's Work®, Beechnut®, Levi-Garrett®, Redman®	Chew, chaw

GENERAL EFFECTS

Stimulants, particularly the stronger ones like cocaine, amphetamines, and amphetamine congeners, increase the chemical and electrical activity in the central nervous system. In low doses, they make the user more alert, active, anxious, restless, and, in general, more stimulated than normal. The major effects of stimulants occur because of the way they manipulate energy chemicals and trigger the reward/pleasure center.

BORROWED ENERGY

Day in and day out, the body releases energy chemicals, hormones, and neurotransmitters, such as adrenaline (epinephrine) and noradrenaline (norepinephrine). More of these chemicals are released while we are awake than when we are asleep, but the average daily output is fairly constant. These energy chemicals can increase heart rate, energize muscles, keep us alert, and help us function normally. In time, they are

The stronger stimulants, such as cocaine, amphetamines, and amphetamine congeners, are shown with the weaker stimulants, like caffeinated drinks and tobacco products.

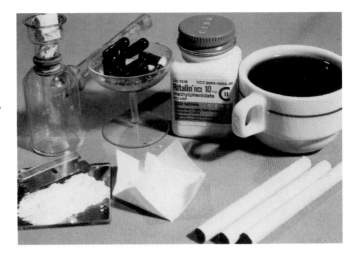

reabsorbed or metabolized and excreted from the body.

Sometimes, though, the body needs extra energy: when it exercises, is scared, is making love, or has to fight. At these moments, the nervous system releases extra amounts of adrenaline and other chemicals. Remember the surge of energy the body receives when frightened? Eventually, the extra energy chemicals are also reabsorbed or metabolized, allowing the body to return to normal.

The normal progression of events is as follows:

- The body demands extra energy.
- Cells release energy chemicals.
- The body receives extra energy.

Stimulants reverse the process.

- When stimulants are ingested, smoked, injected, or snorted, they artificially increase the activity of energy chemicals.
- The body then has extra energy and stimulation it really doesn't need.

Stronger stimulants, such as methamphetamine or "crack" cocaine, keep the chemicals circulating by blocking their reabsorption or metabolism, so the stimulatory effects are greatly exaggerated. If this process continues for hours and even days, the body is infused with tremendous amounts of extra energy which must be released.

"I would stay up three to five days, sleep for a day, and do it again; three to five days, sleep for a day, do it again."

32-year-old recovering methamphetamine abuser

If strong stimulants are only taken occasionally, the body has time to recover. But if they are taken continuously over a long period of time or in large quantities, the energy supply becomes depleted and the body is left without reserves. It is squeezed dry, exhausted. With stronger stimulants, this "crash," its subsequent withdrawal symptoms and depression can last for days, weeks, and in some cases, even months. The severity of the crash depends on the length of use, the strength of the drug, the extent of biochemical disruption, and any preexisting mental or emotional problems.

In the 1960s, stimulants were actually identified in adertisements as "stimulants." This 1968 ad for Ritalin® listed chronic fatigue, drug-induced lethargy, psychoneuroses (e.g., depression), narcolepsy, senile behavior, and finally hyperactivity disorder as conditions that could be treated with the drug. Since many strong stimulants were heavily regulated or banned in the '70s, methylphenidate (Ritalin®) has been advertised mostly for attention deficit/hyperactivity disorder.

* *

"I had a never-ending supply, but there is only so much you can do and after a while you don't get high anymore, no matter how much more you do. You just need to crash and the depression is terrible: the fatigue, not even being able to walk, not being able to get out of bed, and just being desperate to sleep. The depression lasts up to eight days, but it is intensely acute for three or four days in my case."

Recovering methamphetamine user (currently a drug counselor)

It is important to remember that the energy received from stimulants is not a free gift. It is a loan from the rest of the body and must be repaid by giving the body time to recover, to rebuild its supply of stimulatory neurochemicals, and regenerate damaged neurons (as much as possible).

"As soon as you release all that smoke ['crack' cocaine], it makes you feel like you're on top of the world. It gives you a real instantaneous rush." Recovering "crack" user

CARDIOVASCULAR EFFECTS

Many stimulants constrict blood vessels, thus decreasing blood flow to tissues, particularly the skin and extremities. Since blood flow is decreased, tissue repair and healing are slowed. In addition, heart rate is increased and, with the stronger stimulants such as cocaine and amphetamines, various arrythmias including tachycardia can occur. At the same time, blood pressure increases, so a ruptured vessel (a stroke if it's in the brain) is possible.

REWARD/PLEASURE CENTER

Cocaine and amphetamines disrupt the reward/pleasure center. This center, which exists in all mammals as a survival mechanism, gives a surge of pleasure when hunger, thirst, sexual desire, or other need that helps us survive has been satisfied. When cocaine or amphetamines are taken, they stimulate this center and signal the brain that hunger has been satisfied although no food was eaten; that thirst has been satisfied although no liquid has been drunk; and that sexual desire has been satisfied although there has been no sexual activity. This stimulation is perceived as an overall rush, an overall feeling of satiation, well-being, and pleasure. This process is called the reward-reinforcing action of drugs. As the drug is used more and more, the intensity of this rush diminishes, but the memory lingers on.

Since the body is fooled into thinking its basic needs have been satisfied, the user can become dehydrated and malnourished. In fact, many long-term users of stimulants have bad teeth and develop vitamin and mineral deficiencies that can cause other health problems.

WEIGHT LOSS

The ability of stimulants to make the body think it has satisfied hunger and thereby cause the person to lose weight is one of the main reasons they are used. Even tobacco can cause a slight appetite loss because of this effect. The fear of gaining weight causes many cocaine and amphetamine users to maintain their habit.

"I was fat from about the age of 8. My doctor put me on amphetamines when I was 16. Unfortunately, they made my heart race so I gave them up. In my senior year, I took up smoking and that kept the weight off 'cause when I gave them up 10 years later, I gained about 20 pounds. In college, I started drinking coffee to study for exams and that kept my mouth busy doing something instead of eating. It also seemed to lessen my appetite temporarily. Unfortunately, I figure I've screwed up my appestat or whatever controls appetite 'cause I've kept gaining weight over the years." 32-year-old office manager

MENTAL/EMOTIONAL BALANCE

Initially, disruption of neurotransmitters by the stronger stimulants tends to increase confidence, create a certain euphoria, and make users feel they can do anything.

But as use continues, these feelings can quickly turn into irritability, talkativeness, suspiciousness, restlessness, insomnia, paranoia, and even violence.

"It's almost like there's a veneer over the nerves, and it takes off that veneer, that coating, and you are just like a live wire. You'll be on a crowded bus and you might go into a rage very spontaneously, without any real cause." "Meth" user

Everything seems exaggerated under the influence of a strong stimulant.

"It exaggerated almost everything that was going on for me. Initially, it exaggerated excitement or happiness or euphoria. It seemed positive. As it became negative, it became extremely negative. Everything seemed out of proportion to everything else." Recovering cocaine user

COCAINE

Cocaine is extracted from the coca plant, which grows on the slopes of the Andes Mountains in South America (Colombia, Bolivia, Ecuador, and Peru), in certain parts of the Amazon Jungle, and on the island of Java in Indonesia. The *Erythroxylum coca* plant from South America accounts for 95% of the world's production. The United States accounts for 70% of the world's consumption. Although about 300 tons are seized each year on their way to U.S. markets, an estimated 500 to 700 tons still get through.

HISTORY OF USE

The history of cocaine can be viewed in terms of the various changes in the methods of use and the refinement processes that have been developed over the centuries.

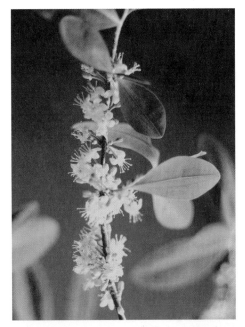

The *Erythroxylum coca* plant.

Chewing the Leaf

Native cultures in South America have used coca leaves for thousands of years for social and religious occasions and to fight off fatigue, lessen hunger, and increase endurance. The South American Indians, the Incas in particular, usually chewed the leaf for the juice, but they also chopped it up and spooned it under the tongue so the active ingredients could be absorbed by the tiny blood vessels in the gums. Even to this day, up to 90% of the Indians living in coca-growing regions chew the leaf. In fact, in many native homes in Bolivia, visitors are ceremoniously offered pieces of coca leaves to chew even before refreshments are served.

Ingesting, Injecting, and Snorting

In 1860, cocaine was isolated from the other chemicals in the coca leaf and extracted as a chemical salt. This extraction from the coca leaf produced pure cocaine

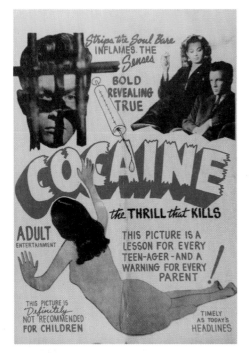

"The Horrors of Cocaine," a movie poster from the late 1930s.

hydrochloride, which causes much more powerful effects than chewing the leaf. Since cocaine readily dissolves in water, users were able to inject it (in solution) directly into the veins, dissolve it in soft drinks (like Coca Cola®) or wine (such as Vin Mariani), or use it in patent medicines. Preparations of cocaine were recommended for asthma, hay fever, fatigue, and a dozen other ailments. It was often used in combination with alcohol and opium.

Injecting cocaine results in an intense rush within 15 to 30 seconds, whereas drinking it results in a milder yet longer-lasting stimulation 30 to 45 minutes after ingestion. Both methods popularized the use of cocaine in the United States by the turn of the century.

The 1920s gave rise to a popular new form of cocaine use, snorting the chemical into the nostrils. Called "tooting," "blowing," or "horning," this method gets the drug to the nasal mucosa (not the lungs), allowing for absorption into the brain within 3 to 5 minutes.

Smoking

In 1914, a pharmaceutical company introduced cocaine cigarettes in America, but the high temperature (198°C or 426°F) needed to convert cocaine hydrochloride to smoke resulted in destruction of many of the psychoactive properties of the drug. Thus, chewing, drinking, injecting, and snorting cocaine remained the principal routes of administration until the mid–1970s when street chemists converted cocaine hydrochloride to freebase cocaine in an effort to make the drug smokable as well as to remove its many cuts or diluting agents. Unlike the cocaine hydrochloride cigarettes introduced in 1914, freebase cocaine could be smoked without destroying its psychoactive properties.

When absorbed through the lungs, cocaine reaches the brain within only 5 to 8 seconds compared to the 15 to 30 seconds it takes when injected through the veins.

The continuing evolution and abuse of this drug in the future are suggested by newer forms of cocaine, like "pasta," "guarapo," and "basay;" a new plant source, the *Erythroxylum coca* variant *ipadu* plant; methods for making new forms of freebase cocaine, like "boulya"; and different combinations of drugs, such as cocaine and marijuana ("champagne," "hubba," "coca puff").

PHYSICAL AND MENTAL EFFECTS

Because cocaine is metabolized very quickly by the body, effects occur and disappear faster than with amphetamines and amphetamine congeners.

1897

WHOLE TOWN MAD FOR COCAINE

Most Prominent Residents of Manchester, Conn, Afflicted with the General Craze for the Drug.

WANT LEGISLATIVE ACTION

Druggist Started the Habit a YearAgo by Preparing a SeductivePreparation of Drugs for use by townspeople.

1927

COCAINE, BROUGHT TO U.S. AS BLESSING, SOON A CURSE

Addict Army Here Grew Rapidly as "Glorious Discovery" of 35 Years Ago Was Boughtfor Base Uses and Became Ally of Crime

by Winifred Black

San Francisco, Feb 12 - Cocaine came into America about 35 years ago.

It was hailed as a glorious discovery and for a long time, no one realized the insidious and cruel danger it brought with it.

1996

Drug agents break cocaine-smuggling ring

By MICHAEL J. SNIFFEN
The Associated Press

WASHINGTON — Federal agents wrapped up more than 150 arrests Thursday designed to break up a coast-to-coast Mexican-Colombian cocaine-smuggling ring that revealed new sophistication and distribution by growing Mexican gangs.

Code-named "Zorro II," the opera-

tion by 10 federal and 42 state and local law enforcement agencies was not disclosed until they were completed Thursday.

Beginning last September, agents traced cocaine produced by Colombia's Cali cartel as it was driven by Mexican couriers across the U.S.-Mexican border in California, Arizona and Texas to the stash houses of wholesalers in Los Angeles. From there, the cocaine was distributed to Colombian street dealers in the

"We have surgically removed an entire operation," said Mike Horn, chief of DEA special operations. "We took out not just the top people — the cell managers and major wholesalers — but we also attacked the violent local organizations. We took everything.".

Horn said the ring moved cocaine with a wholesale value of $100 million during the eight-month investigation.

in drug-trafficking conspiracy indictments unsealed Thursday in Chicago and Midland, Texas.

Fifteen of them were arrested Thursday morning in Los Angeles, Chicago, El Paso, Houston and Midland, and more arrests were under way.

An additional 136 people had been arrested earlier, including 44 alleged members of the Colombian organization taken into custody Feb. 22-25

The current "cocaine epidemic" is nothing new. It seems that almost every generation uses cocaine to excess. They then recognize the problem and try to correct it. When enough people forget that there was a problem, the cycle starts again.

Medical Use

Cocaine is not only a stimulant, it is also the only naturally occurring topical anesthetic. It is used to numb the nasal passages when inserting breathing tubes in a patient, to numb the eye during surgery, and to deaden the pain of chronic sores. (This topical anesthetic effect also numbs the nasal passages when the drug is snorted.) Cocaine will also stimulate the heart muscles directly before it reaches the central nervous system.

"At first, when you put it in your nose, it starts a numbness and you can feel a little drip going down your throat. And then you get hyperactive in 20 minutes. When you smoke it, it's an instantaneous rush."
Cocaine user

Neurotransmitter Disruption

Most of the effects from the use of cocaine, as with all psychoactive drugs, result from the disruption of the neurotransmitter

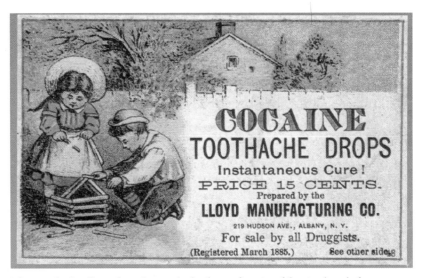

The anesthetic effects of cocaine made the drug a favorite of dentists long before Novocaine® was synthesized.

Courtesy of the National Library of Medicine, Bethesda

balance in the central nervous system. Initially, this stimulation of the body's chemical balance, the increased confidence and energy, and the euphoric rush seem extremely pleasurable.

"I felt real ecstatic, very euphoric. My mind had a great deal of pleasure. I felt like a somebody. I felt like a 'super' person. I could do anything." Recovering cocaine addict

The problem, of course, is that cocaine and amphetamines are not selective about how much they disrupt the natural balance of neurotransmitters. For example, the greatly increased presence of norepinephrine also raises the blood pressure, increases the heart rate, causes rapid breathing, tenses muscles, and induces shaking.

Besides norepinephrine, other disrupted neurotransmitters can have an effect. Over-stimulation of the brain's fright center by dopamine causes most of the paranoia experienced by stimulant abusers. A shadow, sudden movement, or loud voice may suddenly seem threatening.

"A person I know does a shot every 15 to 20 minutes. He fights sleep. He'll go days without sleeping and he'll collapse. He looks for people hiding under mattresses, behind door hinges, and in books. He asks why you're smiling." Intravenous cocaine user

Unbalanced acetylcholine, another common neurotransmitter, can cause muscle tremors, memory lapses, mental confusion, and even hallucinations.

Serotonin helps us sleep and stabilizes our moods, but serotonin depletion by excessive cocaine or amphetamine use results in insomnia, agitation, and severe emotional depression. The lack of epinephrine, norepinephrine, serotonin, and dopamine can also cause severe depression and extreme lethargy.

Formication, another side effect of long-term cocaine and amphetamine use, is extreme itching that feels like hundreds of tiny bugs ("coke bugs," "meth bugs," "snow bugs") crawling under one's skin. Users on "coke" or "speed" runs have been known to scratch themselves bloody trying to get at the imaginary bugs.

Cocaine Versus Amphetamines

Although all the physical and mental effects of cocaine are very similar to the effects of amphetamines, the price of compulsive use is different—a heavy cocaine user spends $100 to $300 a day, whereas a heavy amphetamine user spends about $50 to $100 a day. The other difference between the two drugs is the duration of action (about 40 minutes for cocaine's major effects to wear off compared to several hours for amphetamines). In addition, amphetamines are usually easier to find and buy.

"Cocaine is more euphoric and not as intense as 'speed.' 'Speed' is very intense and you're going, going, going. The 'coke' is shorter lasting. But the cravings are much worse. When I wanted to do 'speed,' it was mainly because I wanted to get things done. I felt 'speed' helped me perform. And the cocaine, I felt like I had absolutely no choice. Cocaine took me down real fast and real hard." "Crack" cocaine smoker

PROBLEMS WITH COCAINE USE

The Crash

Since cocaine is metabolized so quickly by the body, the initial euphoria, the feeling of confidence, the sense of omnipotence,

* * *

When sold legally in the United States, 1 ounce or 28 grams, costs about $80. In Colombia, 1 ounce of illicit cocaine costs about $600 and on the streets of New York or Miami, up to $1,300.
Department of Justice 1995

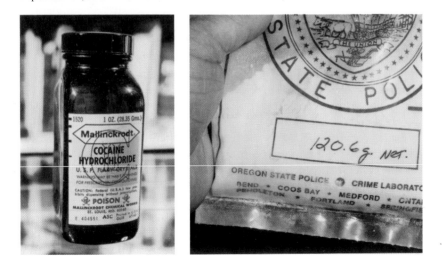

the surge of energy, and the satisfied feeling disappear as suddenly as they appeared, so the crash after using cocaine can be particularly depressing. With cocaine, this depression can last a few hours, several days, or even weeks.

"I really did want to die, and I remember that as being way out of proportion to the actual events of my life although it seemed like my life was over." Recovering cocaine user

Withdrawal, Craving, and Relapse

Contrary to notions held by many researchers until the 1980s, there are true withdrawal phenomena when cocaine is used. Although similar to the crash, withdrawal effects can last months, even years depending on dosage, frequency, length of use, and any preexisting mental problems. The major symptoms are anhedonia, or the lack of ability to feel pleasure; anergia, or a total lack of energy, motivation, or initiative; euthymia, or a temporary elation; and an intense craving for the drug. These symptoms are also common for amphetamine withdrawal. It is these symptoms, particularly craving, which generally cause the compulsive recovering user to relapse.

The time frame for a typical cycle of compulsive cocaine (or amphetamine) use is as follows: immediately after a binge, usually lasting several days, the user crashes, sleeps all day long trying to put energy back into the body, and swears off the drug forever. A few days later, the user starts to feel better and may resolve to go into treatment or thinks he or she doesn't really have a problem. However, about a week to two weeks after quitting, the craving starts to build, the energy level drops, and the user feels very little pleasure from any surroundings, activities, or friends. So, two to four weeks after vowing to abstain,

the craving builds to a fever pitch, and unless in intensive treatment, the user will usually relapse.

"You know, there's no specific time that I can remember where before I went into relapse that I actually decided to go and use again. That's the cunningness of this thing. The next thing you know, you're just there, and you're just doing it. You even ask yourself, 'How the hell did I get into this situation again? What happened?'"
Recovering 28-year-old cocaine abuser

Polydrug Use

One of the problems with cocaine is that the stimulation can be so intense that the user needs a downer to take the edge off or to get to sleep. The most common drugs used are alcohol, Valium®, and heroin, though any downer will do in a pinch. Sometimes, the second drug can be more of a problem than the cocaine.

"After the 'coke' would be gone, you'd be all wired up, and you couldn't sleep, so I'd always have a little bit of heroin on the side and it'd bring me down. And I wouldn't be all jittery all night and grinding my teeth."
23-year-old recovering cocaine and heroin abuser

Adulteration

Adulteration of cocaine involves dilution with such diverse products as baby laxatives, lactose, vitamin B, aspirin, Mannitol®, sugar, Tetracaine® or Procaine® (topical anesthetics), even talcum powder. When the drug is used intravenously, not only are these diluents put into the blood stream, but so are bacteria and viruses from contaminated needles, which can transmit diseases, such as hepatitis, blood and heart infections, and AIDS.

Overdose

An overdose of cocaine can be caused by as little as 1/50th of a gram or as much as 1.2 grams. The "'caine reaction" is very intense and generally short in duration. Most often, it's not fatal. It only feels like impending death. However, in a small number of cases, death can occur within 40 minutes to 5 hours after exposure. Death usually results from either the initial stimulatory phase of toxicity (seizures, hypertension, and tachycardia) or the later depression phase terminating in extreme respiratory depression and coma.

"I have seen a friend go through overdose. His skin was gray-green. His eyes rolled back, his heart stopped, and there was a gurgling sound which is right at death. And I had to bring him back, and that's enough to put the fear of God in anybody."
Intravenous cocaine user

First-time users, and even those who have used cocaine before, can get an exaggerated reaction, far beyond what might normally occur or beyond what they have experienced in the past. This is partially due to the phenomenon known as inverse tolerance or kindling. As people use cocaine, they get more sensitive to its toxic effects rather than less sensitive, as one would expect. With large doses, cocaine can injure heart muscles and blood vessels, making permanent damage to those tissues more likely.

Long-Term Cardiovascular Effects

The elevations and drops in blood pressure caused by cocaine, plus some toxic effects to the vessels themselves, weaken blood capillaries, resulting in a greater risk of stroke. Strokes occur when a weakened blood vessel bursts, causing internal bleeding in the brain. Chronic cocaine use also causes a disorganization in the usual formation of heart muscles, resulting in constriction bands on the heart. This makes chronic users more likely to suffer a cocaine-induced heart attack.

Neonatal Effects

Smoked, snorted, or injected, cocaine and amphetamines are a particular danger to the fetus of a pregnant woman. When a pregnant woman smokes "crack," within seconds her baby will also be exposed to the drug. Because of the stimulatory effects on the cardiovascular system in particular, the chances of miscarriage, stroke, and sudden infant death syndrome (SIDS) are greatly increased.

"I'd been smoking 'crack' for a couple of years, and I had a baby who was born testing positive for 'coke.' Child Protective Services came and placed her in foster care. It took me two years to get my baby back."
17-year-old recovering "crack" user

COMPULSION

Considering all the problems with cocaine—the expense, the dilution, the adulteration, the illegality, the possibility of overdose, the physical and psychological dangers—two questions come to mind, "Why do people use cocaine?" and "Why do they use it so compulsively?"

Why Do People Start Using Cocaine and Amphetamines?

- The drugs mimic pleasurable natural body functions: adrenal energy rush,

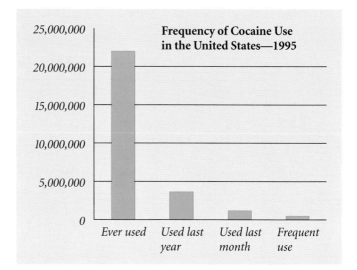

Figure 3–1 •

Of the 22 million Americans who have experimented with cocaine, 16% used it in the past year, 8% used it in the last month, and about 3% (582,000) use it frequently.
NIDA Household Survey 1995

confidence, euphoria, increased sensitivity, and stimulation of the reward/pleasure center.

- It is sometimes easier to get a chemical high instantly than a natural high over a period of time.

- People also use these drugs to combat boredom.

- People succumb to internal or external peer pressure.

- People are curious and the drugs are available.

- People use them as a means of alleviating or forgetting personal problems.

- Some people use the drugs to escape the effects of the poverty, hopelessness, and filth of their surroundings.

Why Are Cocaine and Amphetamines Used So Compulsively?

- Users want to recapture the initial rush (the energy surge and the stimulation of the reward/pleasure center) which is extremely intense. Most find that it's hard to reproduce, but that doesn't stop them from trying.

- They want to avoid the crash that is inevitable after the intense high. In many cases, a user will shoot up or smoke every 20 minutes, or in some cases, every 10 minutes in a binge episode.

- Users want to avoid life's problems, such as difficult relationships, lack of confidence, traumatic events, a hated job, or loneliness.

- Users respond to the environmental cues that remind them of their drug use. Many seemingly innocuous sensory cues in our environment will trigger memories of smoking, snorting or shooting and create an overwhelming desire to use again: seeing white powder, having money in one's pocket, or being in a place where drugs are used.

- Cocaine, in and of itself, changes the neurochemical balance and creates an intense craving that will cause someone to keep shooting, snorting, or smoking until every last microgram is gone, until he or she passes out, or until an overdose occurs.

- People use in response to their hereditary predisposition to use. That is, certain people's natural neurotransmitter balance makes them react more intensely to a drug. They are, in essence, presensitized to the drug.

SMOKABLE COCAINE (freebase, "crack," "rock," "boulya")

Depending on the way it is synthesized, smokable cocaine has been called freebase, "base," "basay," "crack," "rock," "hubba,"

"gravel," "Roxanne," "girl," "fry," and "boulya." Perhaps next month another nickname will appear. Whatever the name, freebase and "crack" are still cocaine and, when smoked, cause all the reactions expected from shooting or snorting the drug.

SMOKABLE COCAINE "EPIDEMIC"

The words "crack cocaine" appeared on the streets and in the media in 1985, tentatively at first, as if society were trying out a new nickname. By 1986, there seemed to be a "crack epidemic" that crossed all social and economic barriers. By the 1990s, it was ingrained in the American psyche as one of

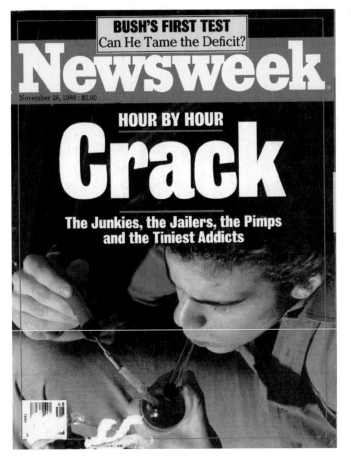

There were thousands of stories in the mid–1980s that sensationalized the "crack epidemic."

the main causes of society's ills: gang violence, AIDS, crime, and addiction.

Some thought that the spread of "crack" to the office, factory, school yard, ghetto, and barrio was generated by media attention. Others thought that the basic properties of smokable cocaine were the cause of the "epidemic." The fact that the use of "crack" continues to be a severe problem, despite vastly curtailed media coverage, speaks to the addictive nature of smokable cocaine rather than to the influence of the media.

PHARMACOLOGY OF SMOKABLE COCAINE

There is a frequent misperception that "crack" and freebase are different drugs from cocaine. They aren't. "Crack" is chemically the same as freebase cocaine. Both substances are simply altered forms of cocaine hydrochloride (snortable or injectable cocaine). Freebase indicates that the base (hydrochloride) is "freed" from the cocaine molecule.

There are two common ways to free the hydrochloride molecule. The first method, freebasing ("basing," "baseballing"), was developed around 1976. It uses highly flammable or toxic chemicals to create smokable cocaine. This is a purer form of the drug since any additives are filtered out by the process. The other simpler technique, called "cheap basing" or "dirty basing," was developed in the early '80s. It does not remove as many impurities or residues as the freebasing technique, so impurities such as talcum powder and, especially, baking soda remain. The lumps of smokable cocaine made by this method are usually called "crack" because of the crackling sound caused by the process, or "rock" because the product looks like little rocks.

The converted freebase cocaine, made by either the "basing" method or the "crack" method, has two chemical properties sought by users. First, it has a lower melting point than the powdered form so it can be heated easily in a glass pipe and vaporized to form smoke at a lower temperature. (Too high a temperature destroys most of the psychoactive properties of the drug.) Second, since it enters the system directly through the lungs, smokable cocaine reaches the brain faster than when cocaine hydrochloride is snorted through the nostrils.

Freebase cocaine is more fat soluble than cocaine that is snorted (cocaine hydrochloride) and so is more readily absorbed by fat cells of the brain, causing a more intense reaction. Users are also able to get a much higher dose of cocaine in their systems at one time because the very large surface area in the lungs (about the size of a football field) can absorb the drug almost instantaneously.

"Crack" and freebase cocaine unbalance the brain's chemicals more quickly than snorted cocaine. Users react in their own ways to the drug depending on how much is used, the purity of the drug, and how long they have been using.

"You get heat energy, heat flashes that go all through your body. You get these pins and needles, depending on the cut, of course." "Crack" cocaine smoker

"Pasta," another form of freebase cocaine which is popular in South America, is an intermediate product of the cocaine refinement process. Being an intermediate product, it contains toxic chemicals, such as kerosene and leaded gasoline. When smoked in a marijuana joint, it is called "basuco."

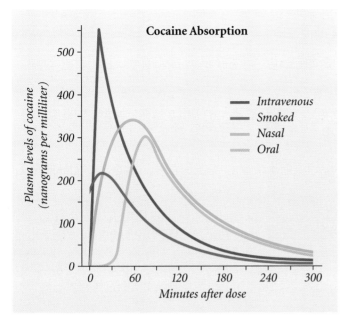

Cocaine Absorption

Plasma levels of cocaine (nanograms per milliliter)

Minutes after dose

— Intravenous
— Smoked
— Nasal
— Oral

Figure 3–2 •

This graph shows the plasma levels of cocaine after equivalent doses were taken through different methods.

NIDA Research Monograph 99, Research Findings on Smoking of Abused Substances

EFFECTS AND SIDE EFFECTS

The effects of "crack," are almost exactly the same as snorting or injecting cocaine, but since smoking cocaine causes more intense reactions, the effects and side effects are usually more intense.

Respiratory Effects

Because a user inhales an extremely harsh substance, smoking cocaine can also cause breathing problems. Smoking "crack" can cause severe chest pains, pneumonia, coughs, fever, and other respiratory complications, including hemorrhage, respiratory failure, and death. "Crack lung" describes the pain, breathing problems, and fever that resemble pneumonia.

"I had a lot of coughing after using it and shortness of breath. I didn't really notice it at the time, but if I went out to ride my bike or lift weights, I would have a really hard time." Recovering 16-year-old boy

"A friend was freebasing heavily, and he started going into convulsions and throwing up blood. It was real awful. I was really scared, and I thought he was going to die. Me and my other friend, we just kept freebasing ... and then when he came out of it, he started freebasing again."
Recovering 16-year-old girl

Polydrug Abuse

As with snorted and injected cocaine, the intensive use of freebase increases the potential for the abuse of other drugs, especially alcohol, heroin, and sedative-hypnotics. Some smokers combine freebase and marijuana in a combination called "champagne," "caviar," "gremmies," "cocoa

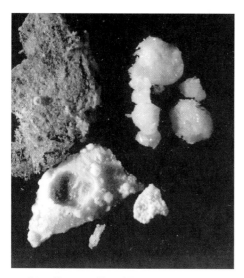

In this collection of "crack" cocaine samples, each "rock" is made in a slightly different manner. The various colors come from the impurities left after heating the mixture.

puff," "hubba," or "woolies." In addition, users are even mixing PCP with "crack" in a nasty mixture called "space basing," "whack," or "tragic magic." Further, there is the addition of freebase cocaine to smokable tar heroin to make a smokable "speedball" called "hot rocks." Finally, "crack" or cocaine hydrochloride is being used with wine coolers for an oral "speedball" known as "crack coolers." When "crack" is not available, users have switched to shooting and even smoking methamphetamine ("speed"). A mixture of "crank" with "crack" smoked together has also appeared recently and is called "super crank."

Overdose

The most frequent type of overdose that people experience when smoking cocaine is on the mild side: very rapid heartbeat and hyperventilation. However, these reactions are often accompanied by a feel-ing of impending death. Although most people survive and only get very sweaty and clammy and feel that they are going to die, several thousand, in fact, are killed by cocaine overdose every year.

REASONS FOR THE WIDESPREAD USE OF "CRACK"

Besides the reasons already mentioned for compulsive use of cocaine, such as the search for the first intense rush or avoidance of the downside, there are several other reasons for the compulsive smoking of cocaine. First, smoking is not as dangerous as using a contaminated needle. (Unfortunately, while avoiding needles would remove one source of infection, lowered inhibitions, bartering sex for drugs, and careless high-risk sexual activities lead to higher rates of sexually transmitted diseases, including AIDS.) Next, smoking a drug is more socially acceptable than injecting it because cigarette, pipe, and cigar smoking are legal and part of our culture.

CONSEQUENCES OF "CRACK" USE

Economic Consequences

The economics of "crack" cocaine have expanded the potential number of users, especially among teenagers. The reason is in the packaging. "Crack" is not cheaper than cocaine hydrochloride; it is just sold in smaller units. One gram of cocaine hydrochloride was the standard amount, going for about $60 to $100. Now, 1/20th of a gram that has been converted to "crack" or "rock" can be bought for $10 to $20, a manageable sum for teenagers and incidentally, about twice the price of cocaine hydrochloride when figured on a per gram basis.

The economics of "crack" cocaine have also created more dealers, and these people have a vested interest in keeping users using. Many housing projects in the inner city have become havens for "crack" houses and dealers. A few young dealers are buying new cars and showing off their wealth, but the majority of the small-time dealers make just enough to support their own habit or get by. Drug-gang homicides are expanding as local gangs, along with gangs from other countries, such as Jamaica and Colombia, expand the trade to smaller cities and towns.

"I know it's jive, I know it's negative. I'm trapped in something here. But, I'm used to the money. What else can I do? You gonna send me to McDonalds? After I'm generating this kind of money everyday, I can't go back to McDonalds for $3.50—what is it?—$4.75 today, which is still insulting."
16-year-old "crack" dealer/user

Unfortunately, this burgeoning drug market is making use of the best sales strategies of a free enterprise system: reduce the price to increase sales; increase the size of the sales force to cover the territory more efficiently; encourage free trade to avoid tariffs and impounding; and create appealing packaging to make the product attractive to a wider segment of the population.

Social Consequences

"It seems like every time I would hit the pipe, my daughter would say, 'Mommy.' And so I would say, 'Why are you bothering me?' It really made me crazy. I mean, my son, he would just pick on things and make noise or something, just to bother me because he knew that I was doing this."
Recovering "crack" user

Because of the compulsive nature of "crack," addictive "crack" use in the United States has had devastating social ramifications which include the single, or even no-parent family, the burned-out grandmother caring for her "crack"-addicted daughter's children, increased rates of abandonment, neglect, and abuse of children, and the formation of an underclass of women who trade sex for "crack." The latter has become a major vector in the spread of AIDS.

"It's two types of women using cocaine. One's a 'tossup' [a woman who trades sex for 'crack']. They're the ones who are down there. They done lost everything they have. They have no self-respect. Me and my sister, we'd work a brother in a minute to get his dope. Once we got his dope— 'Go on, get outta my house.' Me and my sister, we paid our rent, we paid our utilities. We fed our children. We kept clothes on their backs. We kept the house clean. We had not lost our self-esteem. We had not hit rock bottom yet." Recovering "crack" user

For many men (particularly in some inner-city African American communities), the impact on the family and society has occurred because of the high rate of crime associated with "crack" use. There have been high rates of imprisonment, violent deaths, and child abandonment by addicts. In fact, about 75% of all inmates in prisons come from single-parent or no-parent homes (*Bureau of Prisons, 1993*).

"When I talked to one of the groups I work with, we were just asking, 'How many of your friends smoke 'weed'?'
'50%.'
'How many smoke cigarettes?'
'50%.'

'How many drink?'
'60% to 70%.'
'How many smoke 'crack'?'
'Oh, I don't know, 5% or 10%.'
So 'crack' in the sense of the number of adolescents using it is small, but the impact has been disproportionate."

Youth drug counselor

"'Crack' cocaine is not Black or White. 'Crack' cocaine is dope. It doesn't care who it gets, and it has no inhibitions at all. Dope doesn't have a name on it. I have sat down with people up here, and I have sat down with people from down there, and when we do dope, it is all the same."

Recovering "crack" user

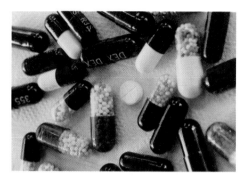

In the past, traditional types of "speed" diverted to street use or manufactured illegally were small tablets of amphetamine or methamphetamine ("crosstops," "whites") originally made in Mexico; Biphetamines®("black beauties"), a combination of several amphetamine compounds; Dexadrine® ("dexys," "beans"), a dextroamphetamine tablet; Benzedrine® ("bennies"), one of the classic "stay awake" amphetamine pills; and Methadrine® (or Ambar®), a methamphetamine.

Courtesy of the Drug Enforcement Administration Laboratory, San Francisco

AMPHETAMINES

CLASSIFICATION

Amphetamines, known variously as "speed," "meth," methamphetamines, "crank," "crystal," "ice," "shabu," and "glass," are a class of powerful, synthetic stimulants with effects very similar to cocaine but much longer lasting and cheaper to use. Amphetamines can be taken orally, but shooting and snorting are the most popular routes of administration. Recently, smoking has gained in popularity.

There are several different types of amphetamines: amphetamine, methamphetamine, dextroamphetamine, and dextromethamphetamine. The effects of each type are almost indistinguishable, the major differences being the method of manufacture and the strength.

HISTORY OF USE

Discovery

Amphetamines were synthesized in 1887, but their medical applications weren't recognized until the 1930s when Benzedrine® was marketed as a stimulant to counter low blood pressure. Amphetamines were also used to dilate constricted bronchial passages to help asthmatics breathe. They were also widely used during World War II by Allied, German, and Japanese forces. (Abuse has continued to be a problem in Japan since the War.) Later on, other amphetamines were used to treat narcolepsy or sleeping sickness, to treat a form of epilepsy, and to try to cure depression. Concurrently, the stimulant effects of amphetamines came to be abused by students cramming for exams, truckers on long hauls, workers laboring long hours, and soldiers or pilots trying to stay awake for 48 hours straight.

Diet Pills

Pharmaceutical companies in the 1950s and 1960s promoted the hunger-suppressing and mood-elevating qualities of amphetamines. Their advertising led to huge quantities of amphetamines, such as Dexedrine®, Methedrine®, Dexamyl®, and Benzedrine®, flooding the market.

"Well, I almost never ate. And when I ate, I ate sugar, colas, cakes, and that was all I ate. I mean, once in a while I'd go to a steak house and treat myself to a fabulous $4.59 steak dinner. I weighed probably 90 pounds and I was anemic and weak, but I always felt up and energized because I was always shooting 'speed.'" "Speed" user

Street "Speed"

The 1960s were the peak of the "speed" craze. Worldwide legal production in 1962 was estimated to be 8 billion tablets. The Controlled Substance Act of 1970 made it hard to buy amphetamines legally in the United States. In addition, prescription use of the drugs was more tightly regulated. The street market expanded to fill the need so, instead of buying legally manufactured amphetamines that had been diverted, people bought "speed" and "crank" that had been manufactured illegally.

"I very seldom ran out in the beginning in the '60s and '70s. It was cheap; people gave it away. It wasn't like using dope. You didn't have to get money together every day."
"Speed" user

The most popular form of street "speed" was the "crosstops." Also called "cartwheels" and "white crosses," these were smuggled into the United States from Mexico, and in the early 1970s, they cost $5 to $10 per 100 tablets. In the '90s, the price is $1 to $5 per tablet if they can be found. As of 1996, what are most often available are bogus (lookalike) "crosstops."

The late 1980s saw a resurgence in the availability and abuse of illicit amphetamines, particularly "crank" (methamphetamine sulfate) and "crystal" (methamphetamine hydrochloride—not to be confused with "krystal" which is PCP). Once stymied by the tight control of chemicals needed to produce illegal amphetamines, clever street chemists learned to alter commonly available compounds to produce "speed" products. However, much of the street "meth" was lookalike drugs, such as phenylpropanolamine (a decongestant), ephedrine, or simply caffeine tablets disguised to look like amphetamine products.

"Ice"

As the 1990s began, a new, highly potent, and smokable form of methamphetamine called dextromethamphetamine ("ice," "glass," "batu," or "shabu") had taken center stage, at least in the press. Besides its smokability, greater strength, and longer duration of effects, "ice" had the appeal of a new fad. As with the spread of smokable "crack" cocaine, "ice" was initially being marketed as a "newer, better amphetamine."

Surprisingly, perhaps because it is so intense, "ice" has not caught on as a common drug of abuse except in Hawaii. In addition, "snot," a skim from heated methamphetamine, has been tried. The reddish brown gel or oil can be smoked in a pipe or in a cigarette.

Several types of methamphetamines are being manufactured illegally including "peanut butter meth" on the left.

Courtesy of Lt. Ed Mayer and JACNET, Jackson County, Oregon

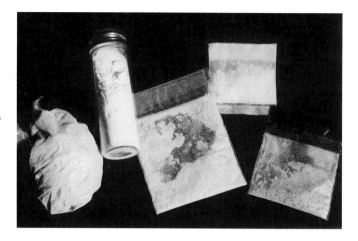

Current Use

The mid–1990s has seen a dramatic resurgence in the use of illicit methamphetamines, predominantly "crank" ("meth"). This resurgence has been signaled by a drastic increase in the number of "meth labs" raided by the authorities, particularly in California, Oregon, and Texas. Over the years, much of the street dealing in methamphetamines had been taken over by biker gangs (Hell's Angels and Gypsy Jokers) because of the money involved and the partiality of bikers to the drug. But there has been an ever increasing involvement of Mexican gangs in the manufacture and distribution of the drug.

While amphetamine use in 1995 is only about one-half the peak level of the early 1980s (*NIDA Household Survey*), the current growth is explosive. At a number of treatment centers in Southern Oregon and California, the majority of those coming in for treatment have "meth" as their primary drug of choice and addiction. An additional worry is that the age of first use has dropped. Some 10–13 year olds are smoking, eating, and snorting "crank." In some high schools, "crank" rather than marijuana, is the drug of choice. Some of the reasons for this upsurge are lower prices, increased availability, and current drug fads.

"A daily supply of 'grass' was about $10 for a mild habit. 'Meth' was $20, except when we were using heavy, it was about $70 a day. Of course we had to do some selling to afford that level of use. We would shoot for three to four days, sleep four or five hours and then start again. After three or four days, no amount of the stuff will keep you up so you have to crash. A lot of the kids I still know in school are more into 'meth'— IV 'meth'—than 'grass.'"

Recovering IV methamphetamine user

"Meth" Manufacture

One of the reasons for the resurgence in the use of methamphetamine is new, somewhat safer, cheaper, and almost odor-free manufacturing techniques. Illicit methamphetamine manufacturing used to be an extremely risky business. The fumes were toxic and explosions could and did occur if the chemicals were handled improperly. Foul odors that emanated from the "cookers" were of great help to law enforcement agencies in locating "meth" labs. Now, methamphetamine can even be manufactured on a stove top. The DEA estimates that there are over 300 ways to manufacture methamphetamine. It is still risky, particularly for amateurs, but not as risky as before. This increase in the number of street chemists means that it is hard to halt the supply and almost impossible for users to know what they are getting until they snort it or shoot it into a vein.

The main ingredient used by street chemists and organized gangs to manufacture methamphetamine is ephedrine. Since it is a controlled substance in the United States, most ephedrine is smuggled to Mexico from China, where it is extracted from the ephedra bush, or from Germany, where it is synthesized. A small portion is converted to methamphetamine in Mexico, but the majority is smuggled into the United States (mainly Central and Southern California) and then converted to "meth." When ephedrine is not available, pseudoephedrine (found in many Over-The-Counter or OTC cold medicines) can be used. The other substances used in the manufacture, particularly hydriodic acid, are also smuggled into the United States or manufactured illegally.

While only 52 of the 419 "meth" labs that were raided in 1994 by the California Bureau of Narcotic Enforcement were run by Mexican gangs, they accounted for five times as much "meth" as the other 367 labs combined. In fact, the Bureau estimates that as of 1996, the Mexican labs manufacture three-fourths of the "meth" consumed in the United States. These Mexican gang-run labs can make 20 to 100 pounds of "meth" every two days. A pound of "meth" wholesales for $4,000 to $18,000 (*NIDA, 1995*).

One other problem with the illegal synthesis of "meth" is the environmental danger of the chemicals, even with the newer manufacturing methods. Toxins and cancer-causing agents, such as acetone, red phosphorus, hydrochloric acid, benzene, toluene, sulfuric acid, and lead acetate, are left behind or secretly dumped into streams and landfills. It costs thou-

Three toddlers die in meth lab blaze
Adults ran away without trying to help, witnesses say
Los Angeles Times

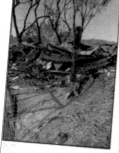

DESTROYED — This is all that remains of a mobile home where three children burned to death in Aguanga, Calif., on Tuesday.

AGUANGA, Calif. — While drug agents sifted through the blackened and melted metal of a mobile home, Art Burnstad remained haunted by the sight of adults fleeing for their lives — and leaving three toddlers for the flames.

The children's mother was screaming and "six or eight men were running away from the fire, and none of those guys were trying to get the kids out," Burnstad said Wednesday. "When we went up to help, one of the guys yelled, 'Get out of here! We can take care of this ourselves.'"

Instead, all the occupants of the home about 60 miles north of San Diego — including the children's mother — sped off, some scattered to the wind, others to local hospitals, leaving the home fully engulfed in fire Tuesday afternoon.

It wasn't until more than 12 hours later that the bodies of three children were recovered, too burned to recognize. The Riverside County coroner's office tentatively identified them as the children of Kathy James, who was critically

burned by the fire: Dion, 3, Jackson, 2, and Megan, 1.

Authorities said the inferno may have started when a pressurized brew of toxic and volatile chemicals to make methamphetamine erupted in flames. But they said there were only a few clues to support their suspicion.

Three adults were hospitalized for burns suffered in the fire and could face criminal charges after investigators piece together what may have been going on inside the home, said Mark Lohman, an investigator with the Riverside County Sheriff's Department.

James, 39, the mother of the three victims, was in critical condition in the burn unit at the San Bernardino County Medical Center, a spokesman there said. Harry Jensen, 42, also was being treated there, in stable condition. A second man, Michael Talbert, 38, was treated for burns and released from a nearby hospital.

None of the three has been arrested because the investigation is in its earliest stages, Lohman said. He said investigators were questioning James' oldest

child, 10-year-old Jimmy, who apparently was pulled from the fire by his mother and taken to family in the area after the fire. The boy was cooperating with the investigation, Lohman said.

Some of the other adults who were seen fleeing from the scene were later identified and questioned by investigators "and they are making statements that corroborate our suspicion, that there was methamphetamine manufacturing going on at the time," Lohman said.

Methamphetamine, considered a bargain substitute for cocaine because it is cheaper to make and has longer-lasting effects, has become the greatest bane to narcotics officers in recent years as its popularity has skyrocketed.

Popularized by outlaw bikers in the 1970s, most of the methamphetamine traded in California today is made in bulk by Mexican drug families who oversee teams of cookers who are dispatched to remote locations throughout the state. They confound law enforcement by making large batches of meth, literally overnight, before dismantling their labs.

sands of dollars to clean up each raided laboratory.

EFFECTS

Routes of Administration

Currently, injecting and snorting "meth" are the most popular methods of use. Snorting "meth" causes irritation and pain to the nasal mucosa and can damage the nasal septum when used to excess. Intravenous use does put large quantities of the drug directly into the bloodstream and causes a more intense "high" than snorting or swallowing; however, it often causes pain in the blood vessels. Also, with injecting, there is the attendant risk of contaminated needles. Because of the extremely bitter taste of methamphetamines, they are often put into a gelatin capsule or in a piece of paper when taken orally.

"I'd already tasted that first high and wanted to get back to it, but it was always different each time I shot up. I started shooting when I was 13, and I was 20 before I learned you could get AIDS from it."
Intravenous "meth" user

Because of the dangers in shooting or snorting "meth," some users have taken to smoking "crank," "crystal," or "ice," a potentially more appealing method of use than the other methods. The technique of smoking "crank" or "ice" is similar to smoking freebase cocaine (in a pipe). Smoking gets the drug to the brain faster. No matter how the drug is taken, amphetamines last 4 to 6 hours compared to only 40 minutes to 1 1/2 hours for cocaine. "Ice," the newest form of methamphetamine, is alleged to last at least 8 hours, some say up to 24 hours, after it is smoked.

Physical Effects

As with cocaine, the physiological effects of small to moderate doses of amphetamines include: increased heart rate, body temperature, respiration, and CNS stimulation; higher blood pressure; extra energy; dilation of bronchial vessels; and appetite suppression.

"I would inject some 'speed' and right after doing it, you get an incredible rush, which some people compare with sexual feelings. And your heart pounds, and I've seen people actually pass out from having too much 'speed.' My heart would pound, and I would sweat, and the rush would pass, and then I would just be very high energy." "Meth" user

A number of athletes have used amphetamines to try to enhance their performance. A review of literature on the subject has shown that the actual performance enhancement is minimal (1% to 2%). The benefits seem to come when counteracting fatigue is desired. The other benefits to athletes are the boost in confidence and aggressiveness. Unfortunately, prolonged use or overreliance begins to reverse these effects.

Users go on binges or "runs," staying up for 3, 4, or even up to 10 days at a time, putting a severe strain on their bodies, particularly the cardiovascular and nervous systems. During these runs, people will try to use their excess energy any way they can—dancing, exercising, cleaning the kitchen at midnight, taking apart a car, or painting the whole house.

"I liked to do little intricate drawings. I would draw for hours. Anything small with a lot of detail. I would clean my apartment

from top to bottom, even doing my floor with Brillo® pads—my wooden floor—vacuuming my ceiling. If I ran out of stuff to do, I would dump out everything in the vacuum cleaner and vacuum it back up. I didn't like to be outside because I would get paranoid." Recovering amphetamine user

Tolerance to amphetamines is pronounced. Whereas 10 milligrams per day is the usual prescribed dose, a long-term user might use 1,000 milligrams over a 24-hour period during a "speed run." This means that extended use (or the use of large quantities) will lead to extreme depression and lethargy.

"If I didn't have 'speed,' if I ran out, I would become depressed, very anxiety-ridden. I had suicidal thoughts, and I would sleep for long stretches of time till I had more 'speed.' And then I would start the whole process over again."

33-year-old recovering "speed" user

Long-term use can also cause sleep deprivation, heart and blood vessel toxicity, and severe malnutrition. This malnutrition, plus the calcium leaching effects of amphetamine overuse, results in bad or rotted teeth. In fact, one of the confirming signs of amphetamine abuse is poor dental health.

Finally, if the user has not built up a tolerance, is unusually sensitive, or takes a very large amount, an overdose can occur (convulsions, hypothermia, and cardiovascular complications).

"I shot some 'speed' once and immediately had a seizure. Apparently my heart stopped beating, and the person I was with was

pounding on my chest. I was real sore and black and blue the next day."

Methamphetamine user

Mental and Emotional Effects

Amphetamines initially produce a mild to intense euphoria and a feeling of well-being, very similar to a cocaine high. But with prolonged use, the unbalanced neurotransmitters (dopamine and norepinephrine) can also induce irritability, paranoia, anxiety, mental confusion, poor judgment, and even hallucinations.

Much like cocaine, amphetamines release neurotransmitters that mimic sexual gratification. Thus, they are sometimes used by those who are sexually active and prone toward multiple partners and/or prolonged sexual activity. The drug has also been heavily used in gay populations for sexual endurance. But again, because of the rapid development of tolerance, there is an eventual decrease of sex drive and performance. For many users, the rush from shooting or smoking "meth" or "ice" becomes a substitute for sexual activity.

Taken to extremes, prolonged use can result in violent, suicidal, and even homicidal thoughts. This amphetamine psychosis (caused by excess dopamine activity) and listless depression (more common with high-dose intravenous use or heavy smoking of "ice") are usually not permanent.

Upon cessation of use, the disturbed user will usually return to some semblance of normality after the brain chemistry has been rebalanced, usually within a week. If there was a preexisting mental condition, recovery can take a lot longer. Since extended use can also damage nerve cells, a number of the changes in long-term users, even without preexisting mental problems, can last a lifetime.

Much of the current interest in "crank," "crystal," and "ice" abuse is concentrated among adolescents and older teenagers, particularly among Asian American and Caucasian American youth. One of the reasons for the popularity of the drug is that initially amphetamines induce qualities which we try to teach to young people— alertness, motivation, self-confidence, socialization, excitement, and the ability to work long hours. Unfortunately, with drug use, these desirable qualities quickly give way to the opposite effects, including depression, paranoia, and antisocial behavior, among others.

In addition, the ability of amphetamines to suppress appetite is one of the main reasons for their current popularity. The projection of an "ideal" thin body in advertisements helps promote current abuse, much as it did in the '60s and '70s before government regulations limited the legal supply of the drug.

Effects of "Ice"

"Ice" is dextromethamphetamine. This form of methamphetamine stimulates the brain to a greater degree than the regular methamphetamine but stimulates the heart, blood vessels, and lungs to a lesser degree. The decrease in circulatory effects (up to 25% less than that of regular "crank") encourages users to smoke more, resulting in more overdoses and a quicker disruption of neurotransmitters. This disruption means more "tweaking," or severe paranoid, hallucinatory, and hypervigilant thinking, along with greater suicidal depression and addictive use. Detoxification from mental and psychotic symptoms of excessive "ice" use usually takes several days longer than detoxifying from regular methamphetamine abuse.

AMPHETAMINE CONGENERS

When the prescription use of amphetamines was severely limited because of Federal legislation, physicians turned to amphetamine congeners to help treat certain problems that had previously been treated with stronger stimulants. Amphetamine congeners are stimulant drugs which produce many of the same effects as amphetamines but are not as strong. They are also chemically related to amphetamines.

METHYLPHENIDATE (Ritalin® and attention deficit/hyperactivity disorder, [AD/HD])

One of the most widely used amphetamine congeners, methylphenidate (Ritalin®), is prescribed as a mood elevator or as a treatment for narcolepsy, a sleep disorder. However, it is most often prescribed to deal with attention deficit/hyperactivity disorder (AD/HD) in both children and adults.

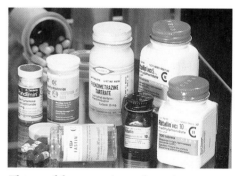

The use of the two main amphetamine congeners, methylphenidate (Ritalin®) and diet pills (e.g., Ionamin®, Pondamin®), has become more widespread in the 1990s.

Salem paper finds 600 kids on Ritalin

The number of children who are being diagnosed with AD/HD has increased dramatically. In Salem, Oregon, about 2% of the 31,700 students take Ritalin®.

The Associated Press

SALEM — A drug to control hyperactivity is given to more than 600 Salem-Keizer School District children every day, a newspaper survey found.

The Statesman Journal found all Keizer schools.

"For me and my life, it has really been a wonder drug," said Patricia Dutkiewicz, Daniel's mother.

Ritalin's growing popularity came as no surprise to Lowell Smith, chief psychologist for Salem-Keizer schools.

This condition is characterized by excessive activity, restlessness, impulsivity, inappropriate behavior in social situations, and difficulty maintaining attention or completing tasks. It seems a contradiction, but many stimulants, in small doses, have the ability to focus attention and control hyperactivity. Amphetamines are also occasionally prescribed for this condition. In addition to drug therapy, other adjunctive or separate therapies that are employed include life style changes, education, environmental engineering, behavior modification, and psychotherapy.

AD/HD is three times as prevalent in boys as in girls: about 10% of boys and 3% of girls in the United States are diagnosed with this disorder. In girls, mood changes, social withdrawal, and fear are more common than the aggressiveness and impulsivity found in boys. If one examines children receiving psychiatric treatment, about 40% to 70% of inpatients and 30% to 50% of outpatients could be diagnosed with AD/HD.

There is an increased risk of alcohol and drug abuse among AD/HD individuals, but the reasons for this relationship are hard to pinpoint. It could be an attempt at self-medication. It could be that AD/HD leads to social alienation and problems with self-esteem, both of which are predictors of problems with alcohol and other drugs. It could be that the preexistence of a mental condition makes one more likely to get into compulsive behavior. Or it could be that the use of psychoactive stimulants makes one more susceptible to drug use because of neurotransmitter disruption or increased acceptance of the idea of taking drugs to alleviate mental problems.

It is estimated that 750,000 school children are receiving psychostimulant therapy, and the figure is growing. These drugs, such as Ritalin®, d-amphetamine, or pemoline (Cylert®), seem to work in about 75% of AD/HD children. Methylphenidate (Ritalin®) is a Schedule II drug which means it has addiction liability. Users that get into compulsive use will develop tolerance quickly and increase dosage. Occasionally, they will even switch to snorting or injecting the drug to try to recapture the original effects. There are grave questions about the long-term effects of strong stimulants on children over extended periods of time and about whether they become psychologically dependent on these kinds of drugs.

Methylphenidate (Ritalin®) is occasionally abused and has been diverted to illegal distribution channels, sold on the street, and used as a party drug. A few teenagers even appropriate their younger brother's or sister's supply to party with or to sell.

DIET PILLS

The other popular amphetamine congeners are diet pills, such as Preludin®, Ionamin®, Redux®, Pondimin®, and Fastin®. The stimulation, loss of appetite, and mood elevation caused by them are similar to the effects of amphetamines with some of the same side effects: excitability, nervousness; and increased blood pressure, heart rate and respiration. If used to excess, heart irregularities, toxic convulsions, and even stroke, coma, and death also occur. Despite their widespread use to control appetite and shed weight—there is significant weight loss in the first four to six months—users usually regain and even exceed their starting weights. Though amphetamine congeners are not as potent as amphetamines, psychological dependence and tolerance develop if used over an extended period of time.

Recently, the combination of fenfluramine (Pondimin®) and phentermin Ionamin®) has become more widely prescribed by physicians. In April of 1996, the FDA approved the prescription use of dexfenfluramine (Redux®) for weight loss. Again, the key to the abuse potential of amphetamine congeners is extended use. These diet pills and amphetamines are only recommended for short-term use, so careful monitoring by physicians and review boards is very important.

LOOKALIKES AND OVER-THE-COUNTER STIMULANTS

LOOKALIKES

The lookalike phenomenon contributed to the abuse of stimulants that began during the 1980s. By taking advantage of the interest in stimulant drugs, a few legitimate manufacturers began to make legal, over-the-counter products which looked identical to prescription stimulants. Their various products contained ephedrine and, occasionally, pseudoephedrine (an antiasthmatic), phenylpropanolamine (a decongestant and a mild appetite suppressant), and caffeine (a stimulant). These were being combined, packaged, and sold as "legal stimulants" in a deliberate attempt to misrepresent the drugs. The same chemicals were also showing up as illicit amphetamine lookalikes, such as street "speed," "cartwheels," and "crank," and as cocaine lookalikes, such as "Supercaine®," "Supertoot®," and "Snow®." The cocaine lookalikes add benzocaine or procaine to mimic the numbing effects of the actual drug.

The problem with the lookalike products is their toxicity when overused, particularly when two or more of the drugs are combined. Also, an amphetamine-like drug dependence developed in users who chronically abused the drugs. The physical problems can be particularly severe since large amounts are required to get a "speed" or cocainelike high. For these reasons, in the early 1980s, the FDA banned the OTC sales of products containing two or more of these ingredients.

OTHER OVER-THE-COUNTER STIMULANTS

Pseudoephedrine and phenylpropanolamine, which have decongestant, mild anorexic, and stimulant effects, are also found in hundreds of allergy and cold medications, often in combination with antihistamines, such as Benadryl®, and in over-the-counter diet pills, like Dexadiet® and Dexatrim®. Individuals who ingest these drugs and drink coffee or other caffeinated beverages often experience anxiety attacks and rapid heartbeats.

OTHER PLANT STIMULANTS

Caffeine is often thought of as the principal plant stimulant other than cocaine, but worldwide, dozens of substances have been discovered that stimulate the user. In fact, in many countries, these substances are much more common than coffee or tea.

KHAT AND METHCATHINONE

Khat ("qat," "shat," "miraa")

When the United States sent troops to Somalia in 1992, they were surprised to find a large percentage of the population chewing the leaves, twigs, and shoots of the khat shrub in order to get a milder amphetamine-like rush and stimulation. In Yemen, another country on the Arabian peninsula, more than half the population uses khat, and it is not unusual for people to spend over one-third of their family income on the drug. It is the driving force of the economy in Somalia, Yemen, and other countries in East Africa, Southern Arabia, and the Middle East. Such drug usage is not a new development in these countries. In fact, references to khat can be found in Arab journals in the thirteenth century. The leaves were used by some physicians as a treatment for depression. Many homes in some Middle East countries actually have a room dedicated to khat chewing.

The khat shrub is 10 to 20 feet tall. The fresh leaves and tender stems are chewed, then retained in the cheek as a ball and slowly chewed or swallowed to release the active drug. Dried leaves and twigs, which are not as potent as the fresh leaves, can be crushed for tea or made into a chewable paste. The main active ingredient, cathi-

Khat is used at many occasions, including this wedding in Yemen.
Reprinted, by permission, Alain Labrousse, Observatoire Geopolitique Des Drogues.

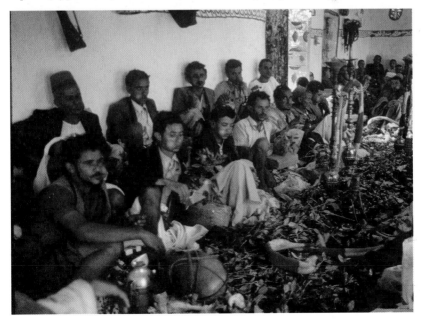

none, is most potent in fresh leaves which are less than 48 hours old.

Cathinone is a naturally occurring amphetamine-like substance that produces a similar euphoric effect along with exhilaration, energy, talkativeness, hyperactivity, wakefulness, and loss of appetite. Unfortunately, side effects include anorexia, tachycardia, hypertension, dependence, chronic insomnia, and gastric disorders. People who use too much khat can become irritable, angry, and often violent. Chronic khat abuse results in symptoms similar to those seen with amphetamine addiction, including physical exhaustion, violence, and suicidal depression upon withdrawal. There are also rare reports of paranoid hallucinations and even overdose deaths.

The constant factional battles in Somalia which devastated the country could be partially due to the effects of khat, along with the struggles to control the money involved in the trade. Hundreds of millions of dollars are spent on the drug, even in poor countries. In Muslim countries where alcohol is banned, khat is used in a number of social situations.

Methcathinone

Recently in the United States, a synthetic version of cathinone called methcathinone has been produced in illegal laboratories, particularly in the Midwest, and sold on the street as a powerful alternative to methamphetamine. Since it is cheap to manufacture, a number of labs have sprung up. By the end of 1994, 34 methcathinone laboratories had been raided in Michigan, and recently, law enforcement officers have found labs in other Midwest states, including 22 in Indiana and 8 in Wisconsin. Labs have also been found in Washington, Texas, Pennsylvania, and a dozen other states. Like methamphetamine manufacture, ephedrine is the main raw ingredient for methcathinone synthesis.

Methcathinone (also known as ephedrone) was originally synthesized in the United States by Parke-Davis Pharmaceuticals but rejected for production due to side effects. The formula became widely known in Russia, and by the early 1980s, methcathinone manufacture was widespread. It has been estimated that 20% of illicit drug abusers in the former Soviet Union use methcathinone.

Like methamphetamines, methcathinone is usually snorted or injected. Using methcathinone instead of khat is similar to using cocaine instead of the coca leaf. Methcathinone is more intense than khat so its addictive properties and side effects are more intense (and quite similar to those of methamphetamines).

BETEL NUTS

References to betel nut use date back more than 21 centuries. They have been widely used in the Arab world, India, Malaysia, the Philippines, and New Guinea. Marco Polo brought betel nuts to Europe in 1300.

Today, more than 200 million people worldwide use betel nuts not only as a recreational drug but also as a medicine. The effects are similar to those of nicotine or strong coffee and include a mild euphoria, excitation, decrease in tiredness, and lowered levels of irritability. Some users chew from morning until night, others use them only in social situations. Some liken the practice to gum-chewing or cola-drinking in the West, but this drug can also produce psychological dependence.

The betel nut (husk and/or meat) is generally chewed in combination with another plant leaf (peppermint, mustard, etc.) and some slaked lime to make it more palatable. The juice of this mixture blackens the teeth over time. In high doses, one of the ingredients, muscarine, can be toxic. However, the principal danger has to do with tissue damage to mucosal linings of the mouth and esophagus. In addition, up to seven percent of regular users have cancer of the mouth and esophagus. There is even a prominent and identifiable set of withdrawal symptoms.

YOHIMBE

Yohimbine, a bitter, spicy extract from the African yohimbe tree, can be brewed into a stimulating tea or used as a medicine. It is reported to be a mild aphrodisiac. It seems to increase the activity of the neurotransmitter acetylcholine, which results in more penile blood inflow. It also increases blood pressure and heart rate. Yohimbine has been reported to produce a mild euphoria and occasional hallucinations, but in larger doses it can be toxic. The bark can be bought at some herbal stores along with a whole series of medicines for "increasing potency," with names like "Male Performance®," "Yohimbe Power®", "Manpower®", and "Aphrodyne®" (prescription only).

EPHEDRA

The ephedra bush, found in deserts throughout the world, contains the drug ephedrine. This drug is a mild stimulant that is used medicinally to treat asthma, narcolepsy, other allergies, and low blood pressure. Many use it to make tea. The Mormons brewed it as a substitute for coffee which was forbidden by their religion. Ephedrine, also known as marwath, has been mentioned as a stimulant tonic in China for over 4,000 years and is still sold in herbalists' shops today. Extract of ephedrine has been used by athletes for an extra boost but can lead to heart and blood vessel problems. A weightlifter's death in Ohio led to the banning of sales of the extract in most stores in that state. Other states, such as Florida, have followed suit and banned the sales of all ephedrine-based products. Many lookalike and over-the-counter products that advertise themselves as MDMA, amphetamine substitutes, or other stimulants contain ephedrine.

Natural ephedra and synthetic ephedrine are also the main ingredients in the synthesis of methamphetamine and methcathinone, and because of the demand for them, a large illegal trade has sprung up.

FDA urges consumers to shun ephedrine high

Newsday

WASHINGTON — Concerned about growing use of herbal stimulants of the kind linked to the death last month of a New York college student, the U.S. Food and Drug Administration Wednesday warned consumers

Kessler said he is awaiting the findings of the medical examiner, but he said that "20-year-olds shouldn't be dying" after using herbal preparations.

Many of the questionable products "bear labels that

Herbal Ecstasy® and Herbal Nexus®

In an attempt to cater to some people's desire for other stimulants and psychedelics, entrepreneurs have introduced new herbal products. These capsules and tablets combine the herbal form of ephedrine (ephedra), an herbal extract of caffeine (possibly from the kola nut), along with other herbs and vitamins, and are advertised as Herbal Ecstasy®, Herbal Nexus®, or other catchy names. The use of herbal substances is an attempt to get around the FDA ban on some combinations of these products and to cash in on the current interest in certain psychoactive drugs including MDMA (ecstasy), nexus (CBR), other stimulants, and even marijuana. Some of these herbal products also contain vitamins and are touted as buffers for the toxic effects of the real ecstasy and nexus. Unfortunately, the problems, even with herbal ephedra, have caused several states to ban products with any form of ephedra or ephedrine and have provoked a warning from the FDA on the use of any substance containing the drug.

CAFFEINE

Caffeine is the most popular stimulant in the world. It is found in coffee, tea, soft drinks, chocolate, and hundreds of over-the-counter or prescription medications.

HISTORY OF USE

Tea was thought to have been present in China as early as the third century B.C., but the first written record dates back to 350 A.D. It was introduced into Europe around the end of the sixteenth century and immediately became quite popular.

Coffee was first cultivated in Ethiopia around 600 A.D., and then spread to Arabia about 800 A.D., and finally to Europe by the thirteenth century. The drink was so

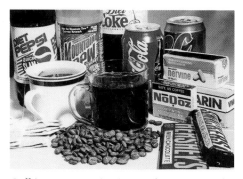

Caffeine concentration in most beverages is only one part in one or two thousand. Pure caffeine extract is a powerful stimulant.

stimulating that many cultures banned it as an intoxicating drug. In colonial America, it was suggested that the use of tea and coffee led to the use of tobacco, alcohol, opium, and other drugs. Fortunately or unfortunately, coffee and tea were also great sources of revenue, and the pressure against prohibition was immense both from governments and the general public. The use of caffeinated beverages continued to expand until today. In the United States alone, each coffee drinker consumes about 20 pounds of coffee per year.

Cocoa was first used in the New World by the Aztecs and Mayan royalty, mostly as an unsweetened drink or as a spice, and brought to Europe by Hernando Cortez in 1528. Widespread use didn't occur until the nineteenth century when the first chocolate bars appeared on the market.

PHARMACOLOGY

Caffeine is an alkaloid of the chemical class called xanthines. It is found in more than 60 plant species such as the *Coffea arabica* (coffee), *Thea sinensis* (tea), *Theobroma cacao* (chocolate), or *Cola nitida* (cola drinks). Caffeine can be used orally, intravenously, intramuscularly, or rectally,

TABLE 3–2   CAFFEINE CONTENT IN VARIOUS SUBSTANCES

Amount of Beverage or Food	Caffeine Content in Milligrams (mg.)	
	Average	Range
1 demitasse espresso	200 mg.	
1 cup freshly brewed American coffee (6 oz.)	100 mg.	90–125 mg.
1 cup of instant coffee	75 mg.	60–100 mg.
1 cup of decaf coffee	3 mg.	2–4 mg.
1 cup of tea	60 mg.	20–100 mg.
12 oz. caffeinated soft drink (e.g., Coca Cola®, Mountain Dew®)	45 mg.	36–60 mg.
4 oz. chocolate bar	800 mg.	15–90 mg.
1 No-Doz® tablet	100 mg.	
1 Vivarin® tablet	200 mg.	
1 Excedrin® tablet	65 mg.	
1 Midol® tablet	32 mg.	

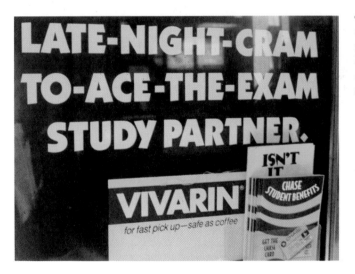

Over-the-counter products that promote their ability to help the user stay awake usually contain 200 milligrams of caffeine.

though most consumption is by mouth. The half-life of caffeine in the body is 3 to 7 hours, so it will take 15 to 35 hours for 95% of the caffeine to be excreted. School-aged children eliminate caffeine twice as fast as adults.

In the United States, per capita consumption of caffeine is 211 milligrams per day; Sweden, 425 milligrams; and the United Kingdom, 444 milligrams. Worldwide, the figure averages about 70 milligrams per day.

PHYSICAL AND MENTAL EFFECTS

Medically, caffeine is used in a number of over-the-counter preparations as a decongestant, an analgesic, a stimulant, an appetite suppressant, and for menstrual pain. Nonmedically, caffeine is most widely known and used as a mild stimulant. In low doses (100–200 milligrams), it can increase alertness, dissipate drowsiness or fatigue, and help thinking. Even at doses above 200 milligrams, there can still be increased alertness and performance, but as with any drug, excessive use can cause problems.

Of the 100 million or so coffee drinkers in the United States, 20% to 30% consume five to seven cups per day. At these doses (250–700 milligrams), anxiety, insomnia, nervousness, gastric irritation, high blood pressure, and flushed face can occur. At doses above 1,000 milligrams, increased heart rate, palpitations, muscle twitching, rambling thoughts, jumbled speech, sleeping difficulties, motor disturbances, ringing in the ears, and even vomiting and convulsions can occur. Caffeine is lethal at about 10 grams (100 cups of coffee).

Consuming 300 milligrams or more per day can lower fertility rates in women and affect fetuses in the womb (higher blood pressure). In addition, it is thought by a number of researchers that some women develop benign lumps in their breasts from drinking too much coffee.

Since excessive caffeine use can trigger nervousness, people who are prone to panic attacks should avoid caffeine. A physician or psychiatrist should ask patients who come in with symptoms of anxiety about their caffeine consumption.

Some researchers also feel that caffeine use makes it harder to lose weight. This difficulty happens because caffeine stimulates the release of insulin. Insulin metabolizes sugar, which then reduces the level of sugar in the blood, triggering hunger in the user.

Coronary heart disease, ischemic heart disease, heart attacks, intestinal ulcers, diabetes, and some liver problems have been seen in long-term, high-dose caffeine users, more often in countries with very high per capita caffeine consumption.

TOLERANCE, WITHDRAWAL, DEPENDENCY

Tolerance to the effects of caffeine does occur, although there is a wide variation among the ways different people will react to several cups of coffee or tea. Coffee drinkers might eventually need three cups to "wake up" instead of the usual single cup with lots of cream and sugar.

Withdrawal symptoms do occur after cessation of long-term use. These symptoms include headaches, fatigue and lethargy, depression, decreased alertness, sleep problems, and irritability, but fortunately, most symptoms pass within a few days, although some users say symptoms can last for a week or more.

"The headache hits me about five in the afternoon of the day I quit and stays around through the next day. Then I feel tired and my ass drags for the next two weeks. I'll stay off it for a while and then I'll start with half-a-cup and pretty soon I got a pot going all the time plus a couple of six-packs of Diet Coke® in the icebox."
20-year coffee drinker

Generally, daily intake levels of 500 milligrams (about 6 cups of coffee, 10 cola drinks, or 8 cups of tea) or more can result in dependence or addiction, although withdrawal symptoms will occur after cessation of long-term use of 100–200 milligrams per day. Coffee creates a milder dependency than that found with amphetamines and cocaine. It interferes less with daily functioning and is not as expensive as the stronger stimulants. However, two-thirds of those treated for excessive caffeine use (caffeinism) will relapse.

NICOTINE (tobacco)

Tobacco comes from the leaves and other parts of a plant species belonging to the genus *Nicotiana,* a member of the deadly nightshade family that also includes tomatoes, belladonna, and petunias. There are 64 *Nicotiana* species, but most commercial tobacco comes from the milder, broadleafed *Nicotiana tabacum* plant and a number of its variants. Though tobacco is available in cigarettes, cigars, pipe tobacco, snuff (oral and nasal), and chewing tobacco, cigarettes account for 95% of all tobacco use in America. In a country such as India, chewing tobacco (and chewing the betel nut) is more popular (85% of all adult men). Whether it is smoked, chewed, absorbed through the gums, or even used as an enema, this stimulant ultimately affects many of the same areas of the brain as cocaine and amphetamines.

HISTORY

Native Americans and then Columbus Discover Tobacco

After several voyages to the New World, Columbus and a number of other French, Portuguese, and Spanish explorers and diplomats introduced tobacco to Europe where it was used for recreation and as a medicine. It was listed as a cure for almost every known disease including ulcerated abscesses, fistulas, and sores. (In this century, it is listed as the cause of many diseases.) Use spread to Europe, Russia, Japan, Africa, and China in the 1600s, and later on to virtually every country in the world. (Note that the smoking of opium and marijuana had been known for thousands of years in Asia, Africa, and Europe but not the smoking of tobacco.)

Growth of Cigarette Smoking

The cigarette market expanded greatly because of improved technology, increased

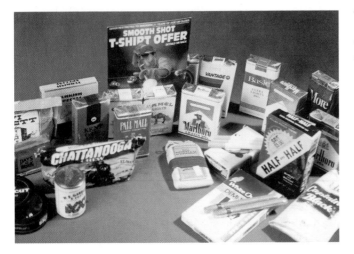

Tobacco is used in cigarettes, cigars, pipe tobacco, snuff, and chewing tobacco.

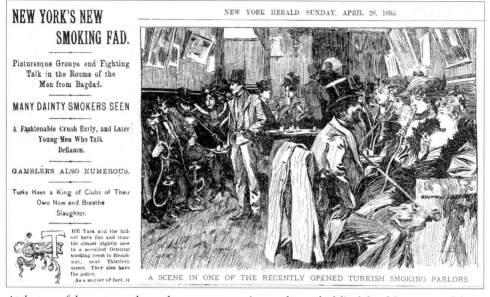

At the turn of the century, tobacco dens were as notorious as the psychedelic clubs of the 1960s and the "rave" clubs of the 1990s.

advertising, and more aggressive marketing techniques. If a user smoked 40 cigarettes a year in the late 1800s, it was not nearly the health problem it is today when the consumption of an average heavy smoker is 30 to 40 cigarettes a day, or more than 10,000 a year. This new popularity of tobacco not only multiplied the number of smokers, it multiplied the number of dollars made from tobacco. Gross sales of tobacco products in the United States in 1995 were approximately $50 billion (*U.S. Commerce Department*). In 1995 in the United States, 46 million Americans, about 1 in 5, smoked cigarettes regularly (more than once a week).

Smokeless Tobacco

Chewing tobacco and snuff became popular in Europe and America in the eighteenth century because a user didn't have to roll a cigarette or carry a means to light it. The other reason was that there was no smoke involved. The use of smoking tobacco didn't exceed the use of chewing tobacco in the United States until the end of World War I.

The two types of smokeless tobacco, moist snuff and loose-leaf, are still popular. A pinch of moist snuff—finely chopped tobacco as found in brands such as Copenhagen® and Skoal®—is stuck in the mouth next to the gums where the nicotine is absorbed into the capillaries. With loose-leaf chewing tobacco, like Beech Nut® and Red Man®, larger sections of leaf are stuffed into the mouth and chewed to allow the nicotine-laden juice to be absorbed.

PHARMACOLOGY

Tobacco

Tobacco and tobacco smoke contain about 4,000 chemicals of which 400 are tox-

TABLE 3–3   SOME INGREDIENTS FOUND IN CIGARETTE SMOKE

Tobacco Smoke	Common Product	Adverse Health Effects
Cadmium	Artists' oil paints	Yellow stains on teeth
Hydrogen cyanide	Gas chamber poison	Breathing difficulty
Vinyl chloride	Garbage bags	Fingers turn white and hurt when cold
Toluene	Embalmers' glue	Inflamed, cracked skin
Benzene	Rubber cement	Drowsiness, dizziness, headaches, nausea
Naphthalene	Paint pigment	Headache, confusion
Arsenic	Rat poison	Pins and needles feeling in hands and feet

(Compiled by the California Department of Health Services)

ins and 43 are known carcinogens. For example, one of the major byproducts of burning tobacco is tar which has direct effects on the respiratory system. Other byproducts are nitrosamines, also carcinogenic.

Nicotine

The most important ingredient in tobacco in terms of cardiovascular and particularly psychoactive effects is nicotine.

Smoking delivers nicotine to the brain in five to eight seconds. Chewing tobacco or snorting snuff delivers it in five to eight minutes. Besides tobacco, nicotine's only commercial use is as a pesticide. However, when tobacco is burned, as in a cigarette, the nicotine is not quite so deadly. The effect of nicotine is the main reason for the widespread use of tobacco.

Nicotine, a central nervous system stimulant, disrupts the balance of neurotransmitters, such as endorphins, adrenaline, dopamine, and particularly acetylcholine. Acetylcholine affects heart rate, blood pressure, memory, learning, reflexes, aggression, sleep, sexual activity,

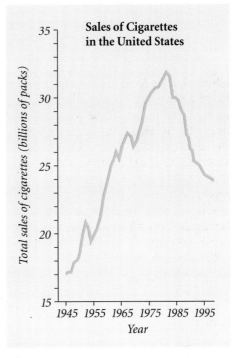

Figure 3–3 •

Sales of cigarettes have climbed from 18 billion packs a year in 1945 to a peak of 32 billion packs a year in 1980. By 1995, U.S. sales had dropped to 24 billion packs.

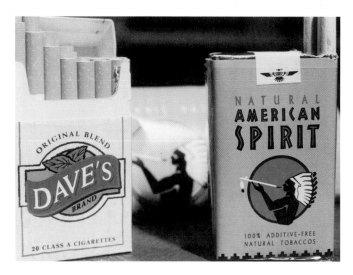

A small but fast-growing segment of the tobacco market includes offbeat brands which advertise that they are not one of the big tobacco companies or that their tobacco is "natural." All the designer brands still contain plenty of nicotine and other chemicals.

and mental acuity. What nicotine does is first mimic acetylcholine by slotting into receptor sites so those stimulatory effects are exaggerated. It also releases the stimulating neurotransmitter, norepinephrine. But the nicotine remains in those acetylcholine receptors, thereby blocking out the natural acetylcholine, limiting its activity, and having a calming effect. Dopamine is also released, exaggerating this calming effect. Nicotine first stimulates, then calms.

- The average cigarette delivers 1 milligram of nicotine. Chain smokers might get their nicotine level up to 6 milligrams; 70 milligrams is fatal.

- In comparison, one chew of tobacco will deliver approximately 4.5 milligrams of nicotine and one pinch of snuff, about 3.6 milligrams.

- The nicotine in the first cigarette of the day raises the heart rate an average of 10–20 beats per minute and the blood pressure by 5–10 points.

Nicotine and Craving

Besides the mildly pleasurable effects that smokers receive from tobacco, some of the reasons for continuing to smoke include:

- the social context, such as drinking and smoking in bars and at a meal;

- the ritual aspects of lighting up and smoking;

- the aura of smoking as an adult activity;

- the desire to lose weight or maintain weight loss;

- the desire to manipulate mood;

- the perception that smoking is sexually attractive;

- the desire to be rebellious.

It is an intense desire to maintain a certain nicotine level in the blood (and therefore in the brain) and to avoid withdrawal symptoms that leads many users to continue smoking all day long and for the rest of their lives.

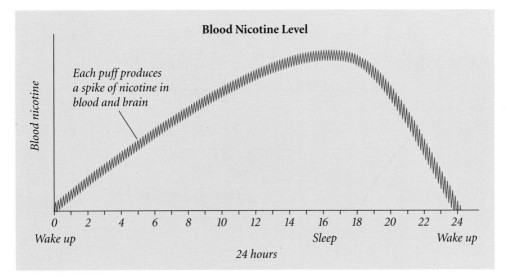

Figure 3–4 •

This chart shows the change in blood nicotine levels in a heavy smoker for a 24-hour period. Notice how the drop in the blood level overnight might lead to that intense craving for a cigarette and a cup of coffee in the morning.

TOLERANCE, WITHDRAWAL, AND ADDICTION

Tolerance

Tolerance to the effects of nicotine develops quite rapidly, even faster than with heroin or cocaine. A few hours of smoking is sufficient for the body to begin adapting to these new, toxic chemicals, particularly nicotine.

"The first time I smoked, it was to impress a girl. When I first started smoking, I got dizzy and high and had to sit down. A year later, my 30th cigarette of the day only gave me a mild stimulation and a nagging cough. Now, all I have left is the cough, a bunch of smoking rituals, and it costs over two bucks a pack." Two-pack-a-day smoker

Withdrawal

Withdrawal from a pack- or two-pack-a-day habit after prolonged use can cause headaches, nervousness, fatigue, hunger, severe irritability, poor concentration, sleep disturbances, and intense nicotine craving. It is a true physical dependence that has been built up. One process that occurs is the creation of more acetylcholine receptors. When a person tries to stop, the activity of acetylcholine is greatly exaggerated by all these extra receptors, thus making the user "restless, irritable, and discontent." Soon, the smoker comes to depend on smoking to stay normal, that is, to avoid these withdrawal effects.

The sense of relaxation and well-being that most smokers receive from a cigarette is, in fact, the sensation of the withdrawal symptoms being subdued.

Smokers will try to maintain a constant level of nicotine in the bloodstream and brain. Even when smokers switch to a low tar and nicotine brand, they often increase the number of cigarettes they smoke just to maintain their nicotine target levels. In fact, nicotine craving may last a lifetime after withdrawal.

"When I wake up at two or three in the morning, I can't go back to sleep without a cigarette. I just can't. If I try, I stay awake and fidget. If I smoke, I go back to sleep. I don't know if I have to smoke or just want to." Two-pack-a-day smoker

Addiction

"I cannot refrain from a few words of protest against the astounding fashion lately introduced from America, a sort of smoke-tippling which enslaves its victims more completely than any other form of intoxication, old or new. These madmen will swallow and inhale with incredible eagerness, the smoke of a plant they call herba Nicotiana, or tobacco."
German Ambassador to The Hague c. 1627

The use of tobacco is a pure example of the addictive process. The pleasure received from the direct effects of smoking is not as intense as the initial pleasure derived from alcohol, cocaine, or almost any other psychoactive drug. Coughing, dizziness, headache, even nausea are experienced by the novice smoker; the cost of a two-pack-a-day habit can run $1,500 a year; the health problems and premature deaths that result from smoking are too numerous to mention; and yet, people continue to smoke.

One of the strongest indications of the addictive potential of tobacco can be seen when you look at the percentage of casual tobacco users who become compulsive users versus the percentage of casual users of other psychoactive drugs who become compulsive users of those drugs.

- Twenty two million people in the United States have tried cocaine. Less than 1/2 million are weekly users, about 2%.
- Sixty-five million people have tried marijuana but only 5 million use it weekly, about 7%.
- One hundred seventy three million have tried alcohol, yet less than 20 million drink on a daily basis, about 12%.
- One hundred fifty two million have smoked cigarettes and about 46 million on a daily basis, about 29%.
(NIDA Household Survey, 1995)

These figures mean that almost one-third of those who ever tried a cigarette became habitual users. And yet, people continue to experiment with cigarettes.

Granted, you might say that people want to keep using cigarettes, that smoking is really pleasurable, that the choice is theirs. Yet, according to one survey, 80% of smokers interviewed say they want to quit, and another 10% say they want to limit the amount they smoke. That means that 9 out of 10 smokers are unhappy with their smoking and yet they continue to smoke.

In many countries, the rate of daily use is even higher than in the United States: 50% in China, 40% in England, 50% in Japan (*World Health Organization, 1994*). In a British study, 90% of teenagers who had smoked just three to four cigarettes at the time of the survey were found to be compulsive smokers years later. This statistic means that even the most casual use of tobacco leads to compulsive use. And yet, people continue to smoke.

It is worth noting here that nicotine craving is much more subtle and less noticeable to the user than the other cravings that occur with drugs like cocaine, heroin, or alcohol. However, the craving is nevertheless extremely powerful and may be associated with what is called a self-determined nicotine state of consciousness or "state dependence." State dependence means that people will try to achieve a certain mental and physical state which may be neither pleasurable nor objectionable, but it is a state with which they are familiar and one that they, and not others, have determined. Many people think that a large part of addiction is created by this desire to be in a familiar physical and mental mood even if it is damaging to the body and mind. In a *USA Today* survey, four out of five smokers and nonsmokers alike believed nicotine is an addictive substance.

EPIDEMIOLOGY

One interesting note: there has been a dramatic decrease over the past 20 years in Black youth who smoke. In 1994, only 5% of Black high school seniors said they smoked on a daily basis compared to 23% of Whites. In focus groups, children said such things as "smoking hurts stamina for sports," "boys don't like girls who smoke," and "we believed the media about the dangers of cigarettes."

TABLE 3–4   CIGARETTE USE IN THE UNITED STATES

By Age	Ever Used	Used Past Year	Used Past Month
12–17	8 million	6 million	5 million
18–25	21 million	13 million	10 million
26–34	28 million	14 million	12 million
Over 35	95 million	35 million	34 million
Totals	152 million	68 million	61 million

(National Institute of Drug Abuse Household Survey, 1995)

TABLE 3–5   SMOKELESS TOBACCO USE IN THE UNITED STATES

By Sex	Ever Used	Used Past Year	Used Past Month
Male	31.5 million	9.0 million	6.3 million
Female	4.4 million	0.6 million	0.7 million
Totals	35.9 million	9.6 million	6.9 million

(National Institute of Drug Abuse Household Survey, 1995)

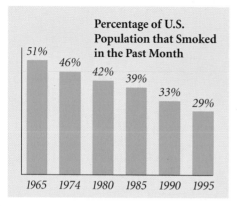

Percentage of U.S. Population that Smoked in the Past Month

51% 46% 42% 39% 33% 29%

1965 1974 1980 1985 1990 1995

Figure 3–5 •

Smoking rates in most other countries are higher than in the United States.

NIDA Household Survey, 1995

EFFECTS

One out of every five premature deaths in the world is caused by the use of tobacco, 390,000 per year in the United States alone. Another 50,000 die from secondhand smoke. The main reason for the extremely high figures is that tobacco takes 20, 30, or even 40 years for its most dangerous effects, such as cardiovascular disease, respiratory impairment, and cancer, to be felt. Most who die from smoking had been smoking more than 20 years. So, the immediate warning signs of overdose—heart palpitations, blackouts, hangovers, rages, paranoia, and nausea—common with other psychoactive drugs are missing. Except for the coughing, dizziness, initial nausea, bad breath, green mucous, lower lung capacity, and lowered energy levels, there are no flashing warning signs. Recognizing the warning signs of cocaine, heroin, or alcohol use is a very visceral, very immediate process. The dangerous side effects weigh directly against the pleasure received. With tobacco, that craving can only be tempered by an intellectual

appreciation of the long-term dangers. In most cases, the craving and fear of withdrawal win out over common sense.

Longevity

"I've smoked two-packs-a-day for 36 years and I'm still alive. I'm active and I'm good at my job. In any case, I'm not going to live forever. So why should I give up smoking?"
54-year-old smoker

The exceptional 75-year-old smoker who is healthy should not be seen as confirmation that smoking won't shorten life span or impair health. One has to look at the overall statistics. They show that, on average, a two-pack-a-day smoker will live eight years less than someone who doesn't smoke. Almost as important as these premature death statistics is the issue of quality of life. Because of breathing difficulties, poor circulation, and a dozen other imbalances caused by smoking, a smoker will have more medical complications, be less able to participate in physical activity, and will not be able to live life to the fullest.

Physical Effects

Smoking or chewing tobacco affects the body by interacting with the organs and tissues directly or indirectly through the central nervous system.

Cardiovascular. Smoking accelerates the process of plaque formation and hardening of the arteries (atherosclerosis), the major cause of heart attacks, by increasing low-density fats, increasing blood coagulability, and triggering cardiac arrhythmias (irregular beatings of the heart). The inhaled carbon monoxide created by tobacco combustion also accelerates the process of athersclerosis. In addition, since nicotine

Smokers More Likely To Contract Leukemia

Study finds 30% greater risk from cigarets

As research continues, the link between smoking and illness becomes overwhelming.

Cancer Deaths Jump In Women Who Smoke

Grim Forecast For World's Smokers

International health group expects 10 million deaths

Smoking Increases Heart-Attack Risk Fivefold for People in Their 30s and 40s

By Ron Winslow
Staff Reporter of THE WALL STREET JOURNAL

People in their 30s and 40s who smoke cigarettes are five times more likely than nonsmokers of the same age to suffer heart attacks, a team of British research-

In the British study, researchers divided the 46,000 participants into two groups — current smokers and those who hadn't smoked regularly in at past 10 years — and compared the rate of heart attacks in each group. They found that smokers aged 30 to 49 had suffered heart

constricts blood vessels, it restricts blood flow and raises blood pressure, increasing the risk of a stroke (ruptured blood vessel in the brain). The combination of nicotine and carbon monoxide also increases the risk of angina attacks (heart muscle spasms).

Respiratory. Eighty five percent of men with lung cancer and 75% of women with lung cancer smoke. The most likely culprits are the tars and other products of combustion that are inhaled by the smoker. Cigarette smokers also have a much higher rate of bronchopulmonary disease, such as emphysema, chronic bronchitis, and chronic obstructive pulmonary disease. In addition, children who live with smokers

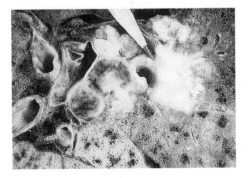

This section of lung tissue is cancerous. Normally, the color should be pink and smooth. More than 100,000 people die prematurely from tobacco-induced lung cancer every year.

Courtesy of Boris Ruebner, M.D.

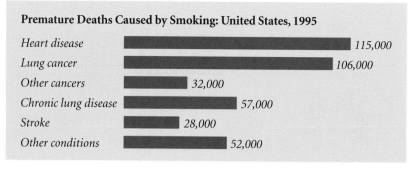

Premature Deaths Caused by Smoking: United States, 1995

Heart disease	115,000
Lung cancer	106,000
Other cancers	32,000
Chronic lung disease	57,000
Stroke	28,000
Other conditions	52,000

Figure 3–6 •
The average life span of a two-pack-a-day smoker is eight years less than a nonsmoker.

have a much higher incidence of asthma, colds, and bronchitis from inhaling secondhand smoke. Finally, environmental pollutants, such as asbestos or volatile chemicals, greatly increase the rates of respiratory illness and cancer above the rates due to exposure from just smoking or breathing dirty air.

Cancer. The increase in lung cancer since the 1930s when the use of cigarettes started to accelerate is startling. The rate in men has gone up 15–fold and in women 9–fold. In the graph (Fig. 3-7), we have juxtaposed the per capita smoking rate from 1930 to the present next to the per capita death rate from lung cancer. As the chart shows, in 1988, lung cancer deaths in women surpassed deaths from breast cancer for the first time in history.

Pipe and cigar smokers are less likely than cigarette smokers to get lung cancer. Pipe and cigar smokers are, however, much more likely than nonsmokers to get not only lung cancer but cancers of the larynx, mouth, and esophagus.

Fetal Effects. Since carbon monoxide and nicotine reduce the oxygen-carrying capacity of a pregnant mother's blood, less oxygen gets to the baby, contributing to a lower birth weight and a higher incidence of "crib death" (sudden infant death syndrome-SIDS).

Weight Loss. Nicotine appears to suppress appetite and increase metabolism. Since withdrawal from smoking is often accompanied by weight gain, the fear of weight gain can cause relapse.

Smokeless Tobacco Effects. Tobacco is almost as addicting in its smokeless form as in its smoked form, even though the nicotine takes 3 to 5 minutes to affect the central nervous system when chewed or pouched in the cheek compared to the 10 seconds it takes when inhaled from a cigarette. Strangely enough, more of the nicotine reaches the bloodstream with smokeless tobacco, and the rush is somewhat more intense. The effects of chewing are almost identical to the effects of smoking, including a slight increase in energy, alertness, blood pressure, and heart rate.

The main advantage of smokeless tobacco over cigarettes is the protection it gives the lungs since no smoke is inhaled. Lung cancer rates and other respiratory problems drop dramatically. Unfortunately, there are other problems with smokeless tobacco.

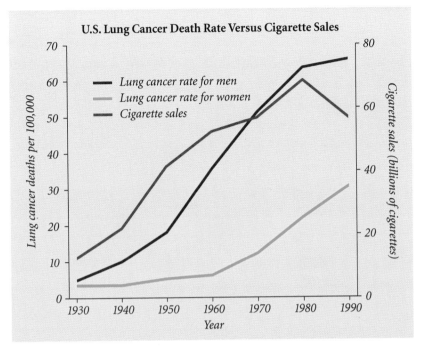

U.S. Lung Cancer Death Rate Versus Cigarette Sales

Figure 3–7 •

Since it takes 10 to 40 years for lung cancer to develop, there is a delay in the decrease of the rate of lung cancer even though cigarette sales among men have already declined.

"I can't think of a more disgusting habit than chewing tobacco. I broke up with my boyfriend because he was always dripping tobacco juice, spitting, and had those awful brown stains on his clothing. Ugh."

High school student

Smokeless tobacco is irritating to the tissues of the mouth and the digestive tract. Many users experience leukoplakia, a thickening, whitening, and hardening of tissues in the mouth. Their gums can become inflamed causing more dental problems, and although the risk of lung cancer is reduced compared to smoking, the risks of oral, pharynx, and esophageal cancers are increased. In addition, since blood vessels are constricted while either chewing or smoking, circulatory problems, the largest

health hazard of smoking, are just as grave with smokeless tobacco.

Mental and Emotional Effects

Nicotine can be stimulating, relaxing, or even depressing, often depending on the mood of the smoker. People use it to get going in the morning, to mellow out after a meal, to get ready for bed, to steady their nerves, and even to conclude sex. Some of the emotional effects are related to the settings where tobacco is used: a person might feel more confident holding a cigarette while starting a conversation or talking on the phone to a client. But after continued use, tobacco's effectiveness at calming and relieving anxiety seems more associated with preventing nicotine withdrawal rather than acting as a true sedative.

BENEFITS FROM QUITTING

A number of beneficial physiologic changes that occur on quitting are the following:

- Within 36 hours, blood carbon monoxide levels return to normal.

- Within 48 hours, nerve endings adjust to the absence of nicotine, and the senses of smell and taste are sharpened.

- Within a week, the risk of heart attack drops, breathing improves, and constricted blood vessels begin to relax.

- Within 2 weeks to 3 months, circulation improves, lung function increases up to 30%, and the complexion looks healthy again.

- Within 1 to 9 months, fatigue, coughing, sinus congestion, and shortness of breath decrease and the lungs increase their ability to handle mucus, thereby helping to clean themselves and reduce infection.

- Within 5 years, the heart disease death rate returns to the rate for nonsmokers.

- Within 10 years, the lung cancer death rate drops almost to the rate for nonsmokers, precancerous cells are replaced, and the incidence of other cancers decreases.

Mentally, there are other beneficial changes:

- Initially, there is anxiety, anger, difficulty concentrating, increased appetite, and craving due to withdrawal.

- After 2 weeks, most of these side effects disappear with the exception of craving and increased appetite.

THE TOBACCO INDUSTRY AND TOBACCO ADVERTISING

The Business of Tobacco

Just a handful of companies control the tobacco market in the United States. Philip Morris (Marlboro®, Virginia Slims®, Basic®), R.J. Reynolds/Nabisco (Winston®, Camel®, Salem®), American Brands (Carlton®, Lucky Strike®, Pall Mall®), British American Tobacco (Kool®), and U.S. Tobacco (Copenhagen®, Skoal®) account for more than 95% of sales ($48 billion in 1994). Over the past 20 years, there has also been an aggressive expansion into foreign markets aided by the weakening and dissolution of state-owned and smaller private tobacco companies. Cigarette smoking is growing at a rate of 3% a year in developing countries.

In the 1980s, because of the ever increasing cost of a pack of cigarettes, many manufacturers came out with generic, cheaper brands that by 1993 accounted for 25% of U.S. cigarette sales. To win back some of that market, the big manufacturers lowered the prices on name brands.

Advertising

Advertising expenditures by the tobacco industry are over $1 billion a year with another $1 1/2 billion in giveaways, premiums, promotional allowances to retailers, and other items. Advertising works. As a result of the Joe Camel advertising campaign, sales of Camels® to teenage smokers from the age of 12–18 more than tripled over a five-year period while the sales to adult Camel® smokers remained the same. The maker of Camels®, R.J. Reynolds Company, claims its campaign is not directed at children. The results seem to contradict its claim.

There is also evidence that, because most smokers acquire their habit before the age of 20, tobacco companies have used advertising to appeal to these new, young smokers. For example, in a confidential memo, one tobacco company advised its advertising department as follows:

"Thus, an attempt to reach young smokers, starters, should be based, among others, on the following major parameters:

- Present the cigarette as one of a few initiations into the adult world.

- Present the cigarette as part of the illicit pleasure category of products and activities.

- In your ads, create a situation taken from the day-to-day life of the young smoker but in an elegant manner have this situation touch on the basic symbols of the growing-up, maturity process.

- To the best of your ability (considering some legal constraints), relate the cigarette to 'pot,' wine, beer, sex, etc.

- **Don't** [their emphasis] communicate health or health-related points."

Antismoking advertising also works. In Massachusetts, when $70 million was spent in an antitobacco campaign on prime time television, sales of cigarettes dropped 20% compared to a national average drop of 3%.

Regulation

Recognizing that regulations and bad publicity could hurt sales, the U.S. tobacco industry created the Tobacco Merchants' Association and later the Tobacco Institute and the Council for Tobacco Research to lobby against laws they didn't like and to mute criticism of tobacco and the tobacco industry with their own research, publicity, and information. This strategy is not unusual in business. Most industries have lobbying and public relations groups. What changed, starting in the 1950s, was the mounting evidence that tobacco was extremely harmful and extremely addicting, highlighted by the first *Surgeon General's Report to the Nation* in 1967 on the dangers of smoking. Since that time, there has been a continuing battle among the tobacco industry, Congress, smokers, and nonsmokers about the legality, availability, and health hazards of smoking.

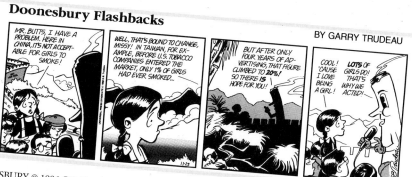

Doonesbury Flashbacks   BY GARRY TRUDEAU

Laws and Lawsuits

Because of the coughing and tearing caused by secondhand smoke, as well as the actual health problems, numerous laws have been passed at the state and federal levels prohibiting the use of tobacco products in a variety of spaces and buildings (e.g., sections of restaurants, airplanes, some businesses, federal and state buildings). From indifference to "other peoples' habits" in the early 1980s to a powerful crusade in the '90s, public opinion has changed. Unfortunately, tobacco has long been exempt from laws protecting the health of Americans. The principal law that has been superseded is the one that states that no substance that causes cancer may be sold for human consumption. A special statute was voted by Congress exempting tobacco from this law. In 1992, 420 out of 535 congressional representatives and 87 out of 100 senators accepted tobacco lobby contributions ($4.7 million). Given the addictive nature of tobacco, some think that such contributions are the equivalent of marijuana or coca growers giving money to politicians to promote drug legalization.

By 1995, the Food and Drug Administration and the Clinton Administration were ready for a full-scale assault on the tobacco industry. The administration said its goal was to cut teenage smoking in half by sharply curtailing "the deadly temptations of tobacco and its skillful marketing" by the industry. The industry said the real aim of the antismoking forces and the new legislation was to outlaw smoking altogether. One of the themes of various tobacco industry campaigns was "the right to choose." Clinton gave the FDA authority to regulate cigarettes because of their nicotine content; that is, because nicotine is addictive, it damages people's abilities to choose freely whether they want to smoke or not. The FDA declared cigarettes a drug, releasing material and memos from the tobacco industry itself showing that tobacco companies have long believed cigarettes are addictive, mainly because of nicotine.

The biggest assault on the tobacco industry has come from a number of state governments that are suing the tobacco companies. Some of the suits are for the extra cost of health care due to smoking. Other suits accuse the tobacco industry of manipulating nicotine levels to keep smok-

Tobacco Firms Sued — Health-Care Costs

Maryland puts costs at $13 billion   1996

Cigarette Firm Settles Suit Claiming Nicotine Is Added

Deal shatters industry's invincible image

ers addicted. Brown and Williamson, the nation's fifth largest manufacturer (Chesterfield®, Eve®), settled a lawsuit in 1996 agreeing to pay 5% of its pretax profits or $50 million a year toward programs that help people stop smoking.

Secondhand Smoke

Besides the issue of the addictive nature of tobacco and nicotine, a main battle over smoking in the 1990s is over the issue of secondhand smoke (the smoke that is inhaled by nonusers in a room with smokers). It is estimated that one person dies from secondhand smoke (mostly from cardiovascular disease) for every eight who die from the direct effects. When the issue was first raised in the early 1980s, the evidence was scant, but since then, the U.S. Surgeon General's Office, the National Research Council, and The International Agency for Research on Cancer have concluded that secondhand smoke does cause lung cancer. Other studies have connected secondhand smoke to other illnesses, including asthma and bronchitis in the children of smokers.

One of the reasons for the danger from secondhand smoke is that the sidestream smoke, mostly from a smoldering cigarette when the user is not inhaling, has higher concentrations of the substances, such as tar, that cause respiratory problems. So, while secondhand smoke has small amounts of nicotine, it has 1 to 40 times the amount of carcinogens found in mainstream (inhaled) smoke.

CONCLUSION

Stimulants seem like All-American drugs because, initially, they mimic virtues which are highly prized: the ability to work hard and stay up late, good appearance,

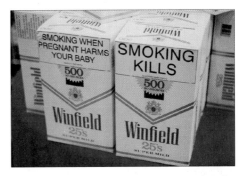

It is interesting to compare the warnings found on American cigarette packages and Australian cigarette packages. The Australians are willing to tell the complete truth about tobacco.

alertness, confidence, aggression, and mental acuity. We want a cup of coffee or a cigarette to wake up; more coffee at work to get going; a cola in the afternoon to carry on; an OTC product or prescription diet pill to hold the appetite down; a snort of methamphetamine to make the class less boring; a daily dose of Ritalin® to hold the kids in line; and a "rock" of "crack" to bring out the party animal. Energy and confidence are needed right away.

Compare the use of stimulants to gain energy and confidence to natural methods where energy supplies are replenished through relaxation, sleep, naps, light morning exercise (e.g., tai-chi), meditation, good nutrition, and a healthy life style. The natural methods first create the energy supplies and then let them be spent. The chemical methods drain the body of its energy supplies so it has to shut down to recover. The natural method works time after time. The chemical method causes tolerance and psychological dependence to develop so the resulting excess use taxes the body's resources and can damage neurochemistry.

Perhaps a new American slogan should be, "If you want to speed up, slow down."

CHAPTER   SUMMARY

General Classification

1. The seven principal stimulants are cocaine, amphetamines ("speed"), amphetamine congeners (e.g., Ritalin® and diet pills), lookalikes or over-the-counter drugs, other plant stimulants, caffeine, and nicotine.

General Effects

2. Uppers are central nervous system stimulants.

3. In general, uppers force the release of energy chemicals (particularly adrenaline), increase electrical activity in the brain, and artificially stimulate the reward/pleasure center.

4. The basic, initial effects of stimulants are restlessness, dilated pupils, talkativeness, irritability, reduced appetite or thirst, increased energy, faster heart rate, higher blood pressure, quicker respiration, and variable euphoria depending on the strength of the stimulant.

5. Most problems with stimulants occur when the body isn't given time to recover from the stimulation and its energy supply becomes depleted.

6. Excessive use of the stronger stimulants can cause neurotransmitter imbalance. A user can become paranoid, have muscle tremors, become aggressive, and fall into a deep mental depression.

7. Another set of problems with the stronger stimulants comes when the stimulated reward/pleasure center does not signal the need for food, drink, or sexual stimulation, resulting in malnutrition, dehydration, or a reduced sex drive.

8. A final set of problems with the stronger stimulants, such as cocaine, comes from overdosing (using too much at one time or having a severe reaction to a small dose). A "'caine" or "speed" reaction can cause uncontrolled heart rhythms, convulsions, ultrahigh blood pressure, heart attacks, strokes, dangerously high body temperatures, psychotic episodes, coma, and even death if not handled quickly by trained or knowledgeable people.

Cocaine

9. Cocaine is noted for the intensity of its stimulation, its high price, and the speed with which it is metabolized in the body. It produces an intense craving and is highly addicting.

10. Cocaine hydrochloride can be snorted, injected, or drunk. Cocaine freebase ("crack," "rock") is smoked. Smoking is the fastest route to the brain, 7 to 10 seconds, compared to IV use which is 15 to 30 seconds, and snorting which is 2 to 5 minutes.

11. Cocaine mimics and intensifies natural body functions and highs. The comedown is equally intense, so the user keeps taking the drug to stay up. And finally, the brain becomes sensitized to the memory of the pleasurable effects.

12. An overdose of cocaine can be the result of as little as 1/50th of a gram or as much as 1.2 grams or more. Most overdose reactions are not fatal, but death can come from cardiac arrest, respiratory depression, and seizures.

Smokable Cocaine

13. Smoking cocaine is more intense than snorting cocaine because, when smoked, the drug reaches the brain more quickly, can be taken more often, and is more fat soluble.

14. "Crack" cocaine causes many problems because of the economics of the drug. It comes in smaller amounts, there's a huge market for it, and the profits are large.

Amphetamines

15. Amphetamines are very similar to cocaine, the main difference being that they are synthetic, longer acting because they take more time to metabolize, and cheaper to buy.

16. Amphetamines were originally prescribed to fight exhaustion, depression, narcolepsy, asthma, and obesity but were taken often for their mood-elevating and euphoric properties.

17. Prolonged use of amphetamines can induce paranoia, heart and blood vessel problems, twitches, increased body temperature, dehydration, and malnutrition.

18. Tolerance develops rapidly with amphetamines. Amphetamine and cocaine withdrawal causes physical and emotional depression, extreme irritability, and nervousness.

Amphetamine Congeners

19. Many diet pills and mood elevators mimic the actions of amphetamines but are not quite as strong. They can still cause many of the problems found with amphetamines and can be as addicting. Ritalin® and Preludin® can be as addicting as cocaine and "speed."

Lookalikes and Over-the-Counter Stimulants

20. Lookalike drugs were popularized to take advantage of the desire for amphetamines and cocaine. They are composed of over-the-counter stimulants. Heavy use can cause heart and blood vessel problems as well as dependence.

Other Plant Stimulants

21. Other plant stimulants, such as khat, betel nut, ephedra, and yohimbe, have been used by hundreds of millions of people, particularly in the Middle East and Africa.

Caffeine

22. Caffeine, particularly coffee, is the most popular stimulant in the world. Tolerance can develop with caffeine, and withdrawal symptoms, such as headaches, depression, and irritability, do occur, particularly if consumption is more than five cups a day.

Nicotine (tobacco)

23. Nicotine (tobacco) is the most addicting psychoactive drug. In the United States, 46 million people are addicted to cigarettes compared to the 15 million addicted to alcohol. Nicotine causes more deaths than all the other psychoactive drugs combined.

24. One of the main reasons for tobacco's addictive nature, besides the slight stimulation it gives, is the need for the smoker's body to maintain a certain level of nicotine in the blood to avoid withdrawal.

25. Besides reducing the number of years of life, tobacco lowers the quality of life.

26. Smokeless tobacco is as addicting and as damaging as tobacco that is smoked.

Downers:
Opiates/Opioids and Sedative-Hypnotics

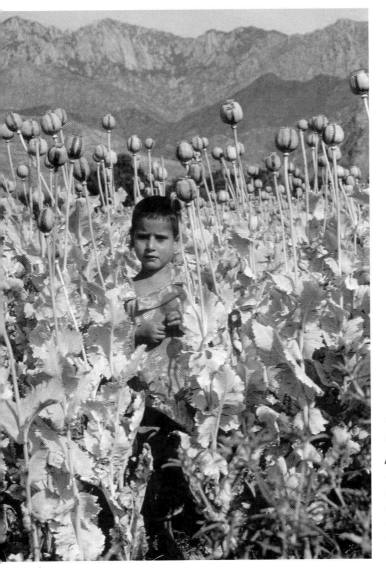

T his Afghani girl is almost lost among the illegally grown opium poppies in the mountains near Kabul.

Reprinted, by permission, Alain Labrousse, Observatoire Geopolitique Des Drogues.

- **General Classification:** The three major downers are opiates/opioids, sedative-hypnotics, and alcohol. The four minor downers are skeletal muscle relaxants, antihistamines, over-the-counter sedatives, and lookalike sedatives.

OPIATES/OPIOIDS

- **Classification:** Opiates/opioids are natural, semisynthetic, and synthetic derivatives of the opium poppy.
- **History of Use:** Changing routes of administration helped determine effects and abuse potential.
- **Effects of Opioids:** These drugs control pain and induce pleasure but create problems because of tolerance, tissue dependence, and severe withdrawal.
- **The Principle Opioids:** Heroin, codeine, and morphine are the major opioids.
- **Problems with Opioid Use:** Drug contamination, dirty needles, high cost, STDs, and a high addiction potential often occur with these drugs.
- **Other Opioids:** Methadone, Demerol®, and other analgesics (painkillers) are also widely used.

SEDATIVE-HYPNOTICS

- **Classification:** Barbiturates and particularly benzodiazepines are the most frequently prescribed sedative-hypnotics.
- **General Effects:** Sedatives are calming drugs, whereas hypnotics are prescribed mainly for insomnia.
- **Barbiturates:** The earliest sedative-hypnotics still prescribed and abused are barbiturates.
- **Benzodiazepines:** These drugs were developed as safe alternatives to barbiturates, but tolerance, addiction, withdrawal, and overdose still occur with them.
- **Other Sedative-Hypnotics:** These drugs, prescribed for anxiety and other problems, are also abused for their psychic effects.
- **Other Problems with Depressants:** Two hundred million doses of prescription drugs are diverted to illicit channels each year in the United States. Besides diversion, there are problems such as polydrug use, synergism, cross tolerance, and cross dependence.

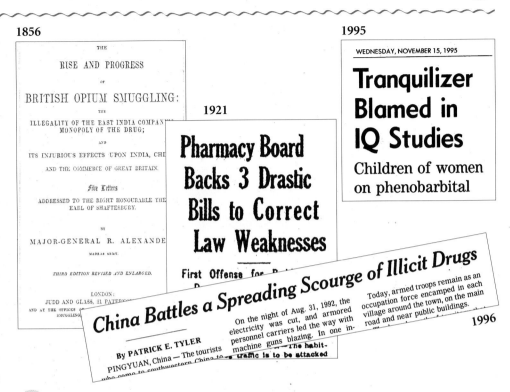

1856

THE
RISE AND PROGRESS
OF
BRITISH OPIUM SMUGGLING:
THE
ILLEGALITY OF THE EAST INDIA COMPANY'S
MONOPOLY OF THE DRUG;
AND
ITS INJURIOUS EFFECTS UPON INDIA, CHINA
AND THE COMMERCE OF GREAT BRITAIN.
Five Letters
ADDRESSED TO THE RIGHT HONOURABLE THE
EARL OF SHAFTESBURY.
BY
MAJOR-GENERAL R. ALEXANDER
MADRAS ARMY.
THIRD EDITION REVISED AND ENLARGED.
LONDON:
JUDD AND GLASS, 31 PATERN...
AND AT THE OFFICES ...
SMUGGLING

1921

Pharmacy Board Backs 3 Drastic Bills to Correct Law Weaknesses

First Offense for...

China Battles a Spreading Scourge of Illicit Drugs

By PATRICK E. TYLER
PINGYUAN, China — The tourists
who come to southwestern China to...

On the night of Aug. 31, 1992, the electricity was cut, and armored personnel carriers led the way with machine guns blazing. In one in-... The habit-... traffic is to be attacked

Today, armed troops remain as an occupation force encamped in each village around the town, on the main road and near public buildings.

1996

1995

WEDNESDAY, NOVEMBER 15, 1995

Tranquilizer Blamed in IQ Studies

Children of women on phenobarbital

GENERAL CLASSIFICATION

Downers (depressants) depress the overall functioning of the central nervous system to induce sedation, muscle relaxation, drowsiness, and even coma (if used to excess). Unlike uppers, which generally release and enhance the body's natural stimulatory neurochemicals, depressants produce their effects through a wide range of biochemical processes at different sites in the brain and spinal cord as well as in other tissues and organs outside the central nervous system.

Some depressants mimic the actions of the body's natural sedating or inhibiting neurotransmitters (e.g., endorphins, enkephalins, GABA), whereas others directly suppress the stimulation centers of the brain. Still others work in ways scientists haven't yet fully understood. Because of these variations, the depressants are grouped into a number of subclasses based on their chemistry, medical use, and legal classification.

The three major classes of depressants are opiates/opioids, sedative-hypnotics, and alcohol. The four minor classes of depressants are skeletal muscle relaxants, antihistamines, over-the-counter sedatives, and lookalike sedatives.

MAJOR DEPRESSANTS

Opiates and Opioids

Opiates and opioids, such as morphine, codeine, heroin, Percodan®, Dilaudid®, methadone, and Darvon®, were developed for the treatment of acute pain, diarrhea, coughs, and a number of other illnesses. Most illicit users take these drugs to experience euphoric effects, to avoid pain, and to suppress withdrawal symptoms.

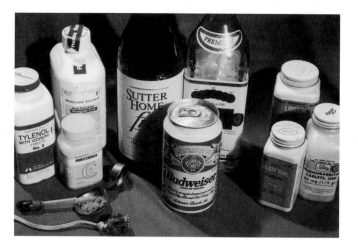

Opiates and alcohol were originally found in nature, whereas sedative-hypnotics were created in laboratories.

Sedative-Hypnotics

Sedative-hypnotics, also referred to as "solid alcohol," represent a wide range of synthetic chemical substances developed to treat nervousness, anxiety, and insomnia. The first, a barbiturate, was created in 1864 by Dr. Adolph Von Bayer. Since then, several thousand different sedative-hypnotics, such as Miltown®, Valium®, Doriden®, Quaalude®, Royhypnol®, and Mandrax®, have been synthesized. All have toxic side effects and can cause tissue dependence.

Alcohol (see Chapter 5)

Alcohol, the natural by-product of fermented plant sugars or starches, is probably the oldest psychoactive drug in the world. It has also been widely used over the centuries for social, cultural, and religious occasions. It is used for a number of medical remedies, from sterilizing wounds to lessening the risk of heart attacks. Because of its overall depressant effect, this liquid sedative has been used to reduce stress and lower inhibitions. Alcohol is also the world's most devastating drug (second in the United States to nicotine) in terms of health consequences, such as cirrhosis of the liver, mental deterioration, ulcers, and impotence. Social consequences of alcohol abuse include violence, crime, absenteeism, marital problems, and automobile accidents. In the United States alone, it is estimated that there are 12 to 14 million active problem drinkers and alcoholics.

MINOR DEPRESSANTS

Skeletal Muscle Relaxants

Centrally acting skeletal muscle relaxants, such as carisoprodol (Soma®) and methocarbamol (Robaxin®), are synthetic central nervous system depressants aimed at areas of the brain responsible for muscle coordination and activity. They are used to treat muscle tension and pain. Whereas the current abuse of these products is rare, their overall depressant effects on all parts of the central nervous system produce reactions similar to those caused by other abused depressants.

Antihistamines

Antihistamines, found in hundreds of cold and allergy medicines, such as Benadryl®, Actifed®, and Tylenol P.M. Extra®, are synthetic drugs which were developed during the 1930s and 1940s for treatment of allergic reactions, ulcers, shock, rashes, motion sickness, and even symptoms of Parkinson's Disease. In addition to blocking the release of histamine, these drugs cross the blood-brain barrier to induce the common and oftentimes potent side effect of depression of the central nervous system, resulting in drowsiness. Even antihistamines are occasionally abused for their depressant effects.

Over-The-Counter Sedatives

Over-the-counter depressants, such as Nytol®, Sleep-Eze®, and Sominex®, are sold legally in stores without the need for a prescription. For years, many brands marketed as sleep aids or sedatives were, in fact, first used as depressants during the 1880s. Scopolamine in low doses, antihistamines, salicylates (a natural form of aspirin), salicylamide, bromide derivatives, and even alcohol constitute the active sedating components in many of these products. As with other downer drugs, these products are occasionally abused for their sedating effects.

Lookalike Sedatives

Lookalike sedatives were advertised along with lookalike stimulants in the early 1980s. The great commercial success of the lookalike stimulants encouraged shady drug manufacturers to sell products which looked like prescription downers. These companies took legally available antihistamines and packaged them in tablets and capsules so they resembled restricted depressants, such as Quaalude®, Valium®, and Seconal®. As with the other antihistamines, lookalike sedatives cause drowsiness as a side effect, thereby mimicking some of the effects of more potent downers.

OPIATES/OPIOIDS

Opiates/opioids, one of the oldest and best documented classes of drugs, have been the source of continual and occasionally explosive worldwide problems (nineteenth century Opium Wars in China, twentieth century drug wars in Mexico, the spread of AIDS from infected needles). Heroin gets the most publicity, but the other opiates/opioids, such as codeine, Demerol® , and fentanyl, also create problems and can be used compulsively.

In the 1970s, the discovery of the body's own natural opiate painkillers, endorphins and enkephalins, significantly changed our understanding of opiates and opioids as well as the whole field of biochemical research, pain management, and drug abuse treatment. This research has provided a new perspective and new models to understand the biochemical mechanisms that govern our thoughts and actions.

CLASSIFICATION

OPIUM, OPIATES, AND OPIOIDS

Opium is processed from the milky fluid of the unripe seed pod of the opium poppy plant (*Papaver somniferum*). There

Many patent medicines and cure-alls contained opium as the main active ingredient. The frontispiece of Book of Antidotes, *c. 1200, contained the prescription for theriac, the opium-based medicine that was first formulated about 100 B.C., 2,000 years before Mrs. Winslow's Soothing Syrup became popular in the United States to calm crying babies.*

Reprinted, by permission, Bibliotheque Nationale, Paris. Courtesy of the National Library of Medicine, Bethesda.

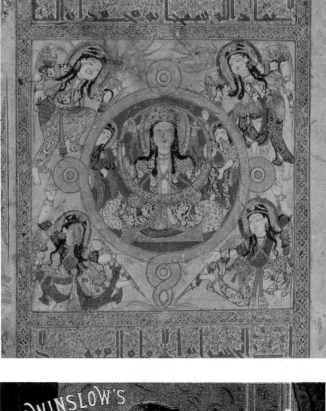

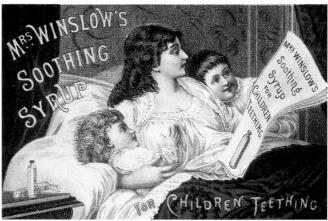

are over 25 known alkaloids in opium but the 3 most prevalent (called opiates) are morphine (4–20% of the milky fluid), codeine (1–5%), and thebaine (less than 1%). Although a small amount of opium is used to make antidiarrheal preparations, such as tincture of opium and paregoric, virtually all the opium coming into this country is first refined into its alkaloid constituents. The popularity of opium has diminished over the last century in the United States with the expansion of the

TABLE 4–1   OPIATES/OPIOIDS

Drug Name	Some Trade Names	Street Names
OPIATES (Opium poppy extracts)		
Opium	Pantopon®, Paregoric® Laudanum®	"O," op, poppy
Codeine (usually with aspirin or Tylenol®)	Empirin® with codeine, Tylenol® with codeine, Doriden® with codeine	Number 4s (1 grain), Number 3s (1/2 grain) Loads, sets, 4s & doors
Morphine	Various	Murphy, morph, "M," Miss Emma
SEMISYNTHETIC OPIATES		
Diacetylmorphine	Heroin	Smack, junk, tar (chiva, puro, goma, puta, chapa-pote), Mexican brown, China white, Harry, skag, shit, Rufus, Perze, "H," horse, dava, boy
Hydrocodone	Hycodan®, Vicodin®	
Hydromorphone	Dilaudid®	Dillies, drugstore heroin
Oxycodone	Percodan®, Tylox®	Percs
SYNTHETIC OPIATES (OPIOIDS)		
Methadone	Dolophine®	Juice
Propoxyphene	Darvon®, Darvocet-N® Wygesic®	Pink ladies, pumpkin seeds
Meperidine	Demerol®	Street derivatives of mepari-dine and fentanyl are mis-represented as China white
Fentanyl	Sublimaze®	Street derivatives are mis-represented as China white
Pentazocine	Talwin NX®	Part of T's and blues
41-acetyl alpha methadol (long-acting methadone)	LAAM	Lam
Buprenorphine	Buprenex®	
Alpha or 3 methyl fentanyl, etc.	Analogues of Sublimaze®	Designer heroin or China white
MPPP, etc.	Analogues of Demerol®	Designer heroin or China white

heroin trade and the availability of prescription opioids. (In 1900, approximately 25% of all Chinese used opium.)

Opium extracts can be slightly modified to form other active semisynthetic opiates, such as heroin, Percodan®, or Dilaudid®. There are also fully synthetic opiate-like drugs called opioids, such as Demerol®, methadone, and Darvon®, and synthetic opioid antagonists (naloxone and naltrexone) which block the effects of opiates and opioids.

HISTORY OF USE

The ancient Sumerians, Egyptians, and Chinese recorded the paradoxical nature of opium in their medical texts, listing it as a cure for all illnesses, a pleasurable substance, and a poison. Over the centuries, experimentation with different methods of use, development of new refinements of the drug, and synthesis of molecules, which act like the natural opioids, have slowly increased not only the benefits of these substances but also their potential for abuse.

ORAL INGESTION AND SMOKING

Opium, from the Greek word *opòs*, meaning juice or sap, was originally chewed, eaten, or blended in various liquids and drunk. Though the drug was used extensively to induce drowsiness as well as to treat many illnesses, the abuse potential of opium was relatively low because it had a bitter taste and the concentration of active ingredients was low. When taken

Morpheus, the son of Hypnos, the Greek god of sleep, is shown with opium poppy flowers strewn at his feet. The word morphine comes from Morpheus.

Sculpture by Jean Antoine Houdon, Louvre Museum, Paris. Reprinted, by permission, Simone Garlaund.

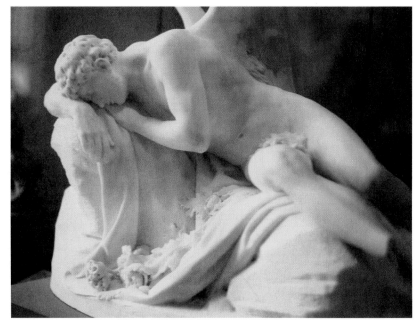

orally, the drug must go through the entire digestive system before it enters the bloodstream and makes its way to the brain 20 or 30 minutes later.

The introduction of the pipe from North America to Europe and Asia in the sixteenth century set the stage for widespread nonmedical use of opium. Smoking puts more of the active ingredients of the drug into the bloodstream faster by way of the lungs. The drug begins to reach the brain in as few as 6 to 8 seconds. The higher concentration of the opiate produces a strong sense of euphoria (mood elevation), relaxation, and well-being, thereby encouraging abuse.

IV USE

In 1806, a German pharmacist, Frederich Serturner, refined morphine from opium and found it to be 10 times stronger. Morphine was a much better pain reliever than opium but its greater strength promoted more compulsive use. In 1832, codeine, the other major component of opium, was isolated and in 1848, the hypodermic needle was invented. These three developments benefited wounded soldiers during the Crimean War and the U.S. Civil War. Unfortunately, they also increased the potential for opiate addiction. At that time in the United States, morphine addiction was called the "soldier's disease."

Intravenous use can inject high concentrations of the drug directly into the bloodstream. It takes 15 to 30 seconds for an injected opiate/opioid to affect the central nervous system. If the drug is injected just under the skin or in a muscle ("skin popping" or "muscling"), the effects are delayed by 5 to 8 minutes.

Just before the turn of the century, morphine was chemically altered to produce diacetylmorphine (heroin) in an attempt to find a more effective painkiller which didn't

have addictive properties. Unfortunately, the opposite proved to be true. Since heroin crosses the blood-brain barrier much more rapidly than morphine, the rush was more instantaneous and intense, thus creating a subculture of compulsive heroin users in the twentieth century.

PATENT MEDICINES, SNIFFING

During the mid– to late–1800s, opiates became so popular that hundreds of tonics and medications came on the market to treat everything from tired blood to coughs, diarrhea, and toothaches. Just before the turn of the century, the use of opioids for pleasure (recreational use) by the middle and upper classes also came into vogue. Whether it was a reaction to the strict Victorian mores and behaviors of the time or simply as an exciting experiment, the numbers of opium dens and the use of opium increased. In addition, new immigrants from Europe brought their habits with them, one of which included sniffing or snorting heroin. Workers from China brought opium and opium smoking.

TWENTIETH CENTURY

Rising concern over the perceived problems caused by use and abuse of opium, morphine, and heroin spurred various governments to action. Casual nonmedical use of opiates was declared illegal at the beginning of the twentieth century, by the international community through The Hague Resolutions in 1912 and then by the United States through The Pure Food and Drug Act in 1906 and The Harrison Narcotics Act in 1914.

Because these restrictions limited supply and made opium and heroin valuable commodities, growing, processing, and distributing opiates/opioids, especially heroin, became major sources of revenue

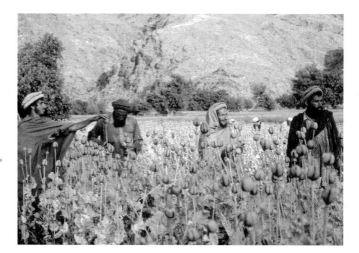

Afghani militia men scrape raw opium from an opium poppy capsule. Many militias around the world fund their military operations with money from growing and trafficking drugs.

Reprinted, by permission, Alain Labrousse, Observatoire Geopolitique Des Drogues.

for criminal organizations worldwide. These groups include the Chinese Triads, the Mafia, Mexican narcoficantes, the Colombian Cartel, African traffickers, and even the Russian "Mafia."

In addition, diversion of legal prescription opiates/opioids, such as codeine and Dilaudid®, through theft, bogus purchases from phony or even legitimate companies, and forged prescriptions, has created an illegal, nearly uncontrolled market of pills and injectables. Currently, an estimated 1.26 million Americans use prescription opiates/opioids illegally every month compared to 300,000 to 800,000 heroin abusers. Approximately 2.45 million Americans have tried heroin.

(Note: For the rest of this chapter, we will use the conventional generic term OPIOID to denote both natural and semisynthetic OPIATES and synthetic OPIOIDS.)

EFFECTS OF OPIOIDS

Medically, physicians prescribe opioids to deaden pain, control coughing, and stop diarrhea. Nonmedically, users self-prescribe opioids to induce euphoria, to drown out their emotional pain, or to try to feel normal by preventing withdrawal symptoms. But to truly comprehend opioids, it is important to understand how pain and pleasure are connected to the nervous system.

PAIN CONTROL

Pain, such as the pain of burned skin or a broken bone, is a warning signal which tells us whether we are being damaged physically. It sends a message to our brain which in turn tells the body to protect itself from further damage. The pain message is transmitted from nerve cell to nerve cell by a neurotransmitter called substance "P."

If the pain is too intense, the body tries to protect itself by softening the pain signals. It reduces pain by flooding the brain and spinal cord with special neurotransmitters, called endorphins. These endorphins attach themselves to receptor sites on the membrane of the sending nerve cell, telling it not to send substance "P" (Fig. 4-1).

However, many signals still get through. If the pain remains unbearable, opioids can

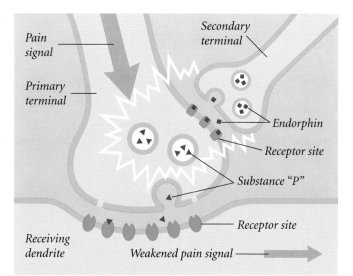

Figure 4—1 •

Natural Pain Suppression.
This diagram of a synapse shows that when pain signals are being transmitted through the nervous system, a secondary terminal releases endorphins which then slot into receptor sites on the primary terminal and limit the release of the pain neurotransmitter, substance "P."

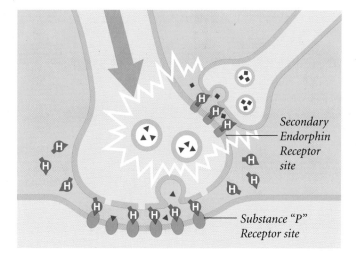

Figure 4—2 •

Artificial Pain Suppression.
Heroin slots into the secondary endorphin receptor sites limiting the release of substance "P." It also blocks most of the substance "P" that gets through by slotting into the primary substance "P" receptor sites on the receiving dendrite of the next neuron.

be used to relieve the agony. These drugs are effective because they act like the body's natural pain-killing endorphins. Opioids not only prevent too much substance "P" from being released, they also help block what little does get through to the receiving neuron (Fig. 4-2).

The effects of the various opioids are similar to each other. The differences have to do with how long the drug lasts, how strong it is per gram, and how toxic it is to the body. For example, heroin, codeine, and Darvon® will affect the user from four to six hours. (Because heroin is relatively short acting, an addict might use it as many as four times a day.) The pain-killing effects of fentanyl, on the other hand, will barely last an hour.

PLEASURE

The other major effect of opioids concerns pleasure. Just as pain is a warning signal to keep us from damaging ourselves, so pleasure is a signal to encourage us to do something that is good for the body and mind. Just as endorphins are released naturally to block pain in a part of the brain called the corpus striatum, so they are released to activate dopamine which in turn triggers the reward/pleasure center in the limbic system, the emotional center of the brain, to tell the body that it is doing well. If the reward/pleasure center is not being activated or if there are not enough endorphins in the system to do the job, a person will not feel good, will not feel rewarded, and will not feel pleasure. Instead, there will be a feeling of emptiness and depression.

Searching for relief or a high, some people try opioids because these drugs, particularly the stronger ones, artificially activate this reward/pleasure center directly by slotting into the receptor sites on the receiving neurons meant for endorphins and artificially trigger signals of pleasure. Heroin, more than any other opioid, has the strongest effect on this area of the brain and for this reason causes more dependence and eventually, a more intense craving.

"The heroin would just have me so mellow and I would feel good. I didn't think about nothing. I didn't want to know nothing. I just didn't care about nothing."
Recovering heroin abuser

The desire for relief from pain and the desire for mood elevation or euphoria, combined with tolerance, tissue dependence, and withdrawal, are the main reasons for the addictive nature of opioids.

"I'm always in pain. I have bad shoulders, arthritis, and all these things, so it was my excuse. This stuff would get me high, so I would take it and I would say, 'Oh, I'm just killing my pain.'"
Recovering codeine/Doriden® user

TISSUE DEPENDENCE AND TOLERANCE

"After a while, they [#4 codeine tablets] didn't really have any effect on me, and the pain was taking over with the drug, so I started taking more codeine. And I took more, and more, and finally, I was going through like two bottles of codeine a week."
Recovering codeine abuser

Tissue dependence and tolerance occur when the body tries to neutralize the opioid by first speeding up the metabolism, then by desensitizing the nerve cells to the drug's effects, and finally by altering the brain chemistry to compensate for the effects of the drug. The body's adjustment requires the user to increase dosage if the same effects are desired. Since tissue dependence and tolerance occur rapidly with opioids, users might need 10 times their initial dose within a month of beginning regular use.

Tolerance and tissue dependence extend to all opioids. That is, if users build a tolerance and a tissue dependence to heroin, they will also have a tissue dependence and tolerance to morphine and codeine. (This cross dependence is the basis for methadone maintenance treatment where one opioid is substituted for another, less damaging one).

WITHDRAWAL

Withdrawal occurs after two to three weeks of continuous use when tissue dependence has developed and the person suddenly stops using. The body has changed enough to trigger this "rebounding" effect as it tries to return (too quickly) to normal.

"You get deep, deep muscle and bone pains. There's no way to get comfortable, and you fluctuate between being chilly and sweating a lot. You can either be constipated or have diarrhea. You're in total body agony that nothing relieves. It's real uncomfortable. I have actually, and this is not a figure of speech, I have been going through withdrawal where I wished I was dead."
35-year-old recovering heroin user

Because opioid withdrawal symptoms can seem so frightening to users, that fear can keep them using. For many long-term users, the fear of withdrawal becomes a greater trigger for continued use than the desire to repeat the "rush."

In general, short-acting opioids, like heroin, morphine, and Dilaudid®, result in more severe yet short-lived (5 to 7 days) withdrawal symptoms. Long-acting opioids, like methadone, will delay the symptoms from 24 to 72 hours, but once they occur, these symptoms can last for weeks and be worse than those seen with short-acting opioids. Other opioids, such as codeine, Percodan®, and Darvon®, have withdrawal phenomena somewhere between those two extremes.

It is important to remember that, although opioid and particularly heroin withdrawal feels like an incredibly bad case of the flu, it is almost never life-threatening, as is withdrawal from alcohol or sedative-hypnotics.

OTHER PHYSICAL AND MENTAL EFFECTS

Opioids affect almost every part of the body: heart, lungs, brain, eyes, voice box, muscles, cough and nausea centers, reproductive system, digestive system, excretory system, and the immune system. Some of the effects of opioids are mild but quite identifiable in the heavier user, particularly if the drug is heroin since it has the ability to relax muscles. Eyelids droop, the head nods, and speech becomes slurred and slowed. The walking gait is also slowed. The pupils become pinpointed and do not react to light. The skin dries out and itching increases.

Other effects are less visible. The cough center in the brain is suppressed, making codeine-based cough medicines some of the most widely used prescription drugs. Opioids also affect the nausea center. In fact, some heroin addicts know a batch of their heroin is good if it makes them vomit.

"It hit from the feet going up to the head. I was yelling at him to take the needle out and I was on the toilet seat. I mean, I hugged that toilet bowl for hours, vomiting." 21-year-old heroin user

Other effects of opioids are even more severe. They stop diarrhea but cause chronic constipation by numbing the intestinal muscles. They also affect the hormonal system. A woman's period is delayed and a man produces less testosterone. Sexual desire is dulled, often to the point of indifference.

"Lots of times I don't want to be bothered by anybody or anyone touching me, like my girlfriend. Like if she wants to hug me, kiss me, I just say, 'Don't touch me.'"
28-year-old heroin user

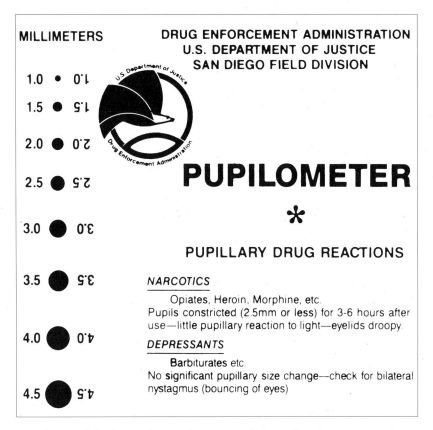

MILLIMETERS

**DRUG ENFORCEMENT ADMINISTRATION
U.S. DEPARTMENT OF JUSTICE
SAN DIEGO FIELD DIVISION**

1.0 • 1.0

1.5 • 1.5

2.0 ● 2.0

2.5 ● 2.5

3.0 ● 3.0

PUPILOMETER

✳

PUPILLARY DRUG REACTIONS

3.5 ● 3.5

NARCOTICS

Opiates, Heroin, Morphine, etc.
Pupils constricted (2.5mm or less) for 3-6 hours after use—little pupillary reaction to light—eyelids droopy.

4.0 ● 4.0

DEPRESSANTS

Barbiturates etc.
No significant pupillary size change—check for bilateral nystagmus (bouncing of eyes)

4.5 ● 4.5

A pupilometer is held up to the eyes of a suspected drug user in order to compare the size of pupils against normal standards. Since opioids contract pupils, pupil size is a strong indicator of drug use. (Cocaine and methamphetamines can dilate pupils.)

Neonatal Effects

Opioids cross the placental barrier between the fetus and the mother, thereby sending large doses of the drug to the developing infant. Pregnant users have a greater risk of miscarriage, placental separation, premature labor, breech birth, stillbirth, and seizures. When a baby is born to an addicted mother, the child is also addicted, and since babies are much smaller than adults, the tissue dependence is more severe. These symptoms can last five to eight weeks, and unlike adults, babies in withdrawal can die.

Overdose

Other effects of opioids in older users can also be life-threatening. Overdose occurs when so much of the drug enters the brain that the nervous system shuts down. Blood pressure drops, the heart beats too weakly to circulate blood, and lungs labor and fill with fluid. The person passes out and, unless quickly revived, will slip into a coma and die.

"You know, people who do heroin aren't worried about dying because like if three people die from a new batch of heroin,

everybody wants to know where they are getting that heroin so they can go get some because it's the best and they figure they will just do a little less."
41-year-old recovering heroin addict

THE PRINCIPLE OPIOIDS

HEROIN (diacetylmorphine)

Since the 1930s, heroin has captured more headlines than any of the other opioids. There are 5 to 10 million heroin users worldwide, and a dozen countries are battling the growth, use, and exportation of heroin on their own soil.

The area of Southeast Asia known as the Golden Triangle (Burma, Northern Thailand, and Laos) is the largest producer and exporter of illegal opium and heroin. It is also one of the largest users. Thailand alone has close to 1/2 million addicts. Golden Triangle heroin, known on the street as "China white" in its exportable form, can be up to 99% pure (in 1995, this region supplied over 40% of the heroin used in the United States). Other Southeast Asian types of heroin include Indian, Cambodian, and Malaysian or Sri Lankan pink heroin (usually around 50% pure). India is the largest grower of opium, but it is highly regulated, and the vast majority of the crop is used for legal medical purposes.

These are just a few of the samples of heroin seized by the Drug Enforcement Administration. Note that many highly diluted samples are dyed to make them appear a purer form of the drug.
Courtesy of Robert Sager, former Drug Enforcement Administration Laboratory Chief

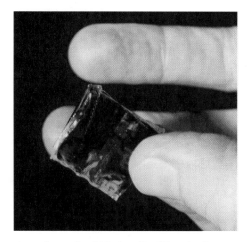

A small sample of Mexican "tar" heroin, the most common type of heroin sold in the United States, is packed in a little plastic bag.

Courtesy of JACNET, Jackson County, Oregon

Since the 1940s, Mexico has been a major supplier of heroin to the United States. In the 1980s, a relatively new form of Mexican heroin, known as "tar" or "black tar," took over most of the market on the West Coast. It is extremely potent, 40% to 80% pure, but also has more plant impurities than the Asian refinement of the drug. A small chunk the size of a match head, which is enough for two to five doses, costs about $20 to $25. "Tar" heroin, also called "chapapote," "puta," "goma," and "puro," is unique in that it's sold as a gummy, pasty substance rather than the usual powder form. It is also more likely to be smoked than other types of heroin. In 1996, an ounce of heroin on the East Coast of the United States was as high as $8,000, while on the West Coast, an ounce could go for as much as $3,000.

"'China white' is real clean. You don't have to heat it at all. It lasts a lot longer too. With 'tar,' it's very filthy. You throw up a lot more

with 'tar.' 'Tar' really makes me sick to my stomach. Unfortunately, on the West Coast that's all you can find anymore."
Heroin dealer/user

There has been a major increase in the production and abuse of heroin in Southwest Asia. From Afghanistan, Iran, Pakistan, Turkey, and Lebanon comes a product that is known as "Persian brown" or "Perze," which can be more than 90% pure. Several of these countries that grow opium now also have exploding addict populations. For example, there are an estimated 1.9 million opioid users in Pakistan.

"Persian heroin is simply raw processed morphine. The process to take raw morphine and turn it into #4 white is a very expensive and lengthy chemical process which takes experts, so dealers are just giving you less quality for ridiculous prices."
Recovering heroin smoker

In addition, several countries have major refining facilities or act as major transshipment points for heroin. These transshipment countries include the Netherlands, Canada, Italy, France, and Nigeria (the latter also grows its own). Also, many ex-Soviet Republics and satellites (e.g., Albania, Armenia, Uzbekistan, Kazakhstan, and Turkmenistan) are involved in production and transshipment of heroin.

Although some homegrown opium exists in the United States, most heroin is imported. A few criminal organizations still control most of the trade and have adapted to changing times. For example, with the return of Hong Kong to the People's Republic of China in 1997, many of the triads (Chinese criminal organizations) based in Hong Kong decided that their headquarters would be wiped out if they stayed. In

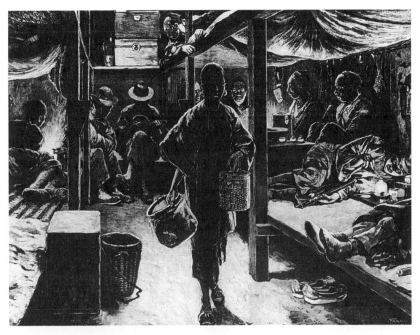

This representation of a turn of the century "opium den" in New York does not exist today, but opium smuggling and smoking are on the rise in the United States.
Courtesy of the National Library of Medicine, Bethesda

response, they increased their presence in other countries and tried to expand their markets and the number of users. This expansion has also led to a large increase in Asian gangs' involvement with heroin trafficking in the United States. These Asian gangs reportedly try to disguise some of their "China white" as "Mexican brown" or "tar," so the authorities won't be as alarmed about their increased presence in the United States.

"Shooting gets to you quicker. You feel it faster, right away in maybe 5—10 seconds. Snorting it, you have to snort more, and then you have to wait to take it in your system. It might take you 10—15 minutes to get loaded. You get sick, your nose runs uncontrollably, and you get stomach cramps." Recovering heroin user

The Asian gangs and the Mafia have also increased the importation of cheaper smokable heroin to encourage many young users to try it in their pipes in order to create a new market, in much the same way that the availability of smokable "crack" cocaine expanded the number of cocaine users. At the present time, injection is the preferred means of abusing heroin in the West, although in most Asian and Middle Eastern countries, it is smoked. Occasionally, it is snorted. Heroin can be smoked in a water pipe or bong. It can be mixed in a regular cigarette or marijuana joint or be heated on foil and the smoke inhaled. This last method is known as "chasing the dragon."

"If anybody has the delusion that smoking's all that much different than shooting heroin, they're in for a big surprise. It's just as easy to get addicted smoking heroin as it is shooting heroin." Heroin smoker

Alarmingly, a number of South American illicit cocaine suppliers have recently begun to grow opium poppies (in addition to their fields of coca shrubs) in an effort to cash in on the growing heroin market.

CODEINE

"For me, codeine is just weak heroin. It doesn't do much for me. Codeine just stops the pain and stops your nose from running. It just gets you able to function enough in order to go get you some heroin."
Recovering heroin user

Codeine is extracted directly from opium or refined from morphine. It is not nearly as strong as morphine and so is generally used for the relief of moderate pain (the most common prescription drugs with codeine are aspirin or Tylenol®) or to control severe coughs (Robitussin AC®, Cheracol®). It is also one of the most widely abused prescription drugs. One of the problems with codeine, as with many opioids, is that it triggers nausea. For this reason, in recent years, many physicians have been prescribing hydrocodone (Vicodin®) for moderate pain because it seems to cause less nausea.

Codeine is sometimes abused in combination with Doriden® (glutethimide), a sleeping pill. This combination, known as "loads," "sets," or "set ups," is taken orally and results in a heroin-like high. The combination has a great overdose potential because it depresses respiration and prolongs Doriden®'s toxic effects.

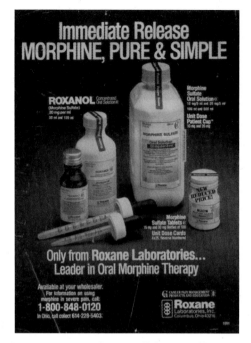

Prescription morphine is still the most effective treatment for acute and severe pain.

MORPHINE

Morphine still remains the standard by which effective pain relief is measured in medicine. Morphine is usually processed from opium into white crystal hypodermic tablets and injectable solutions. This analgesic may be administered orally under the tongue, rectally by suppository, or with a needle into a vein, muscle, or under the skin. From three to six times more morphine must be taken orally to achieve the same effects as an injection. When morphine is used in a hospital setting for pain control, development of addiction is unusual although tissue dependence may develop. In this case, the patient is tapered from the drug to avoid physical withdrawal symptoms.

PROBLEMS WITH OPIOID USE

DILUTION AND ADULTERATION

"The first 'China white' I got came from Vietnam and it looked like a 20 hitter. I know that if I was shooting up, then I probably would have o.d.'d. A 20 hitter means that you could take 1 gram and throw 19 grams of cut on it, and it'd still be good, still get you off. With the 'tar' that's going around now, the most you're going to get is basically a 6 hitter." Vietnam veteran

One of the reasons an overdose occurs is that street drugs can vary radically in strength. Street heroin varies from 0% to 99% pure. So, if a user is expecting 3% heroin and gets 30%, the results could be fatal. Dilution of an expensive item like heroin with a cheap substitute, like powered milk, sugar, baby laxative, aspirin, Ajax®, quinine, or talcum powder is extremely common.

DIRTY AND SHARED NEEDLES

The most dangerous problem with opioids, the one that causes the most illness and death, is dirty or shared needles. Needles are used because they put a large amount of the drug into the bloodstream at one time, but users can also unknowingly inject powdered milk, procaine, Ajax®, or dangerous bacteria and viruses, including the HIV virus that causes AIDS. It is estimated that 50% to 80% of all needle-using heroin addicts in the New York City area carry the HIV virus.

COST

Contrary to popular belief promoted by television and movies, which show heroin addicts as derelicts, criminals, and people who have a mental illness, a majority of heroin users are gainfully employed. However, eventually, a great many users must turn to illegal methods to pay for

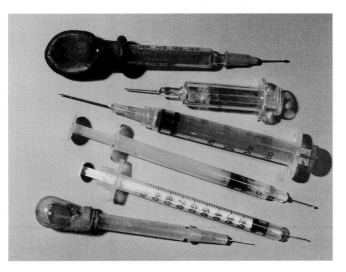

Addicts will use diabetics' syringes, eyedroppers, veterinary needles, and anything else that's handy to inject their heroin or other opioid.

their habits. The cost of a heroin habit can range from $60 to $150 a day depending on the level of use.

"I had two other friends, and one was blackmailing a pharmacist. We'd get outdated drugs they were supposed to throw away. We'd pick them up in the alley and we'd get gallons and gallons of cough syrup and any other narcotics pills."
Ex-heroin user

"Since I worked in the medical field, writing my own prescriptions was no problem except that I committed a felony every time I did it, which was once a week. I never got caught, but I always lived in mortal fear that they would get me."
Recovering Darvon® user

Additional costs to society result from the treatment of HIV infections and other infections contracted through intravenous heroin use.

CRIME

The overwhelming need to support an opioid habit makes antisocial behaviors, such as robbery, prostitution, dealing drugs, and eventual involvement with the legal system, almost inevitable. It is estimated that 60% of the cost of supporting a habit is gotten through consensual crime, such as prostitution and drug dealing, supplemented by welfare payments and occasional work. Some of the remaining 40% comes from shoplifting and burglary.

"As I used drugs more and started putting needles in my arms instead of smoking or sniffing heroin, the friends I associated with became more criminal-like, and they be-

came people who went to jail more often, and I went to jail more often."
Recovering heroin user

POLYDRUG USE

Another danger that comes with the use of opioids is combining them with other drugs. Opioids have additive and synergistic effects when used with most other depressant drugs, such as alcohol and benzodiazepines. These combinations increase the potential for both overdose death and addiction. For example, if another depressant, such as alcohol or a barbiturate, is used at the same time as a shot of heroin or a tablet of codeine, the effects are much greater than one would expect.

"I'd be waiting and waiting, and during the time that I was waiting, I'd be getting drunk. By the time I got around to doing my shot, I was already drunk. I'd hit up and boom, I'd be on the floor." Heroin user

Drug users also combine drugs to enhance the effect of an opioid. In many methadone clinics, addicts use alcohol, Klonopin® (or other sedatives), and even antidepressants like doxepin to enhance the effects of the methadone.

Finally, people use another drug to counter the effects of the opioid. A common opioid combination is the use of cocaine or amphetamine with morphine or heroin. This combination, called a "speedball," utilizes the stimulating effects of the uppers to neutralize the drowsiness experienced from the opioid with an actual enhancement of the pain-killing and euphoric effects.

"As one person said, 'I like going up on 'speed,' and I like taking heroin to

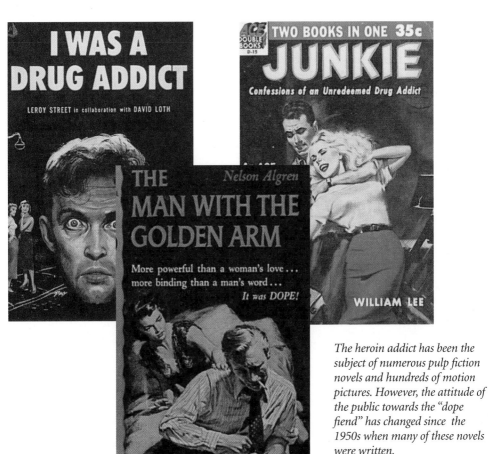

The heroin addict has been the subject of numerous pulp fiction novels and hundreds of motion pictures. However, the attitude of the public towards the "dope fiend" has changed since the 1950s when many of these novels were written.

come down, and I take cocaine to mellow out.'" *Young heroin user*

FROM EXPERIMENTATION TO ADDICTION

Unlike experimentation with alcohol, marijuana, and tobacco which usually begins between the ages of 15 and 17, experimentation with heroin begins about the age of 20. Generally, it takes an average of a year of sporadic use for someone to develop a daily habit, although some users with a predisposition to opioid addiction might jump to daily use within 10 days.

"I'd wake up in the morning and before I'd go to work (when I was working), I'd have to do a hit of dope just to function. I'd have to do a hit of dope just to get out of bed. I'd have to do a hit of dope to go to the bathroom. It wasn't a matter of getting high anymore; it was a matter of getting functional."

Recovering heroin abuser

In addition, the user has to get something from the drug besides just relief from withdrawal symptoms to want to keep returning to the drug. That something could be the rush, a numbing of the emotions, or temporary relief from pain. For example, about 35% of veterans returning from Vietnam had tried heroin, many because of the easy availability of the drug. Half of those who tried it considered themselves addicted to it. However, only one out of eight of those who became addicted stayed addicted to it back home in the United States.

Unfortunately for many users, the onset of tolerance, tissue dependence, and addiction negates many of the benefits that were originally sought. In other cases, the drug works too well.

"After a while, you're not just killing your pain; you start to kill your feelings, any feelings you might have regardless of whether you're having pain. It's not the pain that you're killing. It's never really the pain. It's the feelings that you have."
Recovering heroin abuser

If an opioid user has passed from experimentation to abuse or addiction, treatment becomes a physiological as well as a psychological process. Physically, the addict has to be detoxified from the heroin or other opioid, often with the use of medications, such as Darvon® (a milder opioid than heroin) or naltrexone. Psychologically, the addict has to learn a new way of living.

OTHER OPIOIDS

METHADONE (Dolophine®)

Methadone is the only legally authorized opioid to treat heroin addiction

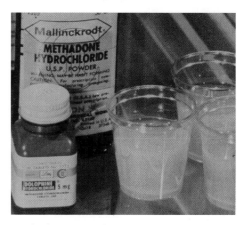

Methadone is mixed with fruit juice, ready to be drunk by heroin addicts at a methadone clinic.

through a program known as methadone maintenance. Under this program, methadone is used as a legally dispensed substitute for heroin. Because this long-acting, synthetic opioid reduces drug craving and blocks withdrawal symptoms for 24 to 72 hours when taken orally, it diminishes the need for heroin, which has a shorter duration of action, causes more intense highs and lows, and is illegal. Like any opioid, methadone also has pain-killing and depressant effects which can be used in clinical situations. The analgesic effects only last 4 to 6 hours. Like heroin, methadone is addicting and must be monitored closely to prevent diversion into illegal uses. Despite heavy regulation of methadone clinics and tight controls of the supply, methadone is still abused and causes a number of overdoses every year. Addicts will combine methadone with other drugs, such as clonazepam (Klonopin®), in order to intensify the high and make it resemble the feeling they get from heroin.

HYDROMORPHONE (Dilaudid®)

A short acting, semisynthetic opioid, hydromorphone, can be taken orally or injected. Hydromorphone is refined from morphine, a process which makes it about eight times more potent and shorter acting than the parent drug. Dilaudid® is used as an alternative to morphine for the treatment of moderate to severe pain. Since it is more potent, it has a higher abuse potential than morphine. Illegally diverted Dilaudid® is becoming increasingly attractive to cocaine users for the drug combination known as a "speedball."

OXYCODONE (Percodan®)

Also used for the relief of pain, oxycodone is most often taken orally, often in combination with aspirin or acetaminophen. By this route, it usually takes about 30 minutes before the effects appear, and these effects last from 4 to 6 hours. Its pain-relieving effect is much stronger than codeine, but weaker than that of morphine or Dilaudid®.

MEPERIDINE (Demerol®)

A short-acting opioid, Demerol® is one of the most widely used analgesics for moderate to severe pain. It is most often injected, though it can be taken orally. Demerol® affects the brain in such a way that it causes more sedation and euphoria than morphine but less constipation and cough suppression. Since it is eliminated by the kidneys, for patients with impaired kidneys, Demerol® should be avoided. Though less potent by weight than morphine, it is often the opioid of choice in the medical community.

PENTAZOCINE (Talwin NX®)

Talwin NX®, prescribed for chronic pain, comes in tablets or as an injectable liquid. Talwin NX® acts as a weak opioid antagonist (a drug that counters the effects of opioids) as well as an opioid agonist (a drug that mimics the effects of opioids). This drug used to be frequently combined and injected with an antihistamine drug ("T's and blues") for the heroin-like high. Increased vigilance and reformulation of Talwin NX® by its manufacturer have almost stopped this problem, although some abusers still take the combination orally or abuse Talwin NX® by itself.

PROPOXYPHENE (Darvon®, Darvocet®, Wygesic®)

Used for the relief of mild to moderate pain, Darvon® is often prescribed by dentists. It is taken orally for moderate pain with the effects lasting four to six hours. Darvon® is occasionally used as an alternative to methadone maintenance and for heroin detoxification, especially for younger addicts, because it has only one-half to two-thirds the potency of codeine. Misuse of this drug makes someone susceptible to overdose or addiction.

"After seven years of doing Darvon®, I started having withdrawals after three to four hours from the last pill that I had taken, so I was addicted to my watch."
Recovering Darvon® abuser

FENTANYL (Sublimaze®)

Fentanyl is the most powerful of the opioids (50 to 100 times as strong as morphine). It is used intravenously during and after surgery for severe pain. It is also available in a skin patch to give steady pain relief for patients with intractable pain. A fentanyl lollipop was introduced in 1994 to be used by children for post operative pain. Unfortunately, fentanyl is popular with some surgical assistants and anesthesiologists due to its availability and strength.

DESIGNER HEROIN

There are street versions of fentanyl (alpha, 3-methyl) and Demerol® (MPPP) manufactured in illegal laboratories. They are extremely potent and can cause drug overdoses and even damage to the nervous system. Sold as "China white," these drugs bear witness to a growing sophistication of street chemists who now can bypass the traditional smuggling and trafficking routes of heroin. Since these "designer drugs" are made without controls on purity or dosage, they represent a tremendous health threat to the opioid-abusing community.

Street fentanyl can be from 100 to 20,000 times stronger than regular heroin. A dose the size of a grain of salt can be powerful enough to kill 30 people. Recently in Baltimore and Vancouver, there were dozens of deaths because of this substitution.

"When I first got out here on the West Coast, I found out that it ['China white'] wasn't white dope at all. It was fentanyl and it wasn't even pharmaceutical fentanyl. It was bathtub fentanyl and people were dying on it." Dealer/heroin user

If improperly made, street Demerol® can contain a chemical, MPTP, which destroys the brain cells that control voluntary muscular movement and mimic the degenerative nerve condition known as Parkinson's Disease. This degeneration causes a condition known as the "frozen addict," when the addict is unable to make any movements.

LAAM
(l-alpha acetyl methadol)

LAAM is another opioid that is still being tested for heroin replacement therapy similar to methadone maintenance. Unlike methadone, its ability to prevent withdrawal symptoms lasts for about three days. In 1993, the U.S. Food and Drug Administration made LAAM available for clinical use.

NALOXONE, NALTREXONE
(Narcan®, Revia®)

Naloxone and naltrexone are opioid antagonists. They block the effects of opioids. Naloxone is effective in treating heroin or opioid overdose, whereas naltrexone is used to prevent relapse and help to break the cycle of addiction. Taking naltrexone daily significantly decreases the effects of heroin or any other opioid. Research is also being conducted on naltrexone's ability to reduce craving in the treatment of alcohol and cocaine addiction as well.

BUPRENORPHINE
(Buprenex®)

Buprenorphine is a powerful opioid agonist at low doses and an opiate antagonist at high doses. In low doses, it is used as an analgesic alternative to morphine. It is being used experimentally in high doses as an alternative to methadone because it limits the supplementary use of heroin or other opiates and opioids by addicts.

SEDATIVE-HYPNOTICS

CLASSIFICATION

More than 150 million prescriptions are written for sedative-hypnotics each year in the United States. These drugs are usually prescribed to diminish the possibility of neurotic reactions in unstable patients, to control anxiety, to induce sleep in chronic insomniacs, and to control hypertension and epilepsy. They are also used as mild tranquilizers and muscle relaxants. The effects of sedative-hypnotics are generally similar to the effects of alcohol (e.g., lowered inhibitions, physical depression,

sedation). The basic difference between the two depressants is the concentration of the drug involved: sedative-hypnotics come in a more concentrated form. Like alcohol, sedative-hypnotic drugs are addictive, and withdrawal symptoms can also be more life-threatening than opioid withdrawal symptoms.

Almost all sedative-hypnotics are available as pills, capsules, or tablets though some, such as Valium® and Ativan®, are used intravenously for instant relief. The two main groups of sedative-hypnotics are benzodiazepines and barbiturates.

. . . .

The market for sedative-hypnotics is in the billions of dollars. Most advertising is directed at physicians who can prescribe these drugs.

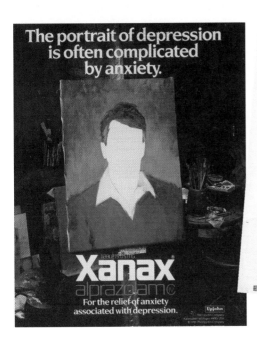

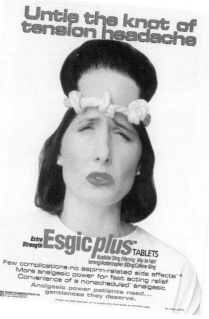

TABLE 4–2 SEDATIVE-HYPNOTICS

Drug Name	Some Trade Names	Street Name
BARBITURATES		
Secobarbital	Seconal®	Reds, red devils, F-40s, seccies, Mexican reds
Pentobarbital	Nembutal®	Yellows, yellow jackets, yellow bullets, nebbies
Equal parts secobarbitol and amylbarbital	Tuinal®	Rainbows, tuies, double trouble
Phenobarbital	(Generic)	Phenos
Amobarbital	Amytal®	Blue heavens, blue dolls, blues
Hexobarbital	Sombulex®	
Thiopental	Pentothal®	
Methohexital		
Butalbital	Esgic®, Fiorinal®	
BENZODIAZEPINES		
Diazepam	Valium®	Vals
Chlordiazepoxide	Librium®, Libritabs®	Libs
Flurazepam	Dalmane®	
Chlorazepate	Tranxene®	
Oxazepam	Serax®	
Triazolam	Halcion®	
Alprazolam	Xanax®	
Lorazepam	Ativan®	
Clonazepam	Klonopin®	
Temazepam	Restoril®	
Halazepam	Paxipam®	
Prazepam	Centrax®	
Flunitrazepam	Rohypnol®	Ruffies, rophies, roofies, rochies
OTHER SEDATIVE-HYPNOTICS		
Methaqualone	Quaalude®, Sope®, Parest®, Optimil®, Somnafac®	Ludes, sopes, soapers, Q
GHB (gammahydroxybutyrate)		Grievous bodily harm
Glutethimide	Doriden®	Goofballs, goofers
Glutethimide & codeine	Doriden® and codeine	Loads, sets, setups, hits, "G & C"
Ethchlovynol	Placidyl®	Green weenies
Chloral hydrate	Noctec®, Somnos®	Jelly beans, Mickeys, knockout drops
Methaprylon	Noludar®	Noodlelars
Meprobamate	Equinil®, Miltown®, Meprotabs®	Mother's little helper

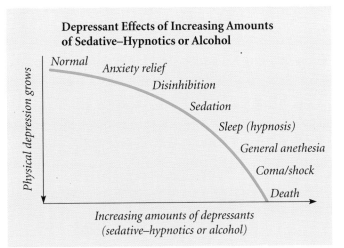

Depressant Effects of Increasing Amounts of Sedative–Hypnotics or Alcohol

Physical depression grows

Normal
Anxiety relief
Disinhibition
Sedation
Sleep (hypnosis)
General anethesia
Coma/shock
Death

Increasing amounts of depressants (sedative–hypnotics or alcohol)

Figure 4-3 •

As this chart shows, sedative-hypnotics can be used to calm, to sedate, or even to anesthetize for surgery. When users self-medicate with sedative-hypnotics and/or alcohol, they often lose track of how much they have used, sometimes with fatal results.

GENERAL EFFECTS

Sedative-hypnotics are quite specific to those sections of the central nervous system they affect. Hypnotics, such as barbiturates, work on the brain stem, inducing sleep along with depression of most body functions, such as breathing and muscular coordination. Sedatives, such as Valium®, Doriden®, Quaalude®, and Miltown®, are calming drugs. They work on a number of sites in the brain and are used as either sleeping aids or as antianxiety agents. Benzodiazepines, for example, act on the neurotransmitter GABA (gama amino butyric acid) to help control anxiety and restlessness. Sedatives are capable of causing relaxation, body heat loss, lowered inhibitions, reduced intensity of physical sensations, and reduced muscular coordination in speech, movement, and manual dexterity. Some sedatives are used as hypnotics, and some hypnotics are used as sedatives, so it is difficult to separate the two functions.

TOLERANCE

Tolerance develops rapidly with sedative-hypnotics. However, tolerance to the mental and physical effects develops at different rates. This difference means that when users increase daily intake to recapture a mental high, they might not be aware that tolerance to the physical effects, such as respiratory depression, develops at a slower rate. Thus, the daily dose taken for the mental effects comes close to the lethal dose for some sedative-hypnotics, particularly the barbiturates, and any accidental overdose can cause respiratory or cardiovascular collapse, killing the user. (This phenomenon is called "selective tolerance.") In time, the intake of sedative-hypnotics might reach 10 to 20 times the original dose.

WITHDRAWAL

After tolerance has developed, withdrawal from sedative-hypnotics can be extremely dangerous. Within six to eight hours after using short-acting drugs (e.g., most barbiturates), users will begin to experience withdrawal symptoms, such as anxiety, agitation, loss of appetite, nausea, vomiting, increased heart rate, excessive sweating, abdominal cramps, and tremulousness. The symptoms tend to peak on the second or third day. With long-acting barbiturates and tranquilizers, such as Valium® or Librium®, the onset of symptoms can be delayed for several days while the peak may not be reached until the second or third week. Severe withdrawal symptoms include seizures, delirium, and uncontrolled heartbeat. These reactions can be fatal.

PREGNANCY PROBLEMS

All sedatives have been associated with a greater incidence of birth defects (e.g., cleft palate syndrome). They can also result in a severe addiction in the fetus when taken by the mother during pregnancy.

OVERDOSING

Symptoms caused by overdosing with sedative-hypnotics, particularly barbiturates, include cold, clammy skin; a weak and rapid pulse; and shallow breathing which can be slow or rapid. Death will follow if the low blood pressure and slowed respiration are not treated. It is particularly dangerous to combine alcohol and any sedative-hypnotic because these combinations can cause an exaggerated depression of the respiratory center in the brain and, therefore, a greater risk of death.

The sedative-hypnotics are commonly involved with both accidental and intentional drug overdose. Actual suicides have decreased with the increased use of benzodiazepines and decreased use of barbiturates and other sedatives since the benzodiazepines have a much greater therapeutic index (the lethal dose of a drug divided by its therapeutic effective dose). However, this margin of safety is lost when benzodiazepines are taken in combination with other sedatives, especially alcohol.

The sedative-hypnotics have additive and synergistic effects with all other de-pressant drugs, antidepressants, and antipsychotic drugs. This means that when used in combination, the effects may simply be the sum of the two effects of the separate drugs or a multiplication of the effects. They may also affect the metabolism of heart medications, blood thinners, and even ulcer medications to either increase or decrease the effectiveness of those agents.

Studies of sedative-hypnotic drug overdose conducted by the *National Institute of Drug Abuse* reveal other factors which contribute to the frequent overdoses seen with these drugs.

- Since sedatives impair memory, awareness, and judgment, individuals fail to realize or forget how many sedatives they have ingested to help them get to sleep or to relieve stress. Rather than waiting long enough for the full dosage of the drug to affect them, they continue to take more of the drug and accidentally reach an overdose state. This effect has been called drug automatism.

- Adolescent attitudes of invulnerability or an unconscious suicidal wish promote risk-taking behavior in respect to the amount of drug ingested.

- Ignorance of additive and synergistic effects resulting from combining these drugs with alcohol or other sedatives is widespread.

- Selective tolerance to some effects of the drug, but not to its toxic effects, results in a narrowing window of safety where the amount needed to produce a high comes closer to the lethal dose of the drug.

In the *Annual Emergency Room Data Survey*, physicians list which drugs cause medical problems severe enough to make people seek medical attention. Table 4–3 shows which drugs are reported most of-

TABLE 4–3 MENTIONS OF DRUG PROBLEMS IN EMERGENCY ROOMS
(In many cases, more than one drug is found in incoming patients)

Drugs	% of Patients Who Tested Positive
1. Alcohol in combination with other drugs	32.6%
2. Cocaine	28.4%
3. Heroin/morphine, codeine, or other opioids	17.3%
4. Acetaminophen, aspirin, ibuprofen	13.9%
5. Benzodiazepines (Xanax®, Valium®, Ativan®, Klonopin®)	10.4%
6. Antidepressants (Elavil®, Prozac®)	8.6%
7. Marijuana	8.6%
8. Methamphetamine/amphetamine	5.1%
9. Antihistamine	1.7%
10. OTC sleeping aids	1.3%

Estimates from the Drug Abuse Warning Network—*1995 Substance Abuse and Mental Health Services Administration*

ten. Alcohol by itself, though probably at the top of the list, is not reported in this survey.

BARBITURATES

Though barbituric acid was first synthesized in 1868, it remained a medical curiosity for 40 years until it was chemically modified to enter the central nervous system, thus becoming psychoactive. Since then, more than 2,500 different barbiturate compounds have been created.

EFFECTS

The slow-acting barbiturates, such as phenobarbital, last 12 to 24 hours and are used mostly as daytime sedatives or as medications to control epileptic seizures.

The shorter-acting compounds, such as Seconal® (reds) and Nembutal® (yellows), last 4 to 6 hours and are used to induce sleep. They can cause pleasant feelings along with the sedation (at least initially), so they are more likely to be abused.

The very short-acting barbiturates, such as Pentothal®, used mostly for anesthesia, can cause immediate unconsciousness. The high potency of these barbiturates makes them extremely dangerous if abused.

Because barbiturates lower inhibitions, they initially seem to have a stimulatory effect, but the drugs eventually become sedating. The effects of alcohol are very similar to the effects of barbiturates. Excessive or long-term use can lead to changes in personality and emotional state, such as mood swings, depression, irritability, and boisterous behavior.

The effects of barbiturates often depend on the mood of the user and the setting

As patents expire on brand name benzodiazepines, such as Xanax®, Valium®, Halcion®, and Klonopin®, other drug companies come out with generic versions: alprazolam, diazepam, triazolam, and clonazepam.

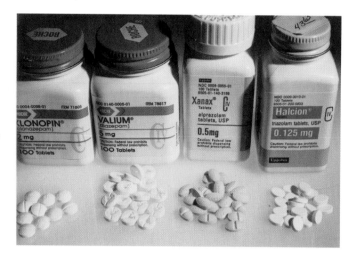

where taken. An agitated barbiturate user might become combative, whereas a tired barbiturate user, in a quiet setting, might go to sleep.

"I'd take Seconals® and they made me feel great. I wouldn't hesitate to say anything; I'd just talk and talk, and sometimes I'd want to fight. It made me very rowdy. But I thought I was on top of the world. I thought I was great, and now when I see other people when they take it, they look like idiots. I guess that's what I was, you know, an idiot." Recovering barbiturate user

Tolerance and Tissue Dependence

Tolerance to barbiturates develops in a variety of ways. The most dramatic tolerance, drug dispositional tolerance, results from the physiologic conversion of liver cells to more efficient cells which metabolize or destroy barbiturates more quickly. This change results in the need to take more barbiturates to reach or maintain the same psychoactive effects originally obtained at lower doses.

"For a long period of time, I would need 3 or 4 Seconals® or Tuinals® to get me straight, just to make me feel normal. And I would take maybe 9 or 10 of them at a time to get high." Recovering barbiturate user

Tissue dependence to barbiturates occurs when 8 to 10 times the normal dose is taken daily for 30 days or more. Withdrawal symptoms resulting from this dependence are very dangerous and can result in convulsions within 12 hours to 1 week from the last dose.

"I'd go into a state of complete unconsciousness, and I'd wake up in the hospital with IVs in me. They'd try to straighten me out, and they would let me go from the hospital, and then I'd do the same thing."
Recovering barbiturate user

BENZODIAZEPINES (Xanax®, Valium®, Halcion®)

Benzodiazepines are the most widely used sedative-hypnotic in the United States.

This class of drugs was developed in the late 1940s and 1950s as an alternative to barbiturates. Starting with Librium®, then Valium®, benzodiazepines came into wide clinical use in the 1960s. By the 1970s, they accounted for more than half of all prescriptions written for sedative-hypnotics. The drugs were considered an innovation in the treatment of anxiety disorders, replacing barbiturates, bromides, opioids, and even alcohol, which were considered too toxic and liable to too many side effects.

"They began to treat my headaches with Valium® because Valium® was 'the wonder drug.' You can't overdose on Valium®. No way you can kill yourself. They were wrong about it." Recovering benzodiazepine abuser

EFFECTS

Benzodiazepines have been shown to exert their sedative effects in the brain by interacting with or acting like a naturally occurring neurotransmitter called GABA. GABA is recognized as the most important inhibitory neurotransmitter. Drugs like diazepam (Valium®) greatly increase the actions of GABA and also influence other sedating neurotransmitters, such as serotonin and dopamine. By increasing the activity of GABA, benzodiazepines increase the inhibition of anxiety-producing thoughts and neural messages.

Several benzodiazepines are used to treat other problems besides anxiety. For example: alprazolam (Xanax®) is used to treat patients subject to panic attacks; triazolam (Halcion®) is used to treat insomnia; diazepam (Valium®) is used to gain relief from skeletal muscle spasms (caused by inflammation of the muscles or joints) or to control seizures, such as those that occur during severe alcohol or barbiturate withdrawal; intravenous Valium® is used as a sedative during some surgeries.

PROBLEMS WITH BENZODIAZEPINES

Benzodiazepines have a fairly safe therapeutic index, meaning that the amount of chemical needed to induce sedation is much lower than the amount that would cause an overdose. Unfortunately, while many health care professionals were hailing the supposedly "safe" new drugs and raving about patient acceptance, they overlooked their peculiarities: the length of time they last in body tissues, their ability to induce addiction at low levels of use, and the severity of withdrawal from the drug.

Benzodiazepines alone can be abused, but they are often abused in conjunction with other drugs. "Speed" and cocaine users often take a benzodiazepine to come down from excess stimulation. Heroin addicts frequently take a benzodiazepine when they can't get their drug of choice, and alcoholics use them to prevent life-threatening withdrawal symptoms, such as convulsions.

Tolerance

Tolerance to benzodiazepines develops as the liver becomes more efficient in processing the drug. However, age-dependent tolerance also occurs with these drugs, meaning that a younger person can tolerate much more of these benzodiazepines than someone older. The effect of a dose on a 50-year-old first-time user can be 5 or 10 times stronger than the same dose on a 16-year-old.

"I started taking Valium® when I went out to parties 'cuz I found that it gives me ... it was the same as drinking. But, liquor gave me headaches, which I was trying to prevent. So I forget when, exactly, it started controlling me. I started taking,

oh, 10 a day, or 5 at a time. Then pretty soon, I'd pop 10 at a time."

Recovering benzodiazepine abuser.

Tissue Dependence

Physical addiction to the benzodiazepine can develop if the patient takes 10 to 20 times the normal dose daily for a couple of months or longer, or takes a normal dose for a year or more. Since many benzodiazepines are slowly deactivated by the body over a period of several days, even low-dose use can lead to addiction when these drugs are taken daily over a number of years. In addition, the pleasant mental effects and "hypnotizing" aspects of the drugs (reinforcement) can result in a mental or psychological dependence.

"If I threw down 10 Valium®, I didn't really feel that much. It wasn't like taking Nembutal® or other barbiturates where you get a real rush. I would have to take an awful lot to feel anything. It relieved certain anxieties; it alleviated depression. You tell the doctor, 'I'm depressed.' 'Okay, take some Valium®.'"

Recovering benzodiazepine abuser

Withdrawal

After high-dose, continuous use for about two months or lower-dose use for a year or more, withdrawal symptoms can be severe. In fact, more people have died from Valium® withdrawal than from Valium® overdoses. The drug is long lasting, so the symptoms are delayed 24 to 72 hours. First, a craving for the drug occurs, followed by more anxiety, sleep disturbances, tremulous movements, and even hallucinations. Some people even allege a temporary loss of vision, hearing, or smell while in withdrawal. The symptoms continue and peak in the first through third weeks. These symptoms can include multiple seizures and convulsions. The severe symptoms will occur in 80% to 90% of the users who stop taking the drug after physical addiction has occurred.

"I stopped taking them and on the third day, I remember, I was sweating. I changed the sheets on the bed. I took a shower. I was fairly relaxed and I went into a convulsion. I don't remember what happened. All I can remember is waking up and all my front teeth were knocked out. I ended up going through about 80 convulsions."

Recovering Valium® abuser

Figure 4-4 •

The delay in the occurrence of withdrawal symptoms can be dangerous to benzodiazepine abusers who stop using abruptly.

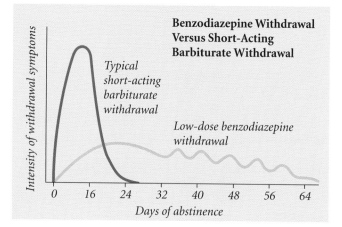

Benzodiazepine Withdrawal Versus Short-Acting Barbiturate Withdrawal

Typical short-acting barbiturate withdrawal

Low-dose benzodiazepine withdrawal

Intensity of withdrawal symptoms

0   16   24   32   40   48   56   64

Days of abstinence

TABLE 4–4   PLASMA HALF-LIFE OF BENZODIAZEPINES
(Length of time various benzodiazepines remain in the body and continue to affect the user)

Chemical (Trade) Name	Half-Life
VERY LONG ACTING	
Flurazepam (Dalmane®)	90–200 hrs.
Halazepam (Paxiapm®)	3–200 hrs.
Prazepam (Centrax®)	30–200 hrs.
INTERMEDIATE ACTING	
Chlordiazepoxide (Librium®)	7–46 hrs.
Diazepam (Valium®)	14–90 hrs.
Clonazepam (Klonopin®)	18–50 hrs.
SHORT ACTING	
Temazepam (Restoril®)	5–20 hrs.
Alprazolam (Xanax®)	6–20 hrs.
Oxazepam (Serax®)	6–24 hrs.
Lorazepam (Ativan®)	9–22 hrs.
VERY SHORT ACTING	
Triazolam (Halcion®)	2–6 hrs.

(Modified from The Journal of Psychoactive Drugs, *15:1–2)*

Overdose

Symptoms of overdose include drowsiness, loss of consciousness, depressed breathing, coma, and death if left untreated; however, it might take 50 or 100 pills to cause a serious overdose. Yet, street versions of the drug, misrepresented and sold as Quaaludes®, are so strong that only 5 or 10 pills can cause severe reactions. The relative safety of benzodiazepines does not extend to mixing them with alcohol or other depressants. People can die from just a few pills and a modest amount of alcohol.

The persistence of benzodiazepines in the body from low or regular doses taken over a long period of time results not only in prolonged withdrawal symptoms but in symptoms that erratically come and go in cycles separated by 2 to 10 days. These symptoms are sometimes bizarre, sometimes life-threatening, and all are complicated by the cyclical nature of the severity. Short-acting barbiturates, on the other hand, follow a fairly predictable course where the symptoms come, and then go, and do not return. Called the protracted withdrawal syndrome, the symptoms of benzodiazepine withdrawal may persist for several months after the drug has been terminated.

OTHER SEDATIVE-HYPNOTICS

METHAQUALONE (Quaaludes®, Mandrax®)

Although widely used at one time as a sleep aid, the heavy abuse of Quaaludes® led to the withdrawal of this product from the legitimate market. This change led to a tremendous increase in the illicit production of Quaaludes®, known as bootleg "ludes," which look identical to the original prescription drug. The active chemical in Quaaludes®, methaqualone, is manufactured by street chemists or smuggled in from Europe, South Africa, or Colombia. In Europe and other countries, Mandrax® (methaqualone and an antihistamine) had great popularity in the 1970s and 1980s. The antihistamine exaggerated the effect of the methaqualone. However, there is no guarantee that the street versions of these drugs contain actual methaqualone, and even when they do, the dosage may vary dramatically, making an overdose more likely. Some street samples analyzed have contained everything from PCP to Benadryl® (an antihistamine) to Valium®. Many of the substitute drugs are more harmful than the Quaalude® itself. The original prescription Quaalude® contained 300 milligrams of the active drug, whereas street "ludes" have contained methaqualone in doses of 0 to 500 milligrams.

The reasons for the popularity of methaqualone are its overall sedative effect and the prolonged period of mild euphoria caused by suppression of inhibitions. This disinhibitory effect is similar to that caused by alcohol.

GHB (gammahydroxybutyrate)

GHB, a metabolite of GABA, an inhibitory neurotransmitter but now synthetically produced, was used as a sleep inducer in the 1960s and 1970s. By the 1990s, this white powder, which is taken orally, had also became popular among body builders because it changed the ratio of muscle to fat. It also induced an effect similar to methaqualone or alcohol intoxication, and so in recent years, it has become popular in "rave" clubs along with other club drugs like LSD, "ecstasy," and Rohypnol®. The side effects are increased dreaming, lack of coordination, nausea, respiratory distress, and occasionally, seizures. The drug was initially available in healthfood stores or by mail order and described as a nutrient rather than a sedative. By the 1990s, the FDA decided there were enough health risks to take it off the market. Street chemists rushed to fill the void.

GLUTETHIMIDE (Doriden®)

Doriden®, a short-acting, nonbarbiturate hypnotic, is used to treat insomnia. Though widely available and somewhat abused in the 1950s, it wasn't until the 1970s and 1980s that Doriden® became popular on the street in a polydrug combination (Doriden® and codeine), variously known as "loads," "sets," "setups," "four by fours," "fours and doors." The effects of this combination are prolonged drowsiness, relaxation, and euphoria over a period of six to eight hours. The combination has led to double addiction to a sedative-hypnotic and an opiate. An additional danger with Doriden® is that the drug is extracted from the blood by the liver, concentrated in the gall bladder, released back into the intestine, and then back into the blood, causing extended, recurring, toxic effects which result in a greater chance of harm.

"'Loads' usually last about 18 hours until you get a habit. Then as long as you don't miss a day, you never get sick. You don't

have to stick them in your arm. Just swallow six pills. They don't leave marks."
Recovering "loads" user

ETHCHLOVYNOL (Placidyl®)

Called "green weenies" on the street, Placidyl® is one of the older sedative-hypnotics. It is still a prescription drug and is subject to limited abuse. Placidyl® is about the equivalent of Doriden® in potency, with similar toxic and addictive effects, but is shorter acting.

MEPROBAMATE (Miltown®, Equinil®)

Meprobamate, popularized in the 1950s, led to the first modern recognition of prescription abuse whereby a legal drug, used by prescription, can lead to addiction. The drug was prescribed excessively and misused in larger than prescribed amounts. It was also the forerunner of a downer cycle dominated by sedative-hypnotics. Miltown® was called "mother's little helper," in part because it was frequently prescribed to young mothers to cope with the stress of raising the baby boomers.

OTHER PROBLEMS WITH DEPRESSANTS

MISUSE AND DIVERSION

As a class, sedative-hypnotic drugs and prescription opioids are frequently misused and diverted to abuse from legitimate prescribing practices. Unfortunately, unscrupulous, addicted, or out-of-date medical professionals also participate in the unethical, criminal, or inappropriate prescribing practices.

Medications from Mexico

Prescription drugs pour into U.S.

By Tim Friend
USA TODAY

Millions of tablets of prescription sedatives, amphetamines and narcotic painkillers are being brought into the U.S. from Mexico, and most appear destined for recreational use or sale on the street, a new study shows.

The 12-month study of U.S. Customs declaration forms suggests serious abuse of federal laws that permit individuals to buy prescription drugs in Mexico and bring them back for personal use, the authors say.

It also suggests U.S. Customs enforcement of controlled substances at the border at Laredo, Texas, is limited.

"It is remarkable what is being brought back across the border," says Marvin Shepherd of the College of Pharmacy at the University of Texas at Austin. "It's a prescription mill down there."

Shepherd set out to determine how many prescription drugs elderly people are buying in Mexico because of the cheaper prices. The study was funded by the National Association of Chain Drug Stores and the Texas Pharmacy Association. They were concerned that unapproved drugs were entering the U.S. and that many elderly were skirting safeguards

The most popular pills

The top 15 drugs declared over a randomly selected 84-day period:

► Valium, anti-anxiety, 928,000 pills.
► Rohypnol, the "date rape" drug banned Wednesday, 338,760 pills.
► Tafil, sedative/hypnotic, 284,130 pills.
► Tenuate Dospan, stimulant, 111,060 pills.
► Asenlix, stimulant, 92,760 pills.
► Diminex, stimulant, 79,140 pills.
► Neopercodan, narcotic analgesic, 42,550 pills.
► Darvon, narcotic analgesic, 37,940 pills.
► Qual, sedative/hypnotic, 20,700 pills.
► Halcion, sedative/hypnotic, 16,470 pills.
► Tylex, narcotic analgesic, 16,230 pills.
► Ativan, anti-anxiety, 15,000 pills.
► Ritalin, stimulant, 13,380 pills.
► Somalgesic, muscle relaxant, 10,890 pills.
► Xanax, anti-anxiety, 7,680 pills.

There is a thriving business across the border in Mexico, where for the cost of a doctor's visit, you can get a prescription for one or more prescription medications. U.S. citizens are allowed to bring back some medications if they say they are for personal use. Other drugs are banned.

One pattern of illicit use with sedatives and/or opioids results when a patient is treated for multiple medical complaints by many different physicians and each prescribes a different sedative or opioid which is then dispensed by different pharmacies. For example, Dalmane® will be prescribed for sleep; Serax® for anxiety; Xanax® for depression; Valium® for muscle spasms; and Librax® for stomach problems. Each prescription, in and of itself, may be at a

U.S. Bans Imports of 'Party' Drug
Strong sedative Rohypnol implicated in date rapes

Reuters

Washington

The United States yesterday banned imports of the powerful sedative Rohypnol — commonly used by teenagers as a party drug — and said it would seize the substance from individuals, in the mail or in commercial shipments.

Considered 10 times stronger than Valium, the compound is being used increasingly by young Americans, especially in Florida and Texas, and has been cited in cases of so-called date rape, where a woman is sexually assaulted by

unit of Roche Holding. It has never been approved for use in the United States.

Food and Drug Administration officials said there is no therapeutic need for the drug in the United States, since many other sedatives are approved and legally available.

Officials in Florida are reported to be investigating cases in which Rohypnol was given to women who were sexually assaulted after the drug had taken effect. It creates a drunk, then sleepy feeling that can last about eight hours. In the past, the drug could be

substance will be confiscated at customs.

The drug has increasingly been brought from Mexico and Colombia and officials said attempts to smuggle it in would treated the same as any other illegal substance, such as cocaine and heroin.

A recently completed Drug Enforcement Agency study found that 101,000 tablets were declared and brought into the country at the border crossing in Laredo, Texas, during a three-week period last July.

"Rohypnol has been called a

The drug Royhypnol® has been called "date rape drug" because, according to anecdotal tales, the inhibition-lowering qualities of the drug make a user more susceptible to rape, and the amnesiac qualities make the crime difficult for the victim to remember.

nonaddictive level, but all these prescriptions combined result in a tissue-dependent dose of benzodiazepines.

"This one doctor, he gave me Nembutal®, Darvon®, a little phenobarbital, Valium®, and Compazine®. I would call the drugstore and get those five drugs, all at one time. And they'd be delivered to my house, free of charge. My medical insurance is paying for them. I mean, luxury, right there."

Recovering sedative-hypnotic abuser

Because of their widespread use for a variety of medical indications, sedative-hypnotics and opioids are also subject to forged prescriptions or prescription manipulations (photocopying or changing dose, amounts, or refills), which provide an abuser with enough drugs for diversion to illicit street sales or to feed an addiction. To

combat this problem, many states have added triplicate prescriptions for benzodiazepines and other stringent mechanisms to prevent diversion, much as they have done for opioids.

Many physicians and psychiatrists see triplicate prescriptions for benzodiazepines as an intrusion in their practice of medicine, whereas many in the chemical dependency treatment community see benzodiazepines as drugs with huge addiction potential or ones which can cause relapse in a recovering addict.

"I couldn't just deal with one pharmacist taking 40 pills a day because they would turn you in to the FDA. They'd turn you in and the doctor would get in trouble, so I had to get several drugstores working for me."

Recovering sedative-hypnotic abuser

Another form of diversion is smuggling drugs which are legal outside the United States. Recently, flunitrazepam (Rohypnol®), a drug which is not sold in the United States, has been illegally making its way into dance and "rave" clubs and into the drug-using community, particularly on the East Coast and in Florida. Flunitrazepam is 10 times more potent, by weight, than Valium® and is short acting (two to three hours). It used to be possible to fill a Rohypnol® prescription in Mexico and then bring it into the United States, but in 1996, the Food and Drug Administration banned all imports of the drug, even if for personal use.

SYNERGISM

If more than one depressant drug is used, the combination can cause a much greater reaction than simply the sum of the effects. One of the reasons for this synergistic effect lies in the chemistry of the liver.

For example, if alcohol and Valium® (diazepam) are taken together, the liver becomes busy metabolizing the alcohol, so the sedative-hypnotic passes through the body at full strength. Alcohol also dissolves the Valium® more readily than stomach fluids, allowing more Valium® to be absorbed rapidly into the body. Valium® exerts its depressant effects on parts of the brain different from those affected by alcohol. Thus, when combined, alcohol and Valium® cause more problems than if they were taken at different times.

Exaggerated respiratory depression is the biggest danger with the use of alcohol and another depressant. That combination also causes more blackouts (a period of amnesia or loss of memory while intoxicated).

"I took my little medication with me one night, drinking in the bar. I played some pool and that's all I remember. This was on a Sunday. When I woke up, it was Wednesday." Recovering polydrug abuser

The synergistic effect causes 4,000 deaths a year. In addition, almost 50,000 people are treated in emergency rooms because of adverse reactions to multiple drug use.

CROSS TOLERANCE AND CROSS DEPENDENCE

Depressant drugs also exhibit cross tolerance and cross dependence between different as well as similar chemical drug classes. Further, some depressants exhibit these characteristics with stimulant, psychedelic, and even with nonpsychoactive drugs.

"I was using a lot of heroin and the heroin wasn't working. I wasn't staying loaded long enough, so I'd make doctors prescribe me barbiturates in order to enhance the heroin." Recovering heroin user

Cross Tolerance

Cross tolerance is the development of tolerance to other drugs by the continued exposure to a drug with similar chemistry. For example, a barbiturate addict who develops a tolerance to a high dose of Seconal® is also tolerant to and can withstand high doses of Nembutal®, phenobarbital, anesthetics, opiates, alcohol, Valium®, and even blood-thinner medication. One explanation of cross tolerance is that many drugs are metabolized or broken down by the same body enzymes. As one continues to take barbiturates, the liver creates more enzymes to rid the body of these toxins. The unusually high levels of these enzymes result in tolerance to all barbiturates as well as other drugs also metabolized by those same enzymes.

Cross Dependence

Cross dependence occurs when an individual becomes addicted or tissue-dependent on one drug, resulting in biochemical and cellular changes that support an addiction to other drugs. A heroin addict, for example, has altered body chemistry such that he or she is also likely to be addicted to an opiate/opioid (Dilaudid®, Demerol®, morphine, codeine, methadone or Darvon®). As in this example, cross dependence most often occurs with different drugs in the same chemical family. A Valium® addict is also tissue-dependent on Librium®, Dalmane®, and Ativan®. A heavy Seconal® user is also tissue-dependent on Nembutal®, Tuinal®, and phenobarbital. Cross dependence has also been documented to some extent with opiates/opioids and alcohol; cocaine and alcohol; and Valium® and alcohol.

CHAPTER SUMMARY

General Classification

1. Downers are central nervous system depressants.

2. The three main groups of downers are opiates/opioids, sedative-hypnotics, and alcohol.

3. Other downers are skeletal muscle relaxants, antihistamines, over-the-counter sedatives, and lookalike sedatives.

OPIATES/OPIOIDS

Classification

4. Opiates (from the opium poppy) and opioids (synthetic versions of opiates) were developed for the treatment of acute pain.

5. Opiates include opium, heroin, codeine, morphine, Dilaudid®, and Percodan®. Opioids include methadone, Darvon®, Demerol®, Talwin®, and fentanyl.

History of Use

6. The change in routes of administration (from ingestion to smoking to snorting to injection), along with refinement and synthesis of stronger opioids (from opium to morphine to heroin to fentanyl), have increased the addiction liability of opioids.

Effects of Opioids

7. Opioids mimic the body's own natural painkillers, endorphins and enkephalins. These analgesic drugs block the transmission of pain messages to the brain by substance "P."

8. Opioids can also cause euphoria, increase nausea, depress respiration and heart rate, depress muscular coordination, and suppress the cough mechanism.

9. A physical tolerance to opioids develops rapidly, increasing the speed with which the body becomes physically dependent on the drug.

10. Withdrawal from opioids is like an extreme case of the flu. People do not usually die from opioid withdrawal although they can die from overdose. However, newborn addicted babies can die from opioid withdrawal.

The Principal Opioids

11. Heroin, morphine, and codeine are the mostly widely used opioids.

12. Heroin can be injected, smoked, or snorted. All three methods of use are very addicting.

13. "China white" heroin from Asia and "Mexican tar" heroin from Mexico are the most widely used in the United States.

14. Codeine is the most abused prescription opioid. A semisynthetic version, hydrocodone, has become a widely used substitute.

15. Morphine, the standard for severe pain relief, can be taken by mouth, by injection, or by suppository.

Problems with Opioid Use

16. Adulteration of drugs, transmission of hepatitis, risk of HIV and other infections through contaminated needles, the high cost of an addiction (up to $200 a day), the dangers of polydrug use, and the high addiction liability of opioids add to the dangers of use.

Other Opioids

17. Methadone is a replacement drug to help addicts avoid the problems of heroin addiction. Other drugs used to treat opioid addiction are LAAM, naloxone, naltrexone, and buprenorphine.

18. A number of synthetic and semisynthetic opioids, such as Dilaudid®, Demerol®, Percodan®, Darvon®, and fentanyl, have made their way to the illicit market. Highly potent synthetic heroin (fentanyl and Demerol® derivatives) have appeared on the street, increasing the danger of overdose.

SEDATIVE-HYPNOTICS

Classification

19. The two main groups of sedative-hypnotics are barbiturates and benzodiazepines.

General Effects

20. Sedative-hypnotics are usually prescribed to control anxiety, induce sleep, relax muscles, and act as mild tranquilizers.

21. Withdrawal from sedative-hypnotics after extended use is dangerous. Overdosing is more common with barbiturates than with benzodiazepines.

22. Tolerance to sedative-hypnotics develops rather quickly.

Barbiturates

23. Barbiturates include Seconal® ("reds"), Nembutal® ("yellows"), Tuinal® ("rainbows"), and phenobarbital.

Benzodiazepines

24. Benzodiazepines include Valium®, Librium®, Xanax®, Halcion® and a dozen more.

25. They work on the inhibitory transmitter GABA as well as serotonin and dopamine.

26. Benzodiazepines can stay in the body for days, even weeks. Withdrawal symptoms can occur many days after ceasing use.

Other Sedative-Hypnotics

27. Nonbarbiturate sedative-hypnotics include Doriden®, Quaaludes®, Miltown®, and Placidyl®.

28. Quaaludes® are only available from illicit sources. The drug causes an overall sedation, mild euphoria, and suppression of inhibitions.

Other Problems with Depressants

29. Hundreds of millions of doses and prescriptions of sedative-hypnotics and prescription opioids are diverted to illicit channels each year.

30. Alcohol and sedative-hypnotics used together can be especially life-threatening. They cause a synergistic (exaggerated) effect which can suppress respiration and heart functions.

31. Cross tolerance and cross dependence occur within the sedative-hypnotic class of drugs and within the opioid class of drugs as well as among sedative-hypnotics, opioids, and alcohol.

Downers:
Alcohol

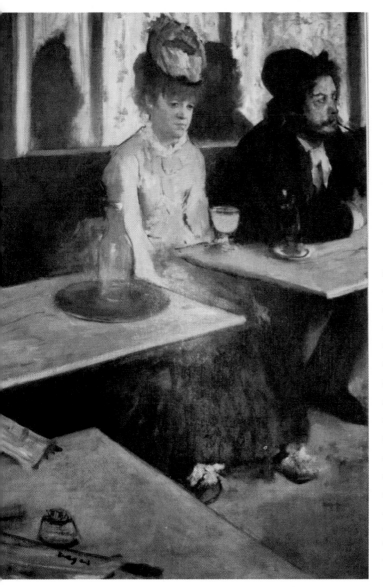

The Absinthe Drinkers by Edgar Degas, 1876. Absinthe, a distilled liquor which is 68% alcohol, was first commercially produced in 1797. It proved so toxic that it was banned in France in 1915 and subsequently by many other countries. Many dissolute artists drank absinthe in the nineteenth century.

Musee D'Orsay, Paris. Photo reprinted, by permission, Simone Garlaund.

- **Overview:** Alcohol is the oldest and most widely used psychoactive drug. It is legal in most countries.

- **Alcoholic Beverages:** Grain alcohol (ethanol) is the main psychoactive component in beer (about 5%), wine (about 12%), and distilled liquor (about 40%).

- **Absorption and Metabolism:** Alcohol is metabolized at a steady rate, mostly by the liver, and it is excreted through urine, sweat, and breath.

- **Effects and Health Consequences:**

  Low-Dose Episodes: If a person is not at risk (e.g., pregnant, in recovery, or with mental or physical health problems) there are some health benefits. In general, sedation, muscle relaxation, and lowered inhibitions accompany low to moderate use.

  High-Dose Episodes: A range of effects occur from decreased alertness and exaggerated emotions up to shock, coma, and death. Effects are directly related to the amount, frequency, and duration of use. They also depend on the tolerance of the user.

  Frequent High-Dose Use: Excessive, chronic drinking causes tolerance and tissue dependence. Withdrawal symptoms can occur upon cessation of drinking. Altered body chemistry can lead to addiction (alcoholism).

  Long-Term Effects: Depending on a drinker's habits and susceptibility, organ damage, particularly liver damage, nutrition deficits, and sexual problems can occur.

- **Other Problems:** One hundred and thirty thousand deaths (e.g., accidents, health problems, suicides, and violence) and 25% of hospital visits are due to alcohol. Alcohol is the leading cause of birth defects.

- **Epidemiology:** Heredity, environment, sex, ethnic group, culture, and age help determine the level of alcohol use from experimentation to addiction. Ten to 12% of drinkers develop problems.

- **Conclusion:** Since alcoholism can take anywhere from 3 months to 30 years to develop, it is important for drinkers to assess their level of use.

Wine industry wants to push health image

The Associated Press

WASHINGTON — American wine makers asked the federal government Monday to let them add a label to their bottles pointing to possible health benefits from wine, in addition to the required one warning of its dangers.

er risk for coronary heart disease in some individuals."

The label would give the address of the National Health Information Center of the Department of Health and Human Services.

Bureau of Alcohol, Tobacco and Firearms officials said they

Scientists Find Clue to Alcoholic Genes

Cocaine-Alcohol Mix And Overdose Deaths

Associated Press

New York

People who drink alcohol while using cocaine create a third brain-targeting substance that may help boost their euphoria and may contribute to a form of overdose death, researchers say.

meeting of the Society for science in St. Louis.

Scientists found that c lene affects a brain-cell c cation system thought to the euphoria that leads t addiction, she said.

La. becomes only state where 18 is drinking age

The Associated Press

NEW ORLEANS — Load 'em up, bartenders: Louisiana's drinking age fell back down to 18 Friday when the state Supreme Court struck down laws making it illegal for people under 21 to buy or consume alcohol.

one 18-to-20 to buy or drink liquor, but it was legal to sell it to them.

After 10 years of lobbying by organizations such as Mothers Against Drunk Driving, lawmakers voted last August by include criminal penalties for the sale of alcohol to 18-, 19- and 20-year-olds.

OVERVIEW

EARLY USE

The mists of prehistory cloak our ancient ancestors' discovery of alcohol. Perhaps it was first found by accident when a bunch of grapes or a basket of plums was left standing in a warm place, allowing the fruit sugar to ferment into alcohol. Perhaps some wild fermented honey was found, diluted with water, and sampled. (The drink would later be called "mead.") Early people enjoyed the taste, the mood-altering effects, or both. Curiosity was followed by experimentation, and it was discovered that the starch in potatoes, rice, corn, fruit, and grains could also be fermented into alcohol.

Eventually, the desire to have ready access to the pleasurable effects of drinking led humans to search out alcoholic beverages and later, systematically produce them. In fact, some historians believe that the first civilized settlements were made to ensure a regular supply of grapes for wine, grain and hops for beer, and poppies for opium-based narcotic drugs.

We know that early societies used alcohol around 7000 B.C., about the same time that agriculture developed. Archeologists have found a recipe for beer along with alcohol residues in clay pots in Iran, dating from 5400 to 5000 B.C. Except for Moslem countries, the use of alcohol is documented in all civilized societies throughout history, in myths, religions, rituals, stories, hieroglyphs, sacred writings, songs, or in commercial records written on papyrus scrolls or clay tablets. The Babylonian *Epic of Gilgamesh* says wine grapes were given to the earth as a memorial to fallen gods. The *Bible* makes reference to wine more than 150 times.

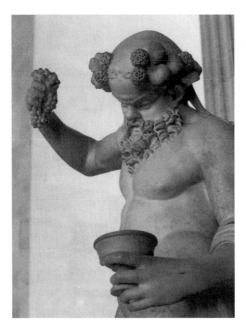

Bacchus, also called Dionysus, was the ancient Greek god of wine and ecstasy. The worship of Dionysus flourished for a long time in Asia Minor by followers called Bacchants. Lodges of Bacchus were suppressed throughout Italy in 186 B.C.

Louvre Museum, Paris. Photo reprinted, by permission, Simone Garlaund.

• •

THE LEGAL DRUG

Because beer, wine, and liquor are so widely available and legal in most societies and are promoted by custom, culture, family traditions, and advertising, many people do not think of alcohol as a drug. Our contemporary society's view of the heavy drinker is more forgiving than its view of a cocaine, heroin, or LSD user. The contradictions surrounding alcohol's accepted place in society and the disfavor in which most other psychoactive drugs are held are not lost on the younger generation.

"Alcohol is heavily social. So one of the problems that I have with prohibition attitudes

is that society drinks as much as we do. And, because it is legal, I feel I am still part of society even when loaded, whereas with illicit drugs like marijuana, I feel I am stepping outside of what is acceptable."
19-year-old college freshman

Although it is legal and widely available, alcohol is nonetheless a powerful psychoactive drug and is classified as a central nervous system depressant. In small doses, it relaxes, sedates, and reduces inhibitions. In moderate doses, even over long periods of time, it continues to relax, sedate, and lower inhibitions in nonsusceptible people. It is, however, a toxin or poison. In large enough doses, a drinker can be killed by acute alcohol poisoning, although a person usually passes out before drinking enough to die.

"I took my 16-year-old brother to a college victory party with my teammates. Three hours later, my friend told me my brother had passed out. We called 911 and they told me at the emergency room they had never seen someone with that high a blood alcohol content who had still lived. He had been drinking straight vodka from a paper cup."
College senior

Taken regularly in large doses over time, alcohol can result in grave physical, psychological, and social problems, including addiction.

ALCOHOLIC BEVERAGES
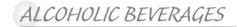

THE CHEMISTRY OF ALCOHOL

Grain alcohol, also called ethyl alcohol (ethanol), is the psychoactive component in alcoholic beverages. There are hundreds

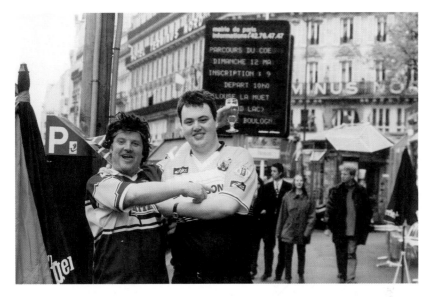

Alcohol is a legal drug in most countries. The preference for beer, wine, or distilled liquors depends on the country's culture, on the availability of certain kinds of beverages, and on the specific occasion. These soccer fans are consoling themselves after their team's defeat. If they had won, they would probably be drinking to celebrate their victory.
Photo reprinted, by permission, Simone Garlaund.

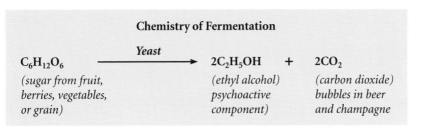

Chemistry of Fermentation

$$C_6H_{12}O_6 \xrightarrow{\text{Yeast}} 2C_2H_5OH + 2CO_2$$

| (sugar from fruit, berries, vegetables, or grain) | (ethyl alcohol) psychoactive component) | (carbon dioxide) bubbles in beer and champagne |

Figure 5-1 •

Yeast feeds on sugar and excretes alcohol and carbon dioxide.

of different alcohols. Some of the more familiar ones include rubbing alcohol, wood alcohol (a toxic industrial solvent), menthol (a flavoring and fragrance base), and ethylene glycol (antifreeze). Grain alcohol is the most intoxicating and the least toxic of the alcohols. Few people drink pure grain alcohol because it is too strong and fiery tasting. By convention, any beverage with a grain alcohol content greater than 2% is considered an alcoholic beverage.

In addition to ethyl alcohol, alcoholic beverages also include trace amounts of other alcohols, such as amyl, butyl, propyl, and methyl, that result from the production process and storage (in wooden barrels, for instance). These organic alcohols, plus other components produced during fermentation, are called congeners. They contribute to the distinctive taste and aroma of beverages. Beer and vodka have a relatively low concentration of congeners; aged whiskies and brandy, a relatively high concentration. It is thought that congeners may contribute to the severity of hangovers, though it is clear that the main culprit is ethyl alcohol.

Alcohol occurs in nature when airborne yeast feeds on the sugars in honey and any watery mishmash of overripe fruit, berries, vegetables, or grain. It then excretes ethyl alcohol and carbon dioxide. Elephants, bears, and deer, as well as birds and insects, have been observed to be intoxicated and exhibit unsteady and erratic behavior after eating fermented mixtures.

TYPES OF ALCOHOLIC BEVERAGES

The principle categories of alcoholic beverages are beer, wine, and distilled spirits. When fruits ferment, the product is wine. When grains ferment, beer is produced. Spirits can be distilled from fermented barley (whiskey), wine, or various other beverages with different alcohol concentrations. Many local drinks exist, including pulque, made from cactus; the Russian drink kvass, made from cereal or bread; the Asian drink kumiss, made from mare's milk; and even a wine made from garlic.

Beer

Beer is produced by adding malt and a sprouted grain, usually barley, that is then roasted and combined with a mixture of water, grain, hops, and yeast. Beer and bread seem to have been invented in the Mesopotamian cultures about the same time. The Mesopotamians taught the Greeks how to brew beer, and Europe learned from the Greeks.

Traditional home-brewed beers were dark and full of sediment, minerals, vitamins, especially B vitamins, and amino acids, and thus had appreciable food value, unlike modern beers which are highly filtered. Varieties of beer such as malt liquor, bock beer, ale, ice beer, and lager generally have more calories and a 1–3% higher alcohol content.

Wine

In some cultures, beer was the alcoholic beverage of the common people and wine was the drink of the priests and nobles, probably because vineyards were more difficult to establish and cultivate, making wine more costly. Wines are made generally from grapes, though some are made from berries or fruit, such as peach or plum wine. (Japanese saké is made from rice.) Grapes are crushed to extract their juices. Either the grapes contain their own yeast or yeast is added and fermentation begins. The kind of wine produced depends on the variety of grape used, the quality of the soil, the ripeness of the grapes, the climate and weather, and the balance between acidity and sugar.

The color and flavor of a particular wine further depend on how long the fermenting liquid is in contact with the grape skins. Red wines are left in contact with skins longer, increasing the amount of tannin in the wine. (Some people are allergic to red wines because of their high tannin and histamine content.) White wines are typically aged from 6 to 12 months and red, from 2 to 4 years. Once bottled, wines continue to age and to improve in taste.

European wines contain from 8–12% alcohol, whereas U.S. wines have a 12–14% alcohol content. Wines with higher than 14% alcohol content are called fortified wines. They have had spirits like pure alcohol or brandy added during or after fermentation.

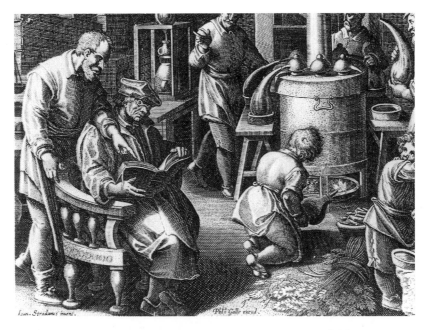

Distillatio *by Philip Galle. Distillation in this sixteenth century Dutch laboratory supplies alcohol for making medicines and for drinking. A clear, colorless, almost 100% pure grain alcohol distillate can be created using this process.*

Courtesy of the National Library of Medicine, Bethesda

Distilled Spirits (liquor)

The alcoholic content of naturally fermented wines is limited to about 14% by volume. At higher levels, the concentration of alcohol becomes too toxic and kills off the fermenting yeast, thus halting the conversion of sugar into alcohol. Drinks with greater than 14% alcohol weren't available until about 800 A.D. when the Arabs invented distillation, which led to the production of distilled spirits, such as brandies, whiskies, vodka, gin, and other liquors.

Brandy is distilled from wine, rum from sugar cane or molasses, vodka from potatoes, whiskey and gin from grains. Distilled spirits can be produced from many other plants including figs and dates in the Middle East, or the agave, yucca, and century plants from which Mexican tequila is made.

One of the results of the invention of distilled beverages is that it became much easier to get drunk. Alcoholism rose in Europe after the introduction of spirits. In England, in the eighteenth century, gin was widely available and cheap. As a result, many poor people suffered during the resulting "London gin epidemic."

Similarly, alcoholism became a major social problem in the early United States with the manufacture of increasing amounts of corn whiskey which was easier and more profitable to transport to market than bushels of corn. Grains and other sugar-producing commodities could be reduced in volume into more potent and higher priced commodities that could be easily transported by wagon or in the holds of ships.

TABLE 5–1 APPROXIMATE PERCENTAGE OF ALCOHOL IN CERTAIN BEVERAGES (by volume)

WINE

Unfortified, natural: red, white, rosé	12%
Fortified, dessert: sherry, port, muscatel	20–21%
Champagne	12%
Vermouth	18%
Wine cooler	6%

BEER

Regular beer	4%
Light beer	4%
Malt liquor	7%
Ale	5%
Ice beer	6%
Low-alcohol beer	2–3%
Nonalcoholic beers (Odoul's®, Sharpe's®)	0.5%

LIQUORS AND WHISKEYS

Bourbon, whiskey, scotch, vodka, gin, brandy, rum	40–50%
Tequila, cognac, Drambui®	40%
Amaretto, Kahlua®	26.5%
Everclear®	95%

(*Note:* To figure the proof of a product, double the alcohol content: e.g., 40% alcohol = 80 proof, 100% alcohol = 200 proof. When a liquid reaches more than 50% alcohol [100 proof], it can be ignited with a match. The match test constituted "proof" of a drink's alcohol content.)

ABSORPTION AND METABOLISM

ABSORPTION

When someone drinks an alcoholic beverage, it is slightly diluted by digestive juices in the mouth and stomach. Because alcohol is readily soluble in water and doesn't need to be digested, it immediately begins to be processed and distributed. Absorption of alcohol into the blood-stream takes place at various sites along the gastrointestinal tract, including the stomach, the small intestines, and the colon.

About 20% of the alcohol is absorbed by the stomach walls through a process of diffusion. About 80% passes into the small intestines where it is absorbed into the bloodstream and is quickly distributed throughout the body. Since alcohol moves easily through capillary walls into surrounding tissues, it can enter any organ or tissue and in the case of pregnancy, can even cross the placental barrier into the fetus. Once it reaches the brain and passes through the blood-brain barrier, psychoactive effects gradually begin to occur.

The highest levels of blood alcohol concentration occur 30–90 minutes after alcohol is drunk. How quickly the effects are felt is determined by the rate of absorption. It is influenced by an individual's weight, body chemistry, and by factors such as emotional state (e.g., fear, stress, fatigue, or anger), state of health, body fat, food taken with the alcohol, and even the outside temperature. Women absorb more alcohol during their premenstrual period than at other times.

Other factors that speed absorption and cause a faster high are

- increasing either the amount drunk or the drinking rate;

- drinking on an empty stomach;

- high alcohol concentrations in drinks, up to a maximum of 40–50%;

- carbonation in drinks, such as champagne, sparkling wines, soft drinks, and tonic mixers;

- warming the alcohol (e.g., hot toddies, hot saké).

Factors that slow absorption and cause a slower high are

- eating before or while drinking (especially meat, milk, cheese, and fatty foods);

- nonalcoholic chemicals in drinks, especially beer and wine, versus spirits such as gin and vodka;

- drinks diluted with ice, water, or fruit juice which lower the amount of alcohol available for absorption.

METABOLISM

Because the body treats alcohol as a toxin or poison, as soon as alcohol is ingested, the body begins to eliminate it from

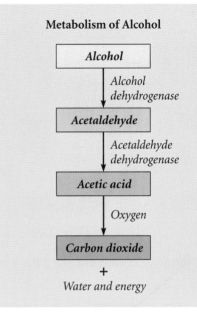

Metabolism of Alcohol

Alcohol

Alcohol dehydrogenase

↓

Acetaldehyde

Acetaldehyde dehydrogenase

↓

Acetic acid

Oxygen

↓

Carbon dioxide

+

Water and energy

Figure 5-2 •

Metabolism is accomplished in several stages involving oxidation. First, the enzyme alcohol dehydrogenase, found in the stomach and the liver, acts on the ethyl alcohol (C_2H_5OH) to form acetaldehyde (CH_3CHO), a highly toxic substance. Acetaldehyde is then quickly acted on by a second enzyme, acetaldehyde dehydrogenase, which oxidizes it into acetic acid (CH_3COOH). Acetic acid is then converted to carbon dioxide (CO_2) and water (H_2O).

the system, directly by exhalation and excretion and chemically through metabolism (oxidation) and excretion.

Approximately 2–10% of the alcohol is eliminated directly. A small amount is exhaled via the lungs while additional amounts are excreted through sweat, saliva, and urine. The remaining 90–98% of alcohol is eliminated by chemical change through metabolism and then by excretion through the kidneys and lungs.

In men, 20% of the alcohol drunk is metabolized in the stomach and the remaining 80% in other organs, principally the liver. In women, almost no alcohol is

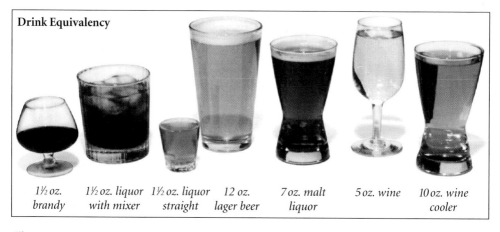

Drink Equivalency

| 1½ oz. brandy | 1½ oz. liquor with mixer | 1½ oz. liquor straight | 12 oz. lager beer | 7 oz. malt liquor | 5 oz. wine | 10 oz. wine cooler |

Figure 5-3 •

One drink is defined as: 1 1/2 oz. brandy, 1 1/2 oz. liquor w/wo mixer, 12 oz. lager beer, 7 oz. malt liquor, 5 oz. wine, 10 oz. wine cooler.

metabolized in the stomach. Given the same body weight, women and men differ in their processing of alcohol. Because women in general have a greater ratio of fat to muscle than men and because muscle contains more blood than fat, women's blood alcohol concentration is higher than men's after the same number of drinks. A woman who weighs the same as a man and drinks the same number of drinks as a man absorbs about 30% more alcohol and feels its psychoactive effects faster and more intensely. Other drugs, such as aspirin, also inhibit metabolism of alcohol and lead to higher blood alcohol concentration.

Weight gain can accompany drinking since the body stores food as fat while it is busy oxidizing alcohol calories. Alcohol provides quick energy and gives the stomach a full feeling. Consequently, another impact of drinking can be a failure to eat enough, leading to malnutrition.

BLOOD ALCOHOL CONTENT (BAC) ✻

Though absorption of alcohol is quite variable, metabolism occurs at a defined

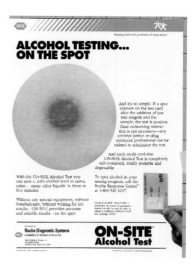

Various modes of detecting alcohol, either exhaled or excreted, have been developed in order to determine a person's degree of intoxication, particularly if caught driving under the influence (DUI). Breath samples can be analyzed by a device such as the Breathalyzer®, or urine and saliva can be tested with a device such as this On-Site® Alcohol Test.

TABLE 5–2 APPROXIMATE BLOOD ALCOHOL CONCENTRATION FOR DIFFERENT BODY WEIGHTS

No. of Drinks	1	2	3	4	5	6	7	8	9	10
MALE										
100 lbs.	.043	.087	.130	.174	.217	.261	.304	.348	.391	.435
125 lbs.	.034	.069	.103	.139	.173	.209	.242	.287	.312	.346
150 lbs.	.029	.058	.087	.116	.145	.174	.203	.232	.261	.290
175 lbs.	.025	.050	.075	.100	.125	.150	.175	.200	.225	.250
200 lbs.	.022	.043	.065	.087	.108	.130	.152	.174	.195	.217
225 lbs.	.019	.039	.058	.078	.097	.117	.136	.156	.175	.195
250 lbs.	.017	.035	.052	.070	.087	.105	.122	.139	.156	.173
FEMALE										
100 lbs.	.050	.101	.152	.203	.253	.304	.355	.406	.456	.507
125 lbs.	.040	.080	.120	.162	.202	.244	.282	.324	.364	.404
150 lbs.	.034	.068	.101	.135	.169	.203	.237	.271	.304	.338
175 lbs.	.029	.058	.087	.117	.146	.175	.204	.233	.262	.292
200 lbs.	.026	.050	.076	.101	.126	.152	.177	.203	.227	.253

If a person drinks over a period of time, use the following table to factor in the time.

TIME TABLE FACTOR

Hours since first drink	1	2	3	4	5
Subtract from BAC	.015	.030	.045	.060	.075

continuous rate. Thus, we can usually predict the amount of alcohol that will be circulating through the body and brain, and how long it will take to be metabolized by the liver and eliminated via urination, sweating, and breathing. However, each person's actual reaction and level of impairment can vary widely, depending on drinking history, behavioral tolerance, and a dozen other factors. It takes about 15 to 20 minutes for alcohol to reach the brain via the blood and cause impairment, but more time for it to enter the urine.

This blood alcohol concentration table (Table 5-2) measures the concentration of alcohol in a drinker's blood. In most states, legal intoxication is .08 or .10. Some think it should be .05 for safety. In general, alcohol is metabolized at the rate of 1/4 to 1/3 oz. per hour.

For example, if a 175 lb. male has 5 drinks in 2 hours, his blood alcohol would be .125 minus the time table factor of .030, so his blood alcohol would be .095, and he would be legally drunk in many states. If his 125 lb. female companion has 5 drinks in 2 hours, her blood alcohol level would be .202 minus the time table factor of .030 or .172, and she would be quite a bit more intoxicated than her companion.

EFFECTS AND HEALTH CONSEQUENCES

There are no conclusive studies that drinking small amounts of alcohol, even over an extended period, has negative health consequences. Nor are there conclusive indications that infrequent, mild intoxication episodes have lasting adverse health consequences for most people. While this statement may be physiologically correct, because of alcohol's disinhibiting effect, intoxication episodes can unfortunately result in unwanted pregnancies, automobile crashes, legal problems, and sexually transmitted diseases (STDs), including HIV/AIDS, from high-risk sexual activity brought on by disinhibition.

Even low-level alcohol use is probably not safe for people who

- are pregnant;
- have certain preexisting physical or mental health problems;
- are allergic to alcohol, nitrosamines, or other congeners and additives;
- have a high genetic/environmental susceptibility to addiction;
- have had abuse and addiction problems with alcohol or other drugs in the past.

Severe effects and both short- and long-term health and social consequences usually result from high-dose use episodes and even more pathological effects are experienced with frequent high-dose use episodes.

LOW-DOSE EPISODES

Physical Effects

Health Benefits. Some people who drink alcoholic beverages think that they taste good and quench the thirst. Consumed in low doses before meals, alcoholic beverages activate gastric juices, improve stomach motility, and stimulate the appetite. After a drink of alcohol, the pulse rate increases and blood vessels dilate, causing increased heat loss from the body.

Because alcohol dilates the blood vessels, moderate drinking (one drink a day for women, two drinks a day for men) has been related to a decrease in heart disease. Another reason for this effect is that alcohol causes a small reduction in fat levels and an increase in good cholesterol.

The doses must be low enough not to cause liver damage or other adverse health effects or to trigger heavier drinking. Of course, any beneficial effects may also be obtained through exercise, low-fat diets, stress reduction techniques, and an aspirin a day.

Sexual Effects. More than any other psychoactive drug, alcohol has insinuated itself in the lore, culture, and mythology of sexual and romantic behavior: a cocktail before sex, beer swilled before a hot date, or champagne to celebrate an anniversary. Alcohol's physical effects on sexual functioning are closely related to blood alcohol levels. In low doses, alcohol usually increases desire in males and females, usually heightening the intensity of orgasm in females and slightly decreasing erectile ability and delaying ejaculation in males.

Psychological Effects

The physical effects of alcohol, as with many psychoactive drugs, are dependent on the amount and frequency of dosage, but the mental and emotional effects are more "conditioned" by the setting in which the drug is used and the mood of the user. In general, alcohol affects people psychologically, at first by increasing self-confidence and promoting sociability. It calms and relaxes, sedates and reduces tension. But for someone who is already lonely, depressed, or suicidal, the depressant effects of alcohol can deepen these emotions. For some drinkers, alcohol may trigger sociability and talkativeness, for others, verbal or physical aggressiveness or violence.

"When I sit down and have a drink, the drink does for me what I want it to. If I'm hyper, it calms me down. If I'm a little in the dregs of life, it picks me up. When I'm having a drink, I don't think that I'm having a drug. That's never crossed my mind."
42-year-old "social" drinker

Disinhibition

Disinhibition is caused by alcohol's action on the higher centers of the brain's cortex, particularly that part of the brain which controls reasoning and judgment. It then acts on the lower centers of the limbic system that rule mood and emotion.

Alcohol's psychological effects stem from the drug's interaction with the brain's neurotransmitters, particularly metenkephalin (which can reduce pain), serotonin (lack of which causes depression and excess of which causes anxiety), dopamine (which can give a surge of pleasure), and gamma amino butyric acid (GABA). GABA is the major inhibitory neurotransmitter in the brain, so, by potentiating the effects of GABA, alcohol lowers inhibitions.

"Drinking is a way of life here. Somebody comes up and you offer them a drink; it's cordial. That's how you break the ice. I like to drink; it makes me happy."
"Social" drinker

HIGH-DOSE EPISODES

Physical Effects of Intoxication

Intoxication is a combination of both psychological mood, expectation, and past experience with drinking as well as the physiological changes caused by elevated blood alcohol levels. In most states, a person is legally intoxicated when BAC reaches a level of .10. But the effects of legal intoxication can be at least partially masked by experienced drinkers. Experiments have indicated that there is a so-called "expectancy effect," such that someone who has not consumed alcoholic beverages, but thinks he or she has, can exhibit signs of intoxication.

However, after enough drinks are consumed, expectation, setting, and the mood of the drinker cease to have determining effects, and the depressant effects of the drug take over. As more alcohol is drunk, blood pressure is lowered, motor reflexes are slowed, digestion becomes poor, body heat is lost, and sexual performance is diminished. In fact, every system in the body is affected. Slurred speech, staggering, loss of balance, and mental confusion are all signs of an increased state of intoxication.

Alcohol Poisoning (overdose)

If truly large amounts of alcohol are drunk too quickly, severe alcohol poisoning occurs, and depression of the various systems can lead to unconsciousness (passing out), coma, and death. Some clinicians use a BAC level of 0.4 as the threshold for alcohol poisoning.

However, even blood alcohol concentration levels of 0.2 or greater can result in severely depressed respiration and vomiting while semiconscious. The vomit can be aspirated or swallowed, blocking air passages to the lung, resulting in asphyxiation and death.

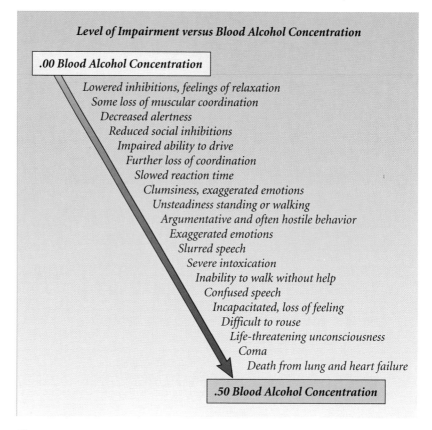

Figure 5-4 •

The actual level of impairment due to a rising blood alcohol concentration (BAC) varies widely from person to person.

Mental and Emotional Effects

Alcohol depresses and slows other functions of the central and the peripheral nervous systems. Initial relaxation and lowered inhibitions at low doses often become mental confusion, mood swings, loss of judgment, and emotional turbulence at higher doses. At a BAC of .05, the thinking and judgment of a drinker become impaired. At a BAC concentration of .10, the level designating legal intoxication in most states, a drinker may demonstrate slurred speech, and beyond that level, progressive mental confusion and loss of emotional

control. Heavy alcohol consumption before sleep may also interfere with the REM (rapid eye movement) or dreaming sleep essential to feeling fully rested. Chronic alcoholics may suffer from fatigue during the day and insomnia at night, as well as nightmares, bed wetting, and snoring.

Hangover

Hangover, a withdrawal syndrome, is the body's response to excessive amounts of alcohol. The effects of a hangover can be most severe many hours after alcohol has been completely eliminated from the system. Typical effects include nausea, vomiting, headache, thirst, dizziness, sensitivity to light and noise, dry, cottony mouth, inability to concentrate, and a generally depressed feeling.

The causes of hangover are not clearly understood. Additives (congeners) in a drink are thought to be partly responsible, although even pure alcohol can cause hangovers. Irritation of the stomach lining by alcohol may contribute to intestinal disorders. Low blood sugar, dehydration, and tissue degradation may also play their parts. Symptoms vary according to individuals, but it is evident that the greater the quantity of alcohol consumed, the more severe the aftereffects.

Sobering Up

A person can control the amount of alcohol in the blood by controlling the amount drunk and the rate at which it is drunk. But the elimination of alcohol from the system is a constant. As was mentioned earlier, the body metabolizes alcohol at about 1/4–1/3 oz. per hour. Until the alcohol has been eliminated and until hormonal, enzymatic, and other systems come into equilibrium, hangover symptoms will persist. An analgesic may lessen the headache pain and fruit juice may help hydrate the body and correct low blood sugar. But neither coffee, exercise, nor a cold shower cures a hangover. Feeling better comes only with rest and enough time for the bodily systems to come back into equilibrium.

FREQUENT HIGH-DOSE USE

Alcoholism

For about 10–12% of the 2/3 of adults in the United States who drink, the use of alcohol has become an addiction. The inci-

dence of alcoholism in men is approximately two to three times greater than in women (14% of male drinkers versus 6% of female drinkers). In addition, onset of alcoholism occurs at a younger age in men. These observations may be misleading, however, in that women are more apt to conceal their alcoholism than men.

"Well, I had an alcoholic father, and I had, as a result of that, a very healthy fear of alcohol all my life, and even do to this day. My father was a Jekyll and Hyde. I really avoided alcohol or treated it with great fear, and that's why I find it hard to believe, even now, that I got so involved in alcohol."
43-year-old recovering alcoholic and cocaine addict

As was discussed in Chapter 2, addiction to alcohol may occur from a genetic predisposition, from the influences of family, workplace, school, community, or other environmental influences, or from the action of the drug itself which can alter the body's neurochemistry and instill craving. Drinkers who become compulsive may have progressed very quickly from experimentation or social drinking to binge drinking and dependence, or it might take decades. As the dependency progresses, both the frequency of their drinking episodes and the amount drunk during each episode increases. For some, it is no longer a matter of simply feeling more comfortable in social situations.

"You can think and say a lot of things that are crass or disgusting or rude when you are drunk. I don't think there is an editing process going on. It's not that you wouldn't have wanted to do some of those things when you were sober, you just wouldn't have gone and done them."
20-year-old college student

For others, drinking is done in solitary settings to overcome boredom or for consolation. Drinking is not done as part of other activities. It becomes an end in itself.

In 1992, a medical panel from the *American Society of Addiction Medicine* and the *National Council on Alcoholism and Drug Dependence* defined alcoholism as follows:

> "Alcoholism is a primary, chronic disease with genetic, psychosocial, and environmental factors influencing its development and manifestation. The disease is often progressive and fatal. It is characterized by impaired control over drinking, preoccupation with the drug alcohol, use of alcohol despite adverse consequences, and distortions in thinking, most notably denial. Each of these symptoms may be continuous or periodic."

"I don't consider myself an alcoholic. I have five drinks a day—and that's an average. It's always three and sometimes it's a lot more, but it's never interfered with my work. I haven't been to the doctor for 15 years. But, since it's never interfered with my work, I see nothing wrong with sitting down and having a drink."
Avowed "habitual" drinker in denial

Blackouts

Some alcoholics suffer blackouts during heavy drinking bouts. During blackouts, a person is awake and conscious and seems to be acting normally, but afterwards cannot recall anything that was said or done. Sometimes even a small amount of alcohol may trigger a blackout. Blackouts, which are caused by an alcohol-induced electrochemical disruption of the brain, are often early indications of alcoholism. They are different from passing out or losing consciousness during a drinking episode, since any drinker can pass out from too much alcohol. A drinker can also have a "brownout" which is a partial recall of events.

Tolerance and Tissue Dependence

As with most depressants, tolerance develops quickly with prolonged use of alcohol. Dispositional tolerance, pharmacodynamic tolerance, and behavioral tolerance are the three ways the body tries to adapt to the effects of alcohol and protect itself.

Dispositional tolerance means the body changes the way it metabolizes alcohol. As a person drinks over a period of time, the liver adapts and changes to create more enzymes to process the protoplasmic poison, alcohol. Unfortunately, since liver cells are also being destroyed by drinking and by the natural aging process, the liver eventually becomes less able to handle the alcohol. A heavy drinker who could handle a fifth of whiskey at the age of 30 can become totally incapacitated by half a pint of wine at the age of 50.

Pharmacodynamic tolerance means brain and body cells become more resistant to the effects of alcohol by increasing the number of receptor sites needed to produce an effect or by just being less responsive to alcohol.

Behavioral tolerance means drinkers learn how to "handle their liquor" by modifying their behavior or by trying to act in such a way that they hope others won't notice they are inebriated.

Withdrawal

A hangover can be a mild withdrawal syndrome after a heavy drinking episode ceases, but with alcoholics, withdrawal can be more serious and can include tremors, sweating, cramps, transitory hallucinations, stomach pains, and, in 10–13% of alcoholics, even seizures or delirium tremens, called DTs.

"I would be more afraid of quitting alcohol than heroin, 'cause with drinking, you go into convulsions and you are really sick. I thought I was going to die from the pain in my stomach; the throwing up, the sweating, and the diarrhea. You don't have any energy, and you know if you just took a drink you'd feel better. And with heroin, you get some muscle cramps and you throw up and you get a little diarrhea, but you're not going to get convulsions. You're not going to die. You can die from kicking alcohol."
Recovering alcohol/heroin abuser

DTs usually begin within a few hours after the last drink in a period of long, heavy drinking and can last for 3 to 10 days. Symptoms include trembling over the whole body or seizures, auditory, visual, and tactile hallucinations, disorientation, and insomnia. DTs is a serious condition requiring hospitalization. Untreated, the mortality rate ranges from 10% to 20%.

Since the main symptoms of severe withdrawal can combine with medical complications, such as malnutrition, pneumonia, depressed respiration, liver problems, or physical damage, medical care for a compulsive drinker or alcoholic needs to be a consideration in any course of treatment.

LONG-TERM EFFECTS

Organ Damage

Liver. Accumulation of fatty acids in the liver, a condition called "fatty liver," can begin to occur after just a few days of heavy drinking, but it is also a preliminary sign of more serious liver diseases. These include necrosis, hepatitis, and, the most serious disease, cirrhosis of the liver. Cirrhosis is, in fact, the leading cause of death among alcoholics. When alcohol kills liver cells, the tissues do not regenerate, they scar. This cirrhosis decreases the liver's ability to metabolize alcohol, thus allowing the alcohol to travel to other organs in its most toxic

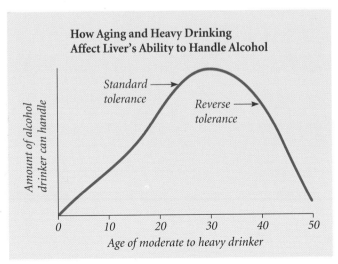

How Aging and Heavy Drinking Affect Liver's Ability to Handle Alcohol

Standard tolerance

Reverse tolerance

Amount of alcohol drinker can handle

0   10   20   30   40   50
Age of moderate to heavy drinker

Figure 5-5 •

This graph shows the decrease in liver capacity to process alcohol as a person ages. As the liver is taxed and poisoned by the alcohol, its capacity is diminished to the point where an older drinker can get tipsy on just one drink.

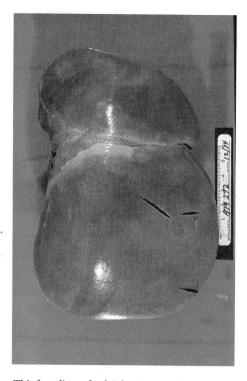

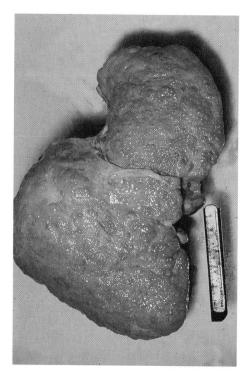

This fatty liver of a drinker is caused by accumulation of fatty acids. When drinking stops, the fat deposits usually disappear.

Both photos courtesy of Boris Ruebner, M.D.

Cirrhosis of the liver takes 10 or more years of steady drinking. The toxic effects of alcohol cause scar tissue to replace healthy tissue. This condition remains permanent, even when drinking stops.

Women's U.S. soccer team advances with 2-0 triumph over Denmark

SPORTS

The Mail Tribune, Friday, June 9, 1995 **1B**

New liver is expected to give Mantle new life

Question of special treatment is raised

Los Angeles Times

DALLAS — Baseball great Mickey Mantle was given an excellent chance for recovery after his diseased liver was replaced Thursday during a 7½-hour transplant operation in Dallas.

"Everything went very, very well," said Dr. Robert Goldstein, the lead surgeon. "He now has an excellent chance for recovery. He's very stable, but still critical."

Goldstein said that Mantle, severely jaundiced and stricken with liver cancer, had to to four weeks to live had he not received a new liver. He said the condition

was caused by a lifetime of heavy drinking and a hepatitis-tainted blood transfusion, possibly decades ago after an athletic injury.

The 63-year-old Mantle, a former New York Yankees center fielder and member of baseball's Hall of Fame, is expected to remain in intensive care for 24 to 48 hours and to be hospitalized for two to three weeks. He entered the hospital May 28 complaining of stomach pains, but his condition worsened to the point that he could neither sit up nor speak at the time of his surgery, Goldstein said.

The drama surrounding Mantle's rapidly deteriorating medical condition and the quick match of a donor liver has rekindled a national debate over the role that celebrity or money plays in organ transplants.

Underscoring the debate were questions raised about Mantle's age and his history of alcoholism and severe medical problems.

Mickey Mantle
Liver functioning

David Mantle
Thankful son

Mantle went on a national waiting list for liver transplants Tuesday, according to Alison Smith of the Southwest Organ Bank, a federally certified nonprofit agency that co-

ordinates organ donations in the Greater Dallas area.

Although the normal waiting period in the transplant program is 130 days, Smith said, patients as critically ill as Mantle, who was classified as Status 2, the second-most urgent status, receive transplants within an average of three days.

The organ bank said that 141 people were waiting for transplants in the Dallas region along with Mantle, but the former ballplayer was the only Status 2-level patient who matched the organ donor in blood type, height and weight.

"When a patient is admitted to the hospital and is suffering as severely as Mr. Mantle, that candidate is given priority because of their extreme need to be transplanted as soon as possible," Smith said. "This is standard practice here and throughout the nation, regardless of age, gender, race or social status."

"His ... condition was worse than any other recipient we had listed from the local area," Smith said. "I'm sure there will be people who refuse to believe there wasn't some special consideration given because of who he is, but that (was) not the case. He was the sickest person with blood Type O in the weight range."

The donor who provided Mantle's liver also donated six other organs to five other people, doctors said. The donor's identity was not revealed and will remain secret unless that person's family and Mantle's family agree to publicize it.

David Mantle, one of the Hall of Fame ballplayer's three remaining sons, said that "later on, down the line, we'd like to meet them. There's always that curiosity, but it will probably take time for them. We lost a brother just over a year ago, so we know it

see MANTLE, Page 5B

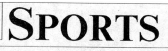

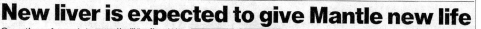

Mickey Mantle's liver failed because of drinking and cancer. He had a liver transplant, but the cancer had spread throughout his body and he died in 1995.

form. Even persistent moderate drinking can begin to damage the liver.

"I would have taken better care of my body if I knew I would live this long."
Mickey Mantle

Heart. Though light drinking can lower the risk of heart disease, chronic heavy drinking is related to a variety of heart diseases, including hypertension or high blood pressure, and cardiac arrhythmias, or abnormal, irregular heart rhythms. One form of irregular heart rhythm is called "holiday heart syndrome" because patients appear in hospitals from Sundays through Tuesdays or around holidays when a large amount of alcohol is consumed.

Brain. Both physical brain damage and impaired mental abilities have been linked to advanced alcoholism. Brain atrophy, loss of brain tissue, has been docu-

mented in alcoholics. Breathing and heart rate irregularities controlled by the brain stem have also been traced to brain atrophy. Dementia, or deterioration of intellectual ability, faulty memory, disorientation, and diminished problem-solving ability are further consequences of prolonged, heavy drinking.

Stomach and Gastrointestinal Tract. Because alcohol stimulates the production of stomach acid and delays the emptying time of the stomach, excessive amounts can cause acid stomach, diarrhea, and peptic ulcers. Gastritis, or stomach inflammation, is common among heavy drinkers, as are inflammation and irritation of the esophagus, pancreas, and small intestine. Serious disorders, such as ulcers and stomach hemorrhage, are also linked to heavy drinking.

Reproductive System. *Female:* Chronic alcohol abuse causes disturbances of the

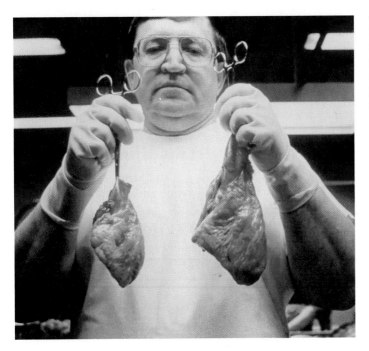

The pathologist compares the heart of a light drinker with the enlarged heart of a heavy drinker.

Reprinted, by permission, George Steinmetz.

menstrual cycle and a greater potential for early menopause. It can cause pathologic changes in the ovaries. Heavy drinking also raises the chances of infertility and spontaneous abortion. After prolonged use, alcohol decreases desire and the intensity of orgasm. In one study of chronic female alcoholics, 36% said they had orgasms less than 5% of the time.

Male: Alcohol abuse impairs gonadal functions and causes a decrease in testosterone (male hormone) levels. Decreased testosterone, in turn, causes an increase in estrogen (a female hormone) which causes male breast enlargement, testicular atrophy, low sperm count, loss of body hair, and loss of sexual desire. About 8% of alcoholics are impotent, and only half can recover sexual function during sobriety. When returning to sexual activity, a recovering alcoholic may experience excessive anxiety, so dysfunction can be intensified by one or two bad performances. Also, alcohol may lead to increased risk-taking behavior, such as unprotected sex or needle sharing, and for those with HIV, a greater risk of lung infections.

Immune System. Excessive drinking has been linked to infectious diseases such as respiratory infections, tuberculosis, pneumonia, and cancer. Heavy drinking may disrupt white blood cells and, in other ways, weaken the immune system, resulting in greater susceptibility to infections.

Nutritional Deficiency Diseases. Alcohol contains calories, about 140 in a 12 oz. beer, but almost no vitamins, minerals, or proteins. Heavy drinkers receive energy, but virtually no nutritional value from their drinking. As a result, alcoholics may suffer from primary malnutrition, including vitamin B_1 deficiency leading to beriberi, heart disease, peripheral nerve degeneration, pellagra, scurvy, and anemia

caused by iron deficiency. In addition, because heavy drinking irritates and inflames the stomach and intestines, alcoholics may suffer from secondary malnutrition (especially from distilled drinks) as a result of faulty digestion and absorption of nutrients, even if they eat a well-balanced diet.

Other Susceptibilities. Alcohol may be a contributing cause to diabetes as well as to cancer of the liver, mouth, throat, and larynx. Chronic drinking can cause atrophied muscle fibers, resulting in flabby muscles. It can also cause weight loss, more so for alcoholic women than alcoholic men.

POLYDRUG ABUSE

Most illicit drug users also drink for a variety of reasons:

- to potentiate or increase the action of a drug (e.g., alcohol with Valium® exaggerates depressant effects);

- to subdue the effects of a stimulant;

- to substitute for another drug they can't get (if heroin supplies are short, the addict will drink to get loaded);

- to stay high (marijuana and alcohol are sometimes used in combination);

- to self-treat withdrawal symptoms from addiction to another drug (alcohol is sometimes used after a methamphetamine or cocaine binge).

Polydrug abuse has become so common that treatment centers have had to learn how to treat simultaneous addictions. Although the emotional roots of addiction are similar no matter what drug is used, the physiological and psychological changes that each drug causes, particularly during withdrawal, often have to be treated differently. For example, if a client of the Haight-Ashbury Detox Clinic has a serious alcohol and benzodiazepine problem, the Clinic

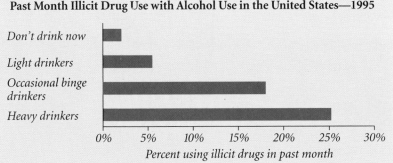

Past Month Illicit Drug Use with Alcohol Use in the United States—1995

Don't drink now

Light drinkers

Occasional binge drinkers

Heavy drinkers

0%   5%   10%   15%   20%   25%   30%

Percent using illicit drugs in past month

Figure 5-6 •

This chart shows that excessive drinking is associated with the use of other illicit drugs. Whether it's the association with other people who drink and use drugs, the lowering of inhibitions that makes other drug use acceptable, or the desire for stronger and stronger experiences, the association is quite clear.

has to be extremely careful detoxifying the client. That is because Librium®, a benzodiazepine, is one of the drugs used to control the symptoms of delirium tremens caused by alcohol withdrawal.

OTHER PROBLEMS

SELF-MEDICATION AND MENTAL PROBLEMS

Often, alcohol is drunk because the person has an existing mental problem or diagnosable disorder such as major depression, schizophrenia, or bipolar illness (manic-depression). The person uses alcohol to try to control the symptoms or to avoid asking for psychiatric help.

"I would pick up some beer to put me out of it. I didn't like the effect that regular psychiatric drugs, such as antidepressants, had on my brain, and I'd rather just put myself out with the booze than face reality."
Patient with major depression and an alcohol problem

Sometimes alcohol is used for other reasons such as overcoming boredom or controlling restlessness, but what happens is that the attempt to self-medicate by drinking takes on a life of its own and creates a new set of problems or aggravates an existing one. For example, a person may use alcohol to escape depression, although chronic alcohol abuse may actually contribute to depression.

"The problems did get worse when I was drinking. That was one reason that I never figured out I was a manic-depressive. I figured I was depressed because I was drunk all the time." Alcoholic with manic-depression

The majority of alcoholics who come into treatment are initially diagnosed as suffering from depression. After detoxification, the figure drops to the 30% to 50% range, still a significant number. In addition, about 1/3 of alcoholics suffer an anxiety disorder.

"The alcohol, that came later on. It intensified my depression and intensified every-

thing. I already felt bad about myself and the alcohol just made it worse. It definitely made it worse."
Recovering 16-year-old alcoholic with major depression.

MORTALITY

Drinking can affect a person's life span. Heavy drinking increases the chances of dying from diseases such as cancer, heart disease, chronic alcoholic liver disease, and cirrhosis. It also increases the chances of dying at a younger age than those who abstain or are light drinkers. For instance, the average life span is shortened 4 years by cancer, 4 years by heart disease, and from 9 to 22 years for alcoholic liver disease. In one study, a difference in life span was found even between abstainers (defined as 12 drinks or less per year) and light drinkers. Another direct link between death and per capita alcohol consumption is with fatal alcohol-related motor vehicle crashes. In one 7-year period, the percentage decrease in fatal crashes paralleled the percentage decrease in per capita consumption. In 1994, alcohol use was implicated in almost half of all fatal traffic crashes.

SERIOUS AND FATAL INJURIES

Alcohol increases the risk of injury in many kinds of human activities. Studies of coroner and medical examiner reports indicate that alcohol was found in approximately 1/2 of the unintentional injury victims and in 35–50% of homicide deaths. Almost 1/4 of suicide victims, 1/3 of homicide victims, and 40% of unintentional injury victims had a BAC over .10, whereas only 20% of those who died from natural causes tested alcohol positive. In one study, 35% of fatalities involving falls and 43% of burn fatalities were linked to alcohol.

Emergency room studies confirm that from 15–25% of emergency room patients tested positive for alcohol or reported alcohol use, with relatively high rates among those involved in fights, assaults, and falls.

Motor Vehicle Accidents

There were relatively high rates of alcohol use for drivers involved in motor vehicle collisions.

- In one study, more than 50% of motor vehicle fatalities indicated alcohol use.

- Projections are that 2 out of every 5 persons in the United States will be in some way involved in an alcohol-related crash during their lifetimes.

- On any weekend night, 3 out of every 100 drivers exceed the legal BAC limit.

- About 40% of first-time DUI offenders and 60% of multiple DUI offenders reported consuming five or more drinks, compared with 10% of the adult male population.

- One in 7 intoxicated drivers involved in a fatal collision had a prior driving-while-intoxicated conviction (DWI), whereas only 1 in 34 sober drivers involved in a fatal collision had a prior DWI conviction.

Suicide

Among adult alcoholics, suicide rates are twice as high as for the general population and from 60 to 120 times greater than the nonmentally ill population, with rates increasing with age. One reason given for increase in suicide with age is that the longer the alcoholism, the more social, health, and interpersonal problems which may increase the risks of suicide. The alcoholic suicide victim is typically white, middle-aged, male, unmarried, and with a long history of drinking. Additional risk factors for suicide include depression, suicidal notes, loss of job, living alone, poor social support, other illnesses, and continual drinking.

TABLE 5–3 SOME ALCOHOL-RELATED CAUSES OF DEATH

DISEASES *(direct causes)*	DISEASES *(indirect causes)*	INJURIES/ADVERSE EFFECTS *(indirect effects)*
Alcoholic psychoses	Tuberculosis	Boating accidents
Alcoholism	Cancer of the lips, mouth	Motor vehicle, bicycle, and
Alcohol abuse	and pharynx	other road accidents
Nerve degeneration	Cancer of the larynx,	Airplane accidents
Heart disease	esophagus, stomach,	Falls
Alcoholic gastritis	and liver	Fire accidents
Fatty liver	Diabetes	Drownings
Hepatitis	Hypertension	Suicides, self-inflicted injuries
Cirrhosis	Stroke	Homicides or shootings
Other liver damage	Pancreatitis	Choking on food
Excessive BAC	Diseases of stomach,	Domestic violence
Accidental poisonings	esophagus, and duodenum	Rapes or date rapes
	Cirrhosis of bile tract	

(Adapted from Alcohol and Health, U. S. Department of Health and Human Services, 1993)

TABLE 5–4 RELATIONSHIP OF BLOOD ALCOHOL CONTENT AND TRAUMA

TYPE OF TRAUMA	ANY ALCOHOL IN BLOOD	BAC GREATER THAN OR EQUAL TO .10%
Homicide	52%	34%
Suicide	40%	24%
Unintentional injury	49%	38%

(Adapted from Alcohol and Health, U.S. Department of Health and Human Services, 1993)

FETAL ALCOHOL SYNDROME (FAS)/FETAL ALCOHOL EFFECTS (FAE)

Maternal Drinking

Alcohol overuse during pregnancy increases the number of miscarriages and infant deaths. There are more problem pregnancies and newborns are smaller and weaker. Specific toxic effects of alcohol on the developing fetus are known as the fetal alcohol syndrome or FAS.

The defects can range widely, from obvious gross physical defects, to retarded growth, to subtle learning disabilities and behavioral problems. Not all women who drink heavily during pregnancy bear children with FAS.

There is as yet no definitive test for confirming FAS at birth and only the most severe cases are able to be diagnosed at birth.

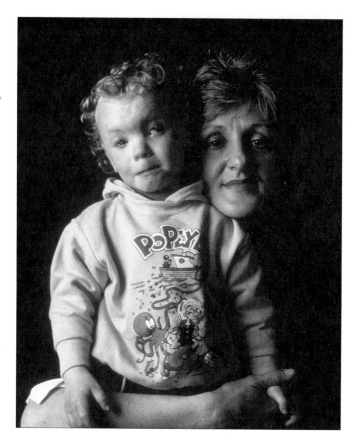

The minimal standards for a diagnosis of FAS are

- retarded growth before and after birth, including height, weight, head circumference, slow brain growth, and small brain size;

- central nervous system involvement, such as delayed intellectual development, neurological abnormalities, behavioral problems, and a malformed skull or brain;

- facial deformities, including shortened eye openings, thin upper lip, a flattened mid face and groove in the upper lip;

- occasional problems with heart and limbs.

In addition, children with FAS are liable to increased risks of other common birth defects, including heart disease, cleft lip and palate, and spina bifida. A weak and irregular sucking response, jitteriness, trembling, and sleep disturbances have been reported in babies exposed to large doses of alcohol. If only a few of these FAS attributes are present, the diagnosis is fetal alcohol effects (FAE) or alcohol-related birth defects (ARBD).

Worldwide studies estimate that FAS births occur anywhere from 0.33 to 1.9 cases per 1,000 live births. In the United States, African Americans have about 6 births per 1,000; Asians, Hispanics, and Whites, about 1 to 2; and Native Americans about 30, although rates from 10 to 120 births per 1,000 have been reported in various Native American and Canadian Indian communities.

Critical period: Because the brain is among the first organs to develop and the last to finish, it appears to be vulnerable throughout pregnancy. The greatest behavioral damage results from early, heavy exposure.

Critical dose: Animal models suggest that peak blood alcohol content rather than the total amount of alcohol drunk determines the critical level above which adverse effects are seen. A pattern of rapid drinking and the resulting high BAC seem to be the most dangerous style of drinking.

How many drinks are "safe" during pregnancy? One study concludes that seven standard drinks per week by pregnant mothers is a threshold level, below which most neurobehavioral effects have not been seen. This might lead some health care professionals to feel that they need not recommend total abstinence. However, seven drinks per week is an average, and if a pregnant woman consumes a large number of those drinks at one sitting, the fetus may be much more at risk. Also, some neurobehavioral tests are so sensitive that effects on the fetus can be found even with extremely low levels of exposure to alcohol.

One approach suggests that one standard drink every 10 days might be "safe," but that there is still the potential for unobservable damage that could impair a child when stressed or when the child reaches old age. The Surgeon General advises that pregnant women not drink while pregnant since there is no way to determine which babies might be at risk from even very low levels of alcohol exposure. Current research simply does not permit us to know at what quantity alcohol begins to damage the fetus.

Paternal Drinking

As we have seen in Chapter 2, genetic transmission of alcoholism by fathers is strongly suspected. There is now growing evidence that the detrimental effects of alcohol on the fetus may also be transmitted by paternal alcohol consumption. Researchers are unable to say definitively whether paternal exposure to alcohol results in FAS or in some other syndrome. In laboratory tests, alcoholic-sired rats produced male offspring with disturbed hormonal functions and spatial learning impairments. Adolescent male rats subjected to high alcohol intake produced both male and female offspring suffering from abnormal development.

Observations of alcoholic-sired human males indicate no gross physical deficits but intellectual and functional deficits in offspring. In addition to the deficits in verbal, thinking, and planning skills of children of alcoholics (COAs), sons of male alcoholics (SOMAs) exhibit further deficiencies in visual/spatial skills, motor skills, memory, and learning.

Preliminary explanations of the causes of these abnormalities suggest that alcohol may either mutate genes in sperm, kill off certain kinds of sperm, or biochemically and nutritionally alter semen and influence sperm.

AGGRESSION AND VIOLENCE

In the past 15 years, almost every major league baseball park and professional football stadium has stopped selling beer in the spectator seats. Alcohol and beer can now be purchased only at the concession stands, where a customer is limited to two drinks at a time, and no sales are allowed after the 7th inning or 3rd quarter. These changes have sharply reduced rowdiness, violence, and fights. In England and other countries

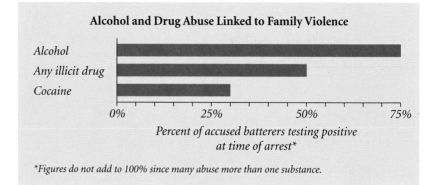

Figure 5-7 •

Three out of four of those arrested for family violence tested positive for alcohol. Half had used some illicit drug and more than one in four tested positive for cocaine.

The National Research Council, 1993

where such a ban doesn't exist, fan violence, especially at soccer matches, is still a major problem.

> *"When you're drunk, you do crazy things, you get violent, and you get self-destructive."*
>
> Recovering alcohol abuser

Interpersonal violence is increasing in the United States which has the highest homicide rate of developed countries. Alcohol itself probably does not cause violence, but it is clear that alcohol works with other factors and contributes to interpersonal criminal violence, including nonsexual assault, sexual assault, domestic violence, robbery, and homicide.

There are some relatively fixed and unalterable pharmacological causal connections between alcohol and violence. Alcohol has been shown to increase aggression by interfering with GABA, the main inhibitory neurotransmitter, in ways that may encourage intoxicated people to become aggressive. Also, in some people, alcohol can increase dopamine which stimulates aggression. And alcohol depletes serotonin which may cause drinkers to use aggression to gain pleasure and avoid punishment and to be less able to stop drinking when once started.

There are also some variable causes of alcohol-related violence that are complex and involve personality, occasion, social and cultural factors, and economic conditions. Also, as the divorce rate increases, more women are victims of alcohol-influenced homicides.

Because alcohol reduces inhibitions, it can encourage someone with a tendency toward violence to release pent-up anger, hatred, and desires forbidden by society, and to act on them. Besides the 50% of all homicides and rapes that occur each year due to alcohol, over 7 million other crimes a year are committed under the influence. Alcohol can also undermine moral judgment and increase aggression. When a person drinks, the common sense that would keep a person out of trouble is often suppressed.

> *"I used to drink with the college friend and we'd go to a bar and we'd be sitting drinking and all of a sudden he would be picking a fight with someone at the other end of the*

Teenage Beer Party Leads to Rape Arrests

By Sandy Kleffman
Chronicle Correspondent

Two Union City teenagers were in custody yesterday for allegedly raping a 15-year-old girl during an afternoon gathering at one boy's apartment.

Police arrested the boys, ages 16 and 14, on Thursday and took

on the be
raped by
who wer

The
in and c
the atta

Packwood Says He Was Drunk in Some Cases

Reuters

Washington

Senator Bob Packwood, facing public hearings over charges of sexual misconduct, said yesterday that he had been so drunk some evenings that he could not remember some of the incidents.

"In some cases I was very

and kissed the women, often sticking his tongue in their mouths, and in one case proposed sex.

Asked whether he denied the charges by the Senate ethics committee, which span three decades, Packwood said: "Some I do. Some I don't. Some I very honestly can't remember."

bar—for no discernible reason. Just, bam—and I'd have to drag him off."
31-year-old ex-drinker

In a controlled experiment with 40 male undergraduates, intoxicated subjects were more likely to accept and approve of violence than placebo-drinking subjects. There is a high correlation between domestic and criminal violence and alcohol. High rates of alcohol use are found among those violent offenders who commit crimes.

EPIDEMIOLOGY

PATTERNS OF ALCOHOL CONSUMPTION

Global Consumption

It is difficult to get accurate, comparable, and consistent data in other countries, but as Table 5-5 points out, most European countries have higher per capita alcohol

TABLE 5–5 WORLDWIDE PER CAPITA USE OF ALCOHOL IN GALLONS OF PURE ETHANOL

France	3.1 gal./*person/year*
Germany	2.8 gal.
Argentina	2.0 gal.
Great Britain	1.9 gal.
United States	1.8 gal.
Japan	1.7 gal.
Canada	1.7 gal.
Cuba	1.0 gal.
Mexico	0.9 gal.
Algeria	0.1 gal.

consumption rates than the United States, while most Asian countries have lower. These differences result from a combination of physiological, cultural, social, religious, and legal factors.

Culture is one of the determinants of how a person drinks. Different drinking patterns are found, for instance, in the so-called wet and dry drinking cultures in Europe. A wet drinking culture, such as those in Austria, Belgium, France, Italy, and Switzerland, sanction daily or almost daily use and integrate social drinking into everyday life. For example, in France, children are served watered down wine at the dinner table. (France also has Europe's second highest per capita consumption of alcohol and more deaths from alcohol-induced cirrhosis of the liver than any other European nation.)

Dry drinking cultures, such as Denmark, Finland, Norway, and Sweden, restrict the availability of alcohol and tax it more heavily. Wet cultures consume more wine and beer, 5 times the amount of wine drunk in dry cultures. Dry cultures consume more distilled spirits, almost 1.5 times the amount in wet cultures, and are characterized by binge style drinking, particularly by males on weekends. Countries like Canada, England, Ireland, the United States, Wales, and Germany exhibit combinations of wet and dry or "mixed" drinking cultures where patterns such as binge drinking in social situations are common. A relatively higher incidence of violence against women is found in mixed drinking cultures than in dry or wet cultures, probably because binge drinking occurs in social situations.

Chinese families generally don't drink much because of cultural pressures. However, in Japan and South Korea, social pressures to drink are very powerful. In Japan, most of the men and half the women drink, yet their alcoholism rate is half of that in the United States.

In Russia, vodka is traditionally drunk between meals in large quantities. Alcoholism had become so rampant in Russia (40,000 died each year from alcohol poisoning) that in 1985, Premier Gorbachev severely restricted the availability of alcohol, almost to the point of prohibition. Illegal stills and the consumption of anything with alcohol in it, such as shoe polish and insecticides, soared.

In England, a trip to the pub for warm beer and darts is a tradition, so 70% of Britons drink regularly. In a recent campaign to stem alcoholism, Britons were urged to reduce their average daily consumption to three drinks a day.

In the United States, a land of many different cultures and life styles and a mixed drinking culture, a variety of culturally influenced drinking customs are present. However, much drinking is done away from the lunch and dinner table.

United States Consumption

Even though the per capita consumption of alcohol is less in the United States than in many countries, the statistics in the United States are still startling.

Last month

- About 110 million Americans, or about 52% of the population over 12 years old (211 million), had a can of beer, a glass of wine, or a cocktail.
- One-half of the 2.8 million high school seniors had a drink.
- About 3/4 of the 6 million college students had a drink.

In the last two weeks

- About 30% of high school seniors had 5 or more drinks at one sitting.
- About 45% of college students had 5 or more drinks at one sitting.

Yesterday

- About $200 million were spent at bars, restaurants, and liquor stores for those drinks.
- Champagne toasts were made to 7,000 brides and grooms.

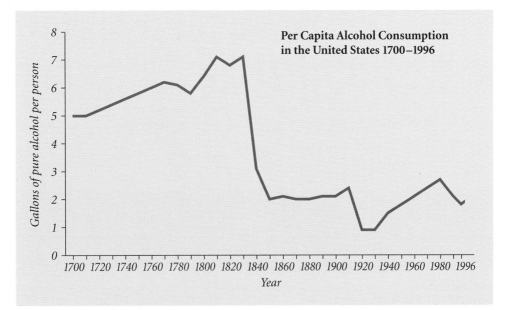

Figure 5-8 •

In the United States, the annual per capita consumption of pure alcohol at present is 1.8 gallons, but as this chart shows, the rate has varied wildly with the rise and fall of prohibition movements, health concerns, and the availability of a good water supply.

Adapted from David F. Musto's *Alcohol In American History* in *Scientific American*, April 1996.

Also yesterday, unfortunately

- From 25% to 30% of all hospital admissions were due to direct or indirect medical complications from alcohol.

- About 1/2 the people who were murdered were drinking, as were 1/2 the murderers.

- More than 1/2 of the 300 rapes that occurred involved alcohol.

- About 20,000 of the crimes that occurred involved alcohol or other drugs.

ALCOHOL AND POPULATION SUBGROUPS

Men

In all age groups, men drink more per drinking episode than women do, regardless of country. Much of this difference has to do with the cultural acceptability of male drinking and the disapproval of female drinking in almost every country. The other reason for the difference reflects the ability of men to be able to more efficiently metabolize higher amounts of alcohol.

Unfortunately, men also have more adverse consequences and develop problems with alcohol abuse or alcohol dependence (alcoholism) at a higher rate.

Women

For women, alcohol problems become greater in their 30s, not in their 20s as for men. Women as a group drink less than men and have fewer problems. However, individual women can have quite serious

TABLE 5–6 ALCOHOL ABUSE OR DEPENDENCE WITHIN PAST YEAR

	MALES	FEMALES	
Abstainers	28%	38%	
Light Drinkers	50%	32%	(At least once a month)
Heavy Drinkers	29%	15%	(At least once a week)
Abusers/Alocoholics	12–13%	2–4%	(5 or more drinks per day during 5 or more days in the last 30 days)

(NIDA Household Survey, 1994)

TABLE 5–7 WOMEN AND ALCOHOL PROBLEMS

MORE LIKELY TO HAVE DRINKING PROBLEMS	LESS LIKELY TO HAVE DRINKING PROBLEMS
Younger women	Older women (60+)
Loss of role (mother, job)	Multiple roles (married, stable, work outside home)
Never married	Married
Divorced, separated	Widowed
Unmarried and living with a partner	Children in the home
White women	Black women
Using other drugs	Hispanic women
Experiencing sexual dysfunction	Nondrinking spouse
Victim of childhood sexual abuse	

(NIDA Household Survey, 1994)

problems, and if they are pregnant, alcohol can severely affect the fetus.

Negative health consequences develop faster for women than for men. Proportionally, more women than men die from cirrhosis of the liver, circulatory disorders, suicide, and accidents. Female alcoholics have a 50–100% higher death rate than male alcoholics. But just as health problems develop after sustained heavy drinking, health disorders, especially reproductive problems, and depression may precede heavy drinking and even contribute to it.

In terms of treatment, studies show that society has a double standard which more readily accepts the alcoholic male but disdains the alcoholic female. Thus, women are less likely to seek treatment for alcoholism than men but are quicker to utilize mental health services when, in fact, their real problem is alcohol or other drugs.

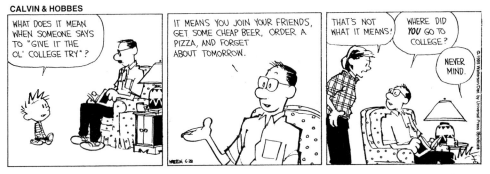

TABLE 5–8 AVERAGE NUMBER OF DRINKS PER WEEK, LISTED BY GRADE AVERAGE

GRADE AVERAGE	DRINKS PER WEEK		
	MALES	FEMALES	OVERALL
A	5.4	2.3	3.3
B	7.4	3.4	5.0
C	9.2	4.1	6.6
D or F	14.6	5.2	10.1

(Core Alcohol and Drug Survey of 56 four-year and 22 two-year colleges by Southern Illinois University-Carbondale, 1993)

Alcohol, Students, and Learning

It used to be that only college students, away from the control of their parents, began heavy drinking. But in the late 1980s and '90s, the age of first use and heavy use has been dropping to where many students have "done it all" by the time they finish their senior year in high school. The problem is that since so much maturing and developing takes place during high school and college years, drinking can negatively affect learning and maturation.

"Often, it's the style of drinking, not experimentation, that gets college students (as well as high school kids and young adults) in trouble. Many think the name of the game is to get drunk. They drink too fast, they drink without eating, they play drinking games or contests, or they binge drink. They drink heavily and hard on "hump day" [Wednesday] or over the weekend. But because they drink heavily only once or twice a week, they think that there is no problem. But there usually is a problem: lower grades, disciplinary action, or behavior they regret, which usually means sexual behavior. And both males and females talk to me

about having been drunk and regretting the person they were with or their conduct with that person."
College drug and alcohol counselor

Forty percent of college students admit to binge drinking at least once a week. Binge drinking is defined as having five or more drinks at one sitting for males, four for females. About half the students in one study who admitted to binge drinking also admitted that their grades fell in the "C" to "F" range as opposed to the "A" to "C" range of most students. Many missed classes on a regular basis. In a national study, there was a startling, dramatic, and direct correlation between the number of drinks consumed per week and the grade point average.

Notice that women's grades start to deteriorate at slightly less than half the level it takes for men's marks to go down. The college Core Survey (Fig. 5–8) indicates that the higher the level of educational attainment, the more likely was the current use (not necessarily abuse) of alcohol. This seems a contradiction with the statistics about grade performance; however, the rate of heavy alcohol use in the 18 to 34 age group among those who had not completed high school was twice that of those who had completed college. In general, college students learn to moderate their drinking before they graduate.

Older Americans

Studies indicate that patterns of drinking persist into old age and that amount and frequency of drinking are a result of general trends in society rather than the aging process. However, about 1/3 of elderly alcohol abusers are of the late onset variety. Some older people may increase their drinking because of isolation, retirement, more leisure time, financial pressures, depression over health, loss of friends or a spouse, lack of a day-to-day structure, or simply the availability and access to alcohol in the home or at friends' homes. This increased drinking can lead to abuse and addiction problems. The elderly alcohol abuser is less likely to be in contact with the workplace, the criminal justice system, or treatment providers than those experiencing the more visible, mainstream problems. Thus, it may be more difficult to identify elderly abusers and get help to them.

However, even with all the reasons and pressures to drink, people 65 and older have the lowest prevalence of problem drinking and alcoholism. There are several reasons for the lower rates.

- People who become alcohol abusers or alcoholics usually do so before the age of 65, suggesting a high degree of self-correction or spontaneous remission with age.

- Cutting down on drinking or giving up drinking may be related to the relatively high cost of alcohol for those on a fixed income, to adverse health consequences, or to the fear of adverse health consequences.

- The body is less able to handle alcohol since liver function declines with age. The general aging process also decreases tolerance and slows metabolism, so the older drinker often has to limit intake.

- Since effects are increased if someone is ill or is taking medications, more severe side effects and greater toxic effects are other reasons given for cutting back or quitting as people age.

Minority Populations

Biological and neurochemical differences between different ethnic groups account for some of the different patterns in different communities. However, diverse

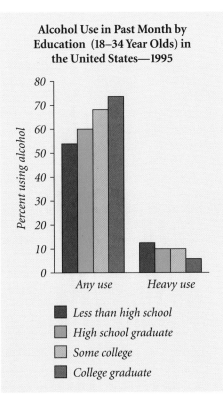

Alcohol Use in Past Month by Education (18–34 Year Olds) in the United States—1995

Percent using alcohol

Any use   Heavy use

■ *Less than high school*
▨ *High school graduate*
□ *Some college*
▨ *College graduate*

Figure 5-9 •

This chart compares the use of alcohol versus the level of education and the abuse of alcohol versus the level of education.

NIDA Household Survey, 1995

Heavy Alcohol Use in Past Month by Ethnic Group in the United States—1995

Percent heavy alcohol use

5.5%   5.7%   4.6%   6.3%

Total   White   Black   Hispanic

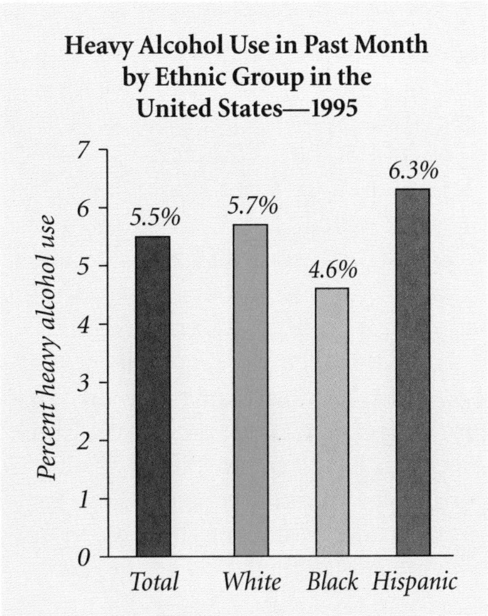

Figure 5-10 •

Perceptions of a problem versus the reality are often at odds.

NIDA Household Survey, 1995

cultural traditions represented in the ethnic minorities seem to make a greater contribution to alcohol use and abuse patterns, as do the degree of assimilation into the drinking patterns of the dominant culture. Sensitivity to ethnic traditions and degrees of assimilation can help us understand how alcohol use affects the health, family life, and social interactions of various cultures and in turn, can contribute to more effective treatment and prevention.

African American Community. Black men abstain at a higher rate than White men (43% versus 30%). The same patterns hold for abstention by Black women versus White women (67% abstention versus 50%). On the other hand, even though more Black women abstain than White women, there is greater heavy drinking among those Black women who do drink. Peak drinking for Blacks occurred after the age of 30, whereas drinking among Whites peaked at a younger age. Two reasons for the higher rate of abstention and the lower rate of heavy drinking is the long history of spirituality in the African American community, along with a matriarchal family structure.

One disturbing fact is that medical problems brought on by heavy drinking among African Americans are more severe due to less access to health care facilities, insurance programs, and prevention programs as well as a delayed entrance into treatment for alcoholism compared to Whites.

Hispanics. According to a 1984 national alcohol survey which provided an in-depth survey of the Hispanic population in the United States, Hispanic men drink more than Hispanic women. In middle age, five times more men than women exhibit abuse or dependence. Drinking increases with both sexes as education and income increase. Among Hispanics, Mexican American men and Puerto Rican men were more likely to abstain, but Mexican American men had more alcohol-related problems. Cuban American men were least likely to abstain and had few drinking problems. The heaviest and most frequent drinking occurs among males in the 30–39 age group.

Asian Americans. A rapidly increasing component of the population of the United States, Asian Americans currently make up about three percent of the total population. However, because the label "Asian American" encompasses dozens of cultures throughout the Pacific basin, such as Japanese, Chinese, Filipino, Korean, Vietnamese, Thai, Indonesian, Burmese, and Pacific Islanders, the diversity of Asian cultures is much greater than the differences between European cultures.

Asian Americans have the lowest rate of drinking and drinking problems among the population. There are possibly genetic factors that may help deter heavy drinking among Asians, but the biggest influence seems to be cultural. Surveys confirm that there are significant differences in drinking patterns among different national Asian American groups. (Note that there are sometimes large differences between Asian and Asian American drinking patterns for the same country.)

Filipino Americans and Japanese Americans were twice as likely to be heavy drinkers as Chinese Americans, but Chinese Americans were less likely to be abstainers. The Korean Americans have the highest number of abstainers. In general, Asian American males under 45 who are educated and in the middle class are most likely to drink, but there is relatively little problem drinking even among this group.

Native Americans and Alaskan Natives. Stereotypes and old western movies seem to have influenced much thinking about Native Americans and drinking. The picture of the "Indian who can't hold his liquor" has been perpetuated for generations. One explanation is that although the rate of abstinence is quite high in many tribes, it is the pattern of heavy drinking that accounts for the highly visible Native American alcoholic. A more cru-

TABLE 5–9 DRINKING PATTERNS OF 1,100 LOS ANGELES ASIAN AMERICANS

GROUP	HEAVY DRINKING	MODERATE DRINKING	ABSTAINING
Japanese Americans	25%	42%	33%
Chinese Americans	11%	48%	41%
Korean Americans	14%	24%	62%
Filipino Americans	20%	29%	51%

(Alcohol Health & Research World, *Vol. II, No. 2*)

cial reason for the stereotype stems from a common pattern of heavy binge drinking among males in various tribes, especially on reservations. (However, in a survey of Sioux tribes, the women drank as much as the men.) The grinding poverty found on many tribal reservations is also a strong causative factor in heavy drinking.

Generally, the abuse of alcohol accounts for 5 of the leading 10 causes of death in most tribes. Alcohol-related motor vehicle deaths are 5.5 times higher than for the rest of the U.S. population. Cirrhosis of the liver is 4.5 times higher; alcoholism, 3.8 times higher; homicide, 2.8 times higher; and suicide, 2.3 times higher. Although Native American women drink less than men, they are especially vulnerable to cirrhosis and account for almost half of the deaths.

In general, drinking patterns vary widely among the more than 300 tribes of Native American and Alaskan peoples who make up about 1% of the population of the United States. Some tribes are mostly abstinent; some drink moderately with few problems; and some have high rates of heavy drinking and alcoholism. One study in Oklahoma found alcohol-related causes of death varied from less than 1% up to 24% among the 11 tribes surveyed, compared with 2% for Blacks and 3% for Whites.

Homeless

There is a wide variety to the homeless population. There are

- the situationally homeless who, because of job loss, spousal abuse, poverty, or eviction, find themselves on the street;

- the street people who have made the streets their home and have made an adjustment to living outside;

- the chronic mentally ill who have been squeezed out of inpatient mental facilities in the last three decades due to a reliance on outpatient health facilities;

- the homeless substance abusers, particularly alcohol abusers, whose lives center around their addiction which has made them incapable of living within the boundaries of normal society.

Within the last two groups are seen the mentally ill person who has begun to use drugs, often to self-medicate, and the drug user/abuser who has developed mental/emotional problems as a result of drug use. One of the keys to all these groups is to understand their lack of affiliation with any kind of support system. Services to identify substance abuse or mental problems are hard to come by or shunned by the homeless person.

TABLE 5–10 PREVALENCE OF CHRONIC MENTAL ILLNESS AND SUBSTANCE ABUSE IN 379 HOMELESS INDIVIDUALS ON THE LOS ANGELES SKID ROW

Chronically mentally ill	12%
Substance abusers	34%
Chronically mentally ill substance abusers	16%
No mental or drug problem	38%

(Alcohol Health & Research World, *Vol. II, No. 2*)

A comprehensive program to alleviate the drug and mental problems of the homeless usually involves outreach that will bring services to the clients and eventually bring the clients to where the services are located. Many cities try to locate services at shelters and gathering places for the homeless, but since many services are needed to meet the wide variety of problems, budget constraints often become the deciding factor.

CONCLUSION

When surveys are done on the incidence of alcoholism and drinking problems, what is often lost is the idea that first, alcoholism is a progressive illness that will prove fatal if not treated. Second, and just as important, is that, although the progression from experimentation to addiction can take 3 months or 30 years, if one continues to drink heavily and frequently, the biochemical and psychological changes become extremely difficult, if not impossible, to reverse.

LEVELS OF USE

Abstention

"It's simple. I don't like the taste and I don't like the feeling. There's no reason for me to drink anything stronger than a Coke®"
22-year old senior

Experimentation

"My brother experimented with Puerto Rican rum on New Year's Eve when he was 15. He threw up on me on the way to the

toilet. That took care of his drinking for 5 years and mine for about 10."
54-year-old nondrinker

Social/Recreational Use

"We know which dorm has the drinkers, so when we feel like a bit of a party and a few drinks, that's where we go. They're more serious about their drinking; they like '40s [40 oz. malt liquor bottles or cans] but I can take it with a grain of salt."
20-year-old college sophomore

Habituation

"In New Rochelle where we are, we get together every weekend at whoever's turn for barbecue it is. We BYO the wine, but the barbecuer supplies the vodka and cheap scotch." *38-year-old suburbanite*

Abuse

"In the service overseas, the drinks at the club were 50¢. About half the time I would wake up in the morning sleeping on the pool table or on the couch in the rec room, and it wasn't till noon or later that my head stopped throbbing."
33-year-old veteran with a medical discharge

Addiction

"I would drink till closing at 2:00 in my bar, then I'd have a few beers with me, drink them, and then fall asleep or pass out about 3:00. I'd wake up at 5:30 looking for a drink and even though 'my bar' opened at 6:30

A.M., I would go four blocks to the one that opened at the legally allowable 6:00."
33-year-old recovering alcoholic

DETERMINING LEVELS OF USE

The most widely used direct assessment test is the Michigan Alcoholism Screening Test (MAST) Questionnaire. It was developed in 1971 (Selzer) and updated in 1980 and 1981 (see page 212).

Traditionally, the cutoff score for determining alcoholism was 5 but this seemed to result in a high false positive rate of 33% to 59%. By using a cutoff of 12, the false positive dropped to 5% to 8%. Scores between 5 and 10 are suggestive of an alcohol problem, not necessarily alcoholism. Each clinician giving the test determines the cutoff best for his or her clients or patients. A person self-administering the test also has to judge whether a score of between 5 and 12 is reason for concern.

Several other assessment tools have been developed to evaluate individuals for alcohol problems. In recent years, an intensive and comprehensive instrument known as the Alcohol Severity Index is gaining popularity. (See Chapter 9.)

CHAPTER SUMMARY

Overview

1. Since the process of fermentation occurs naturally, alcohol was discovered by chance. Over the centuries, alcohol has become the most widely used psychoactive drug and the one that causes the most problems (although cigarettes cause more deaths).

Alcoholic Beverages

2. Grain alcohol (ethyl alcohol or ethanol) is the most intoxicating of the various alcohols.
3. When yeast is added to certain fruits, vegetables, or grain, they ferment into alcoholic beverages.
4. When grains ferment, beer is the result. When fruits ferment, wine is the result. More highly concentrated spirits are distilled from the original fermentation.
5. Most wine is 12% alcohol; most beer is 4–7% alcohol; and most liquors and whiskeys are about 40% alcohol.

Absorption and Metabolism

6. When alcohol is drunk, it is first absorbed, metabolized, and then excreted.
7. The rate of absorption depends on body weight, sex, health, and a dozen other factors. Women usually absorb alcohol faster than men.

TABLE 5–11 THE MICHIGAN ALCOHOLISM SCREENING TEST (MAST) QUESTIONNAIRE

POINTS	QUESTIONS
2*	1. Do you feel you are a normal drinker?
2	2. Have you ever awakened the morning after some drinking and found that you could not remember a part of the evening before?
1	3. Does your wife (husband), girlfriend (boyfriend) and/or parents ever worry or complain about your drinking?
2*	4. Can you stop drinking without a struggle after one or two drinks?
1	5. Do you ever feel guilty about your drinking?
2	6. Do your friends or relatives think you are a normal drinker?
2	7. Do you ever try to limit your drinking to certain times of the day or to certain places?
2*	8. Are you always able to stop drinking when you want to?
5	9. Have you ever attended a meeting of Alcoholics Anonymous (AA) because of your own drinking?
1	10. Have you gotten into fights when drinking?
2	11. Has drinking ever created problems with you and your wife (husband) or girlfriend (boyfriend)?
2	12. Has your wife (husband), girlfriend (boyfriend), or other family member ever gone to anyone for help about your drinking?
2	13. Have you ever lost friends because of your drinking?
2	14. Have you ever gotten into trouble at work because of your drinking?
2	15. Have you ever lost a job because of drinking?
2	16. Have you ever neglected your obligations, your family, or your work for two or more days in a row because you were drinking?
1	17. Do you ever drink in the morning?
2	18. Have you ever been told you have liver trouble? Cirrhosis?
5	19. Have you ever had delirium tremens (DTs), severe shaking, heard voices, or seen things after heavy drinking?
5	20. Have you ever gone to anyone for help about your drinking?
5	21. Have you ever been in a hospital because of drinking?
2	22. Have you ever been seen at a psychiatric hospital or on a psychiatric ward of a general hospital where drinking was part of the problem?
5	23. Have you ever been seen at a psychiatric or mental health clinic, or gone to any doctor, social worker, or clergyman for help with an emotional problem related to drinking?
2 (for each arrest)	24. Have you ever been arrested, even for a few hours, because of drunk behavior?
2	25. Have you ever been arrested for drunk driving?

Scoring: For each "yes" for all questions except 1, 4, and 8, give yourself the points indicated. For questions 1, 4, and 8 (marked with an asterisk) give yourself the points indicated if you give a "no" answer and zero points for a "yes" answer. A score of 12 or more indicates in most cases, that the client/patient has alcoholism.

8. Two to 10% of alcohol is excreted directly through the urine and lungs, the rest is metabolized and then excreted as carbon dioxide and water.

9. Alcohol is metabolized at a defined, continuous rate so it is possible to determine what level of drinking will produce a certain blood alcohol concentration.

Effects and Health Consequences

10. Small amounts of alcohol or occasional intoxication episodes are usually not harmful except for accidents, unwanted pregnancies, STDs, or legal problems.

11. Women who are pregnant or who have preexisting physical or mental health problems, allergies to alcoholic beverages, high genetic/environmental susceptibility to addiction, and preexisting abuse problems should avoid alcohol.

12. Low-dose use can help digestion, promote relaxation, and lower the risk of heart attacks.

13. The psychological effects depend on the mood of the drinker and the setting where the alcohol was consumed.

14. Since alcohol is a disinhibitor, low-dose use can increase self-confidence, sociability, and sexual desire.

15. As the amount consumed increases, the initial desirable effects are often offset by unwanted side effects, such as physical and mental depression.

16. Intoxication is a combination of blood alcohol concentration, psychological mood, expectation, and drinking history.

17. As the blood alcohol concentration rises, effects go from lowered inhibitions and relaxation, to decreased alertness and clumsiness, to slurred speech and inability to walk, to unconsciousness and death.

18. About 10% to 12% of drinkers progress to frequent high-dose use, 2 to 3 times more men than women have a problem.

19. Heredity, environment, and frequency of consumption help determine if a person will have a problem with drinking.

20. Tolerance and tissue dependence occur as the body, especially the liver, attempts to adapt to ever increasing amounts.

21. Withdrawal after cessation of frequent high-dose use can be life-threatening.

22. The liver is the organ most severely affected. Problems include a fatty liver, hepatitis, and cirrhosis (which is a scarring of the liver and is eventually fatal).

23. Enlarged heart, high blood pressure, brain damage, and impaired mental abilities are seen with frequent high-dose use.

24. Most drug abuse involves more than one substance, especially alcohol, so the problems can be synergistic, that is, greater than just the sum of the effects of the individual drugs.

Other Problems

25. Many people use alcohol to self-medicate but as drinking continues, it can induce depression.

26. A large percentage of homicides, suicides, and accidents involve alcohol.

27. Heavy drinking during pregnancy can cause birth defects, most notably fetal alcohol syndrome (FAS), that involve abnormal growth and mental problems. It is not known what level of drinking is safe during pregnancy.

28. Alcohol is heavily involved in aggression, violence, and sexual assault, mostly from the lowering of inhibitions. The mood of the drinkers and the setting can also cause violence.

Epidemiology

29. Alcohol consumption varies from 3.1 gallons of pure alcohol a year in France to 1.8 gallons in the United States, down to 0.1 gallons in a Moslem country, such as Algeria.

30. About 28% of high school students and 45% of college students have five or more drinks at one sitting.

31. Men drink more per episode than women and have more drinking problems. This results from of a combination of physiological differences and cultural mores.

32. The amount and frequency of alcohol consumption directly affects academic performance and grades.

33. Each ethnic group in the United States has unique problems due to physiology and culture. Heavy drinking is lower in the African American community than the Caucasian or Hispanic communities. The Asian community has so many components that it is hard to make generalizations. There is also a wide variation in the Native American communities, although in some, 5 of the 10 leading causes of death are due to alcohol.

Conclusion

34. The road to alcoholism can take 3 months, 30 years, or alcoholism may never occur. One has to recognize that alcohol is a strong psychoactive drug and can cause irreversible physiological changes that make one susceptible to alcoholism.

All Arounders

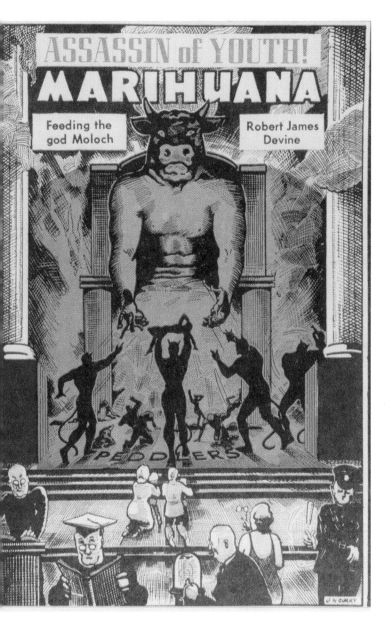

A ntimarijuana propaganda, popular in the late 1930s and 1940s, depicted the drug as the devil (Moloch) incarnate and its peddlers as servants of the devil. Note, learned men and judges are shown with their backs turned to the problem, ignoring or denying its existence.

- **Classification:** The most commonly used psychedelics are marijuana, LSD, MDMA, PCP, peyote, and psilocybin mushrooms.

- **General Effects:** Psychedelics cause intensified sensations, mixed-up sensations (visual input becomes sound), illusions, delusions, hallucinations, stimulation, and impaired judgment and reasoning.

- **LSD, Mushrooms, and Other Indole Psychedelics:** LSD is very potent, stimulating, and can cause illusions. Psilocybin mushrooms cause nausea and create hallucinations. Ibogaine and yage are also indole psychedelics.

- **Peyote, MDMA, and Other Phenylalkylamine Psychedelics:** Peyote cacti (mescaline), used in sacred rituals and ceremonies, cause more hallucinations than LSD. Designer psychedelics like MDMA ("ecstasy") are similar to amphetamines but also have calming and psychic effects.

- **Belladonna and Other Anticholinergic Psychedelics:** Plants such as belladonna, jimsonweed, and henbane have been used for more than 3,000 years in ancient cultures, often in rituals and ceremonies.

- **PCP and Other Psychedelics:** PCP, an animal tranquilizer, causes mind-body dissociation and a sensory-deprived state. Ketamine is becoming more popular. Amanita mushrooms, nutmeg, and mace are rarely used.

- **Marijuana and Other Cannabinols:** Marijuana is the most popular illicit psychoactive drug. It magnifies existing personality traits of users. Effects often depend on the mindset of the user and the setting where used.

CLASSIFICATION

Uppers stimulate the body and downers depress it. All arounders (psychedelics) can act as stimulants or depressants but mostly they distort the perception of the world and create a world in which logic takes a back seat to intensified confused sensations. From alphabet soup psychedelics (LSD, PCP, MDMA) to naturally occurring plants used socially or in religious ceremonies (marijuana, peyote, mushrooms, belladonna), all arounders represent a diverse group of substances.

Historically, amanita mushrooms were eaten in India and pre-Columbian Mexico, belladonna was drunk in ancient Greece and medieval Europe, marijuana was inhaled and eaten in ancient China and Egypt, and poisonous ergot, found in rye mold (a natural form of LSD), was accidentally eaten in Renaissance Europe.

In the twentieth century, even though psychedelics can be found in every country,

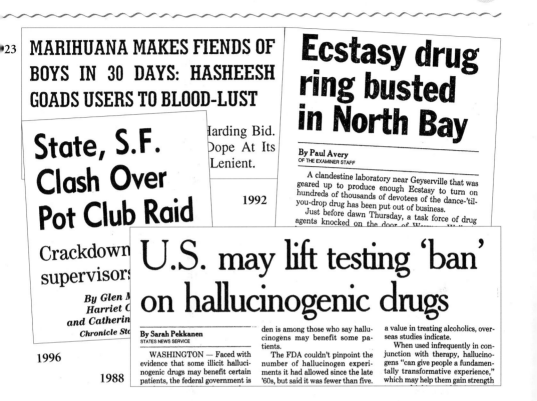

MARIHUANA MAKES FIENDS OF BOYS IN 30 DAYS: HASHEESH GOADS USERS TO BLOOD-LUST

Ecstasy drug ring busted in North Bay

By Paul Avery
OF THE EXAMINER STAFF

A clandestine laboratory near Geyserville that was geared up to produce enough Ecstasy to turn on hundreds of thousands of devotees of the dance-'til-you-drop drug has been put out of business.

Just before dawn Thursday, a task force of drug agents knocked on the door of W_____ H___

Harding Bid.
Dope At Its
Lenient.

1992

State, S.F. Clash Over Pot Club Raid

Crackdown
supervisors

By Glen
Harriet
and Catherin
Chronicle St

1996

1988

U.S. may lift testing 'ban' on hallucinogenic drugs

By Sarah Pekkanen
STATES NEWS SERVICE

WASHINGTON — Faced with evidence that some illicit hallucinogenic drugs may benefit certain patients, the federal government is

den is among those who say hallucinogens may benefit some patients.

The FDA couldn't pinpoint the number of hallucinogen experiments it had allowed since the late '60s, but said it was fewer than five.

a value in treating alcoholics, overseas studies indicate.

When used infrequently in conjunction with therapy, hallucinogens "can give people a fundamentally transformative experience," which may help them gain strength

---

the majority of these drugs are grown and used in the Americas and Africa (the major exception is marijuana which is grown in most countries). Hundreds of primitive tribes in the Americas, such as the Aztecs and Toltecs in the past and the Kiowa and Huichols in the present, have used peyote, psilocybin, yage, morning glory seeds, and dozens of other substances for social, ceremonial, and medical reasons.

Recently, there has been an upsurge of interest in psychedelics, such as LSD, MDMA ("ecstasy," "rave"), and even psychedelic mushrooms ("shrooms") containing psilocybin. The percentage of high school seniors who used LSD in the past month has doubled since 1992 (4% in 1995) and is greater than those who used cocaine in the past month (1.8% in 1995). Interest in marijuana, the most widely used psychedelic, had been declining since 1979 but in the past few years, use has begun to

rise again (21% of high school seniors used in the past month in 1995, double the amount in 1992).

The five main classes of psychedelics are the indole psychedelics, such as LSD and psilocybin; the phenylalkylamines, such as mescaline and "ecstasy"; the anticholinergics, such as belladonna; those in a class by themselves such as PCP; and the cannabinols, found in marijuana (Cannabis) plants.

GENERAL EFFECTS

Unlike stimulants and depressants which have been well researched, psychedelics are manufactured or grown illegally, so, with the exception of marijuana, much of the information about the effects is anecdotal or the result of surveys rather than extended scientific testing. Since many

TABLE 6–1 ALL AROUNDERS–PSYCHEDELICS

Common Names	Active Ingredients	Street Names
INDOLE PSYCHEDELICS		
LSD (LSD 25 & 49)	Lysergic acid diethylamide	Acid, sugar cube, window pane, blotter, illusion
Mushrooms	Psilocybin, psilocin	Shrooms, magic mushrooms
Tabernanthe iboga	Ibogaine	African LSD
Morning glory seeds or Hawaiian woodrose	Lysergic acid amide	Heavenly blue, pearly gates, wedding bells
DMT (synthetic or from yopo beans, epena or Sonoran Desert toad)	Dimethyltryptamine	Businessman's special, cohoba snuff
Yage, ayahuasca, caapi	Harmaline (also mixed with DMT)	Visionary vine, vine of the soul, vine of death
PHENYLALKYLAMINE PSYCHEDELICS		
Peyote cactus	Mescaline	Mesc, peyote, buttons
STP (DOM) (synthetic)	4 methyl 2,5, dimethoxy-amphetamine	Serenity, tranquility, peace pill
STP-LSD combo	Dimethoxy-amphetamine with LSD	Wedge series, orange and pink wedges, Harvey Wallbanger
Designer Psychedelics, e.g., MDA, MDMA (MDM), MMDA, MDE	Variations of methylene-dioxy amphetamines	Ecstasy, rave, love drug, XTC, Adam, Eve
2CB	4 bromo, 2,5 dimethoxy phenethylamine	
U4Euh	4 methyl pemoline	Euphoria

psychedelics contain more than one active ingredient, it is hard to say which chemical is causing certain effects. Also, many drugs which are sold as one psychedelic may actually be another cheaper psychedelic, so even the anecdotal information can be incorrect. Some common examples of misrepresentation are PCP sold as THC (the active ingredient in marijuana) or regular mushrooms sprinkled with LSD and sold as psychedelic mushrooms.

Generally, psychedelics interfere with neurotransmitters such as dopamine, acetylcholine, anandamide, noradrenaline, and especially serotonin. Serotonin, which affects mood, is particularly influenced by the indole psychedelics, such as LSD.

The effects of many psychedelics are uncommonly dependent on the size and toxicity of the dose. A drug like LSD is thousands of times more powerful by weight than a similar amount of peyote.

TABLE 6–1   (continued)

Common Names	Active Ingredients	Street Names
ANTICHOLINERGICS		
Belladonna, mandrake, henbane, datura, (jimson weed, thornapple), wolfbane	Atropine, scopolamine, hyoscyamine	Deadly nightshade
Artane	Trihexypheneidyl	
Cogentin	Benztropine	
Asmador cigarettes	Belladonna alkaloids	
OTHER PSYCHEDELICS		
PCP	Phencyclidine	Angel dust, hog, peace pill, krystal joint, ozone, Sherms, Shermans
Ketamine	Ketajet®, Ketalar®	Special K
Nutmeg and mace	Myristicin	
Amanita mushrooms (fly agaric)	Ibotenic acid, muscimole	Soma
Kava root	Alpha pyrones	Kava-kava
CANNABINOLS		
Marijuana	Δ-9-tetrahydrocannabinol (THC)	Grass, pot, weed, Acapulco gold, joint, reefer, dank, dubie, blunt, honey blunt
Sinsemilla	High potency, seedless flowering tops of female marijuana plant	Sens, skunk weed, ganja
Hashish, hash oil	THC (pressed resin of marijuana)	Hash

The effects of a 25-microgram dose of LSD are quite different than the effects of a 250-microgram dose.

Experience with the drug, the basic emotional makeup of the user, the mood and mental state at the time of use, and the surroundings in which the drug is taken are also crucial to the kind, duration, and intensity of the effects. For instance, a first- or second-time psychedelic user may become nauseous, extremely anxious, depressed, and totally disoriented, whereas an experienced user may only experience euphoric feelings or some mild illusions. A user with a tendency towards schizophrenia or major depression could get a severe reaction from LSD because it might trigger any unstable tendencies. Someone who is basically aggressive might become violent when using PCP, whereas a young and immature user of marijuana could become more childlike.

Figure 6–1 •

Chemical models of MDMA (methylenedioxymetham-phetamine), PCP (phencyclidine), Δ-9-THC (tetrahydrocannabinol), and LSD (lysergic acid diethylamide). There is a wide variation in the chemical structures of the different classes of psychedelics.

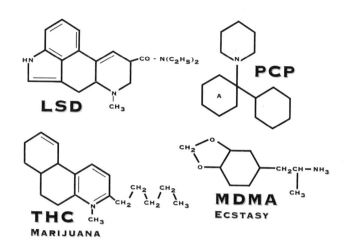

This 1760 painting of Shudja-Quli Khan shows a water pipe that is used to smoke hashish. It was most popular in the Middle East but has been used in Europe and the West to reduce the harshness of the hash smoke.

Courtesy of the Bibliotheque Nationale, Paris

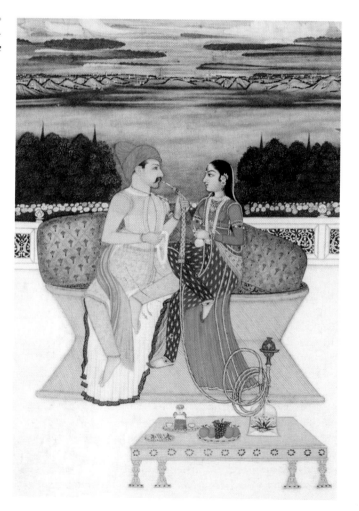

PHYSICAL EFFECTS

LSD and most other hallucinogens stimulate the sympathetic nervous system. This stimulation results in a rise in pulse rate and blood pressure. Many psychedelics can produce sweating and palpitations or trigger nausea. The stimulation of the brain stem, and specifically the reticular formation, can overload the sensory pathways, making the user very conscious of all sensation. Disruption of visual and auditory centers can cause effects ranging from flashes of light to melting walls. An auditory stimulation such as the sound of music might jump to a visual pathway, causing the music to be "seen" as shifting light patterns, or visual impulses might shift to audio ones, resulting in strange sounds. This crossover or mixing of the senses is known as synesthesia.

EMOTIONAL EFFECTS

Psychedelics have a strong effect on mood by affecting the emotional center (the limbic system). They also often suppress the memory centers and other higher cerebral functions, such as judgment and reason.

It's important to note the differences among an illusion, a delusion, and a hallucination. An **illusion** is a mistaken perception of a real stimulus. For example, a rope can be misinterpreted as a snake or smooth skin as silk. A **delusion** is a mistaken idea that is not swayed by reason. An example is someone who thinks he can fly or thinks he has become deformed or ugly. A **hallucination** is a sensory experience which doesn't relate to reality, such as seeing a creature or object which doesn't exist. With LSD and most psychedelics, illusions and delusions are the primary experiences. With mescaline, psilocybin, and PCP, hallucinations are the primary experience.

LSD, MUSHROOMS, AND OTHER INDOLE PSYCHEDELICS

LSD (lysergic acid diethylamide)

History

"Acid," "blotter," "barrels," "sunshine," "illusion," and "window panes" are just some of the street names for LSD, a synthesized form of an ergot fungus toxin which infects rye. Tested and developed in the late 1940s at Sandoz Pharmaceuticals by Dr. Albert Hoffman, LSD was investigated as a therapy for mental illnesses and as a weapon for chemical warfare. It was popularized by Dr. Timothy Leary, originally a professor at Harvard University who did LSD research, and by others in the 1960s as a way to explore consciousness and feelings. Dr. Leary's slogan, "Tune in, turn on, and drop out" was used in endless newspaper articles and TV news shows leading to the suspicion that the media was as much responsible for the rise and fall of LSD as was its identification as the drug of the hippie generation. Scientific research virtually ceased in the early 1970s and it wasn't until recently that any research on LSD or psychedelics in general has been renewed.

Epidemiology

Currently, LSD is being used by younger and younger Americans. Studies indicate that LSD is often abused by junior high and high school students while they are sitting in class. LSD is popular because it results in less detectable physical symptoms than alcohol or marijuana and because the drug is relatively inexpensive, costing one dollar to five dollars a hit. In the 1960s, "acid heads" were usually in their early twenties, and

TABLE 6–2   30-DAY PREVALENCE OF LSD AMONG 8th, 10th, AND 12th GRADERS

	1991	1993	1995
8th Grade	0.6%	1.0%	1.4%
10th Grade	1.5%	1.6%	3.0%
12th Grade	1.9%	2.4%	4.0%

The use of LSD by high school students started climbing in 1991 after years of decline.

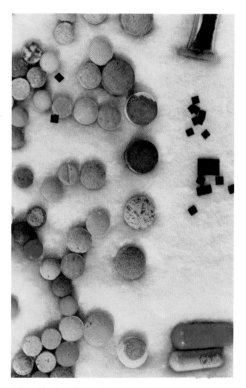

The effective dose of LSD is so small that it can be delivered in many guises. Tablets and impregnated blotter paper or sugar cubes can be swallowed or saturated bits of gelatin can be put in the eye.

many were searching for a quasi-religious experience. In the 1990s, younger teenagers said they mostly just wanted to get high.

Besides the usual reasons for using a drug like LSD (experimentation, peer pressure, availability, and curiosity), there are three others that have spurred current usage. One is the proliferation of "rave" clubs and parties where MDMA, LSD, and amphetamines are used. Another reason is that standard drug testing usually does not test for LSD and even when tested for, the effective dose is so small that it is almost impossible to detect. Finally, low-dose "blotter acid," 30–50 micrograms of LSD, results in less toxic reactions than in the past, so many users take it on a daily basis.

Manufacture of LSD

The majority of LSD is manufactured in northern California, mostly in the San Francisco Bay area. The labs are hard to find since the quantities of raw material needed to make the drug are very small. Indeed, the entire U.S. supply for one year could be carried by one person. Crystalline LSD is dissolved in alcohol and drops of the solution are put on blotter paper or in a

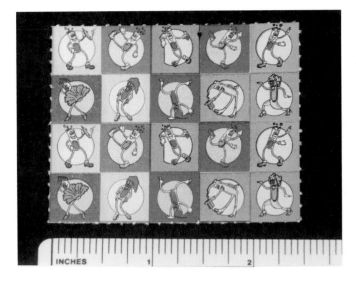

On a sheet of "blotter acid" (LSD), each perforated square contains a drop of LSD, anywhere from 30–50 micrograms of the drug. In the 1960s and '70s, they each contained 100–300 micrograms.

sugar cube and chewed or swallowed. It has also been put into microdots or tiny squares of gelatin and eaten or dropped onto a moist body tissue and absorbed.

To reach the younger group of potential users, illegal manufacturers even use Mickey Mouse, Donald Duck, a teddy bear, and other characters printed on the blotter paper. In 1995, about 10% of high school seniors said they had tried LSD at least once. About 4% said they use it on a monthly basis.

Pharmacology

LSD is remarkable for its potency. Doses as low as 25 micrograms (mics) or 25 millionths of a gram, can cause mental changes (spaciness, decreased perception of time, mild euphoria) and mild stimulatory effects. Effects appear 15 minutes to 1 hour after ingestion and last 6–8 hours. The usual psychedelic dose of LSD is 150–300 micrograms. Low-dose use of 30–50 micrograms acts more like a stimulant than a psychedelic. Tolerance to the psychedelic effects of LSD develops very rapidly. Within a few days of daily use, a person can tolerate a 300 microgram dose without experiencing any major psychedelic effects. Cross tolerance can also develop to the effects of mescaline and psilocybin.

Several years ago, a new version of the drug called LSD-49 (instead of the old designation, LSD-25) appeared on the streets. Called "illusion," it seems to give more intense visual effects than an equal amount of the original LSD-25.

Physical Effects

LSD can cause a rise in heart rate and blood pressure, a higher body temperature, dizziness, dilated pupils, and some sweating, much like amphetamines. Users see many light trails, like after-images in cheap televisions where there is always an after-image of whatever is happening on camera (this aftereffect is known as the trailing phenomena).

Mental Effects

Mentally, LSD overloads the brain stem, the sensory switchboard for the mind, causing sensory distortions (seeing sounds, feeling smells, or hearing colors), dreaminess, depersonalization, altered mood, and impaired concentration and motivation.

"In a real strong 'acid'—the old kind— you'll see the walls melting like candles and water running down the wall. That kind of distortion is not a complete hallucination or anything real solid like a bottle where you wonder whether it's there or not. The thing that got me really crazy was hearing a dog or airplane or passenger car miles away and you didn't know whether that was real or an illusion. There was also what we called the psychedelic hummmmmm that we thought we heard."
Recovering LSD and marijuana user

It becomes difficult to express oneself verbally while on LSD. Single word answers and seemingly nonassociated comments (non sequiturs) are common. A user might experience intense sensations and emotions but find it difficult to tell others what he or she is feeling.

One of the greatest dangers of LSD is the loss of judgment and impaired reasoning. This, coupled with slowed reaction time and visual distortions, can make the driving of a car or a simple camping trip risky.

"I stuck my hand in this flame and then I went, 'Uh-oh, my hand is in the flame,' and I pulled it out and I thought it didn't burn but later that night, my hand started blistering and I'm going, 'Oh no, I got burned.'"
Ex-LSD user

Bad Trips (acute anxiety reactions). Because LSD affects the emotional center in the brain and distorts reality, a user, particularly a first-time user, is subject to the extremes of euphoria and panic. Depersonalization and lack of a stable environment can trigger acute anxiety, paranoia, fear over loss of control, and delusions of persecution or feelings of grandeur leading to dangerous behaviors. One survivor of a jump from the Golden Gate Bridge claimed he was jumping through a golden hoop. (See Chapter 9 concerning treatment for bad trips.)

Mental Illness and LSD

Much of the early research, as well as enthusiasm for LSD as an adjunct to psychotherapy, has decreased over the years. Proponents of psychotherapeutic use claim that drug-stimulated insights afford some users a shortcut to the extended process of psychotherapy where uncovering traumas and conflicts from the unconsciousness helps to heal the patient. Opponents of this kind of therapy say that the dangerous side effects of LSD more than outweigh any benefit.

The popular picture of someone using LSD just one time and becoming permanently psychotic or schizophrenic is incorrect. It is an unusual occurrence. What usually happens is that in people with a preexisting mental instability, LSD use nudges those tendencies into more severe mental disturbances. Use can also cause people to experience their mental illness at an earlier age or it may provoke a relapse in someone who has previously suffered a psychotic episode or disorder.

"I got pretty involved in the Grateful Dead scene and that was when I was doing 'acid.' And the whole thing started with my

schizophrenia. That always plays a part. And any time I get too involved in the scene, the acid starts to trigger the schizophrenia, like flashbacks, and sometimes it makes me want to use. But I'm drawn to it like a moth drawn to a light."
Recovering LSD user with schizophrenia

Also, some otherwise normal users can be thrown into a temporary but prolonged psychotic reaction or severe depression that requires extended treatment. In addition, prolonged trips (extended LSD effects) devoid of other psychiatric symptoms have also occurred. Though very rare, these reactions can be emotionally crippling and may last for years.

A small number of users experience mental flashbacks of sensations or a bad trip they had under the influence of LSD. The flashbacks, which can be triggered by stress, the use of another psychoactive drug, or even exercise, recreate the original experience (much like the posttraumatic stress phenomenon). This sensation can also cause anxiety and even panic since it is unexpected and the user seems to have little control over its recurrence. Most flashbacks are provoked by some sensory stimulus: sight, sound, odor, or touch.

PSILOCYBIN AND PSILOCIN ("magic mushrooms")

Psilocybin and psilocin are the active ingredients in a number of psychedelic mushrooms found in Mexico, the United States, South America, Southeast Asia, and Europe. These mushrooms, called Teonanacatl (divine flesh) by the Aztecs, were especially important to Indian cultures in Mexico and some other areas in the pre-Columbian Americas and were used in ceremonies dating as far back as 1000 B.C. They are still used today, although persecu-

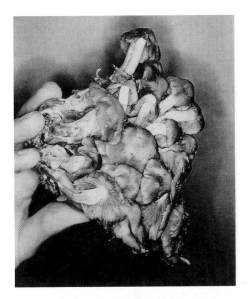

One of the 75 species of mushroom containing psilocybin. The "shrooms" can be used fresh or dried. Courtesy of Allan Richardson

tion by the Spaniards, who conquered much of Central and South America in the sixteenth and seventeenth centuries, drove the ceremonial use of mushrooms underground for hundreds of years. It wasn't until the 1950s that much was known about the ceremonies conducted by shamans or curandera (medicine women or men). The ceremonies include eating or drinking the psychedelic substances in order to get intoxicated, along with hours of chanting in order to have visions which will help treat illnesses, solve problems, or get in contact with the spirit world.

Pharmacology

Psilocybin and psilocin, the active psychedelic ingredients of the mushrooms, are found in about 75 different species from three genera: *Psilocybe*, *Panaeolus*, and *Conocybe*. Fifteen species have been identified in the U.S. Pacific Northwest. Psychic effects are obtained from doses of 10 milligrams to 60 milligrams and generally last for five to six hours. Both wild and cultivated mushrooms vary greatly in strength so 1 potent plant might have as much psilocybin as 10 weak ones. When ingested, the psilocybin is converted to psilocin, also present in the mushrooms. However, psilocybin is almost twice as potent as psilocin and crosses the blood-brain barrier more readily. Its chemical structure is similar to that of LSD.

Effects

Most mushrooms containing psilocybin cause nausea and other physical symptoms before the mental effects take over. The mental effects include visceral sensations, changes in sight, hearing, taste, and touch, and altered states of consciousness. There seem to be less disassociation and panic than with LSD. Prolonged psychotic reactions are rare. However, the mental effects are not consistent and depend on the setting in which the drug is taken.

"We ate some of the dried mushrooms and didn't feel anything for a while. Then all of a sudden, we were into the sensations. We got the giggles and visually it was like watching a strobe light show. Our vision was slowed like something would happen and then we would see it. After the first time, the trips were never as good."
Former "shroom" eater

There is a small market in mail order kits containing spores for growing mushrooms in a closet or basement. Some users also tramp the countryside looking for a certain species. The major danger in "shroom" harvesting is mistaking poisonous mushrooms for those containing psilocybin. Some poisonous mushrooms (e.g., *Amanita phalloides*) can cause death or permanent liver damage within hours of ingestion. Further, grocery-bought mushrooms laced with LSD or PCP are often sold to those seeking the "magic mushroom" experience.

OTHER INDOLE PSYCHEDELICS

Ibogaine

Produced by the African *Tabernanthe iboga* shrub, ibogaine is a long-acting psychedelic and stimulant. In low doses, it acts as a stimulant while in higher doses, it can produce psychedelic effects and a self-determined catatonic reaction which can be maintained up to two days. It is rarely found in the United States although it has been synthesized in laboratories. Its use is generally limited to native cultures in western and central Africa such as the Bwiti tribe of Gabon. They use it to help them stay alert and motionless while hunting. They also claim ancestral visions while using it.

Recently, there has been research into the use of ibogaine to treat heroin addiction. Anecdotal reports, as well as a few limited studies, claim that just a few treatments eliminated withdrawal symptoms and craving for opioids. The theory is that ibogaine prevents the increase in dopamine caused by use of heroin and cocaine and that many of the changes are permanent. Since dopamine stimulation of the brain's reward/pleasure center is one of the reasons for compulsive use of drugs, the use of ibogaine in treatment deserves further research.

Morning Glory Seeds (ololiuqui)

These seeds from the *Turbina* plant (morning glory plant also called the Hawaiian woodrose) contain an LSD-like substance, lysergic acid amide, in low concentration. Used by Indians in Mexico before the Spanish arrived, several hundred seeds have to be taken to get high, so the nauseating properties of the drug are magnified. In sufficient quantities, the seeds cause LSD-like effects but they are not particularly popular among those who use psychedelics. Morning glory seeds are sold commercially but to prevent misuse, many of these seeds are dipped in a toxic substance. The seeds have street names such as "heavenly blue" and "pearly gates."

DMT

Dimethyltryptamine is a naturally occurring, easily synthesized psychedelic substance. Since digestive juices destroy the active ingredients, the drug is usually powdered and snorted or occasionally smoked. South American tribes have used it for at least 400 years. They prepare it from several different plants as a snuff called yopo, cohoba, vilca, cebil, or epena. They blow it into each other's noses through a hollow reed and then dance, hallucinate, and sing. The synthetic form is usually put into a joint or cigarette and smoked. Occasionally, it is injected.

DMT causes intense visual hallucinations, intoxication, and often a loss of awareness of surroundings lasting about 30 minutes or less. The short duration of action gave rise to the nickname "businessman's special" for the synthetic version.

Recently, newspaper reports have sensationalized a new source of a variant of DMT, 5-MeO-DMT, the venom of the Sonoran Desert toad. Contrary to anecdotes about people licking the toad to get high, the substance is milked onto cigarettes, dried, and smoked.

Yage

Yage, a psychedelic drink made from an Amazonian vine (*ayahuasca* or vine of the soul), causes intense vomiting, diarrhea, and then a dreamlike condition which usually lasts up to 10 hours. The active ingredient is thought to be harmaline, an indole alkaloid found in several other psychedelic plants, such as the Syrian rue herb from China. Native cultures often mix yage with many DMT-containing plants in order to intensify the effects of their psychedelic drink. It has been recently discovered that harmaline protects the DMT from being deactivated by gastric enzymes thus allowing DMT to be effective when taken orally.

PEYOTE, MDMA, AND OTHER PHENYLALKYLAMINE PSYCHEDELICS

This class of psychedelics is chemically related to adrenaline and amphetamines although many of the effects are quite different. Whereas the effects of amphetamines will peak within half an hour, much sooner if smoked, the phenylalkylamines take several hours to reach their peak. Effects of phenylalkylamines also take longer to reach their peak than effects of indole psychedelics, such as LSD.

PEYOTE (mescaline)

Mescaline is the active component of the peyote and the San Pedro cacti. Synthetic mescaline, which was isolated in 1890, is a thin needlelike crystal which is sold in capsules. Peyote cacti are still eaten in ritual ceremonies by the northern Mexican tribes, such as the Huichol, Tarahumara, and Cora, and by the Southwest Plains Native American tribes, such as the Comanches, Kiowas, and Utes. In addition, the Native American Church of North America, with a claimed mem-

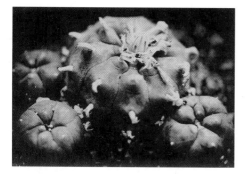

A mature peyote cactus (Lophophora williamsii) *is ripe for harvesting. Each button (the top of the cactus) contains about 50 milligrams of mescaline. It can take from 2–10 buttons to get high.*

bership of 250,000, also uses the peyote cactus as a sacrament.

The use of peyote stretches as far back as 300 B.C. Over the centuries, the Aztecs, Toltecs, Chichimecas, and several Meso-American cultures included it in their rituals. When the Spaniards invaded the New World and encountered the use of peyote, they regarded it as evil and the hallucinations as an invitation to the devil. They tried to abolish it but never succeeded. In the 1800s, its use spread north to the United States where about 50 North American tribes were using it by the early 1900s.

Effects

The tops of the peyote cactus are cut at ground level or uprooted. They are eaten fresh or dried into peyote or mescal "buttons" and then ingested. The bitter nause-ating substance is either eaten (seven to eight buttons is an average dose) or boiled and drunk as a tea. They can also be ground and eaten as a powder. The effects of mescaline (which was isolated in the lab-oratory about 1890) last approximately 12 hours and are very similar to LSD with an

emphasis on colorful visions. Users term it the "mellow LSD" but real hallucinations are more common with mescaline than with LSD. Each use of peyote is usually ac-companied by a severe episode of nausea and vomiting although some users can de-velop a tolerance to these effects. As with most psychedelics, tolerance to the mental effects can also develop rapidly.

A peyote ceremony might consist of in-gesting the peyote buttons, then singing, drumming, chanting hymns, and trying to understand the psychedelic visions in order to have spiritual experiences. Many partic-ipants also have hallucinatory visions of a deity or spiritual leader whom they are able to converse with for guidance and under-standing.

Since the reaction to many psychedelics depends on the mindset and setting almost as much as on the actual properties of the drug, use of a mind-altering substance in a structured ceremonial setting will induce more spiritual feelings than if it's used at a rock concert. Some people would liken the difference to taking wine during the sacra-ment of Communion in a Catholic Mass or during Passover as opposed to drinking a pint at a tail-gate party.

Many challenges have been made con-cerning the legality of using a psychedelic substance for a religious ceremony. In 1990, the U.S. Supreme Court ruled that the use of a psychoactive drug, such as pey-ote, during religious ceremonies is not pro-tected by the Constitution and that states can ban its use. For this reason, many cere-monies are held in secret.

DESIGNER PSYCHEDELICS (MDA, MDMA, MMDA, MDM, MDE, and others)

This set of synthetic drugs uses labora-tory variations of the amphetamine mol-ecule. First discovered over 70 years ago, the drugs can cause feelings of well-being and euphoria along with some stimulatory effects, side effects, and toxicity similar to amphetamines. The differences among the drugs have to do with duration of action, extent of delusional effects, and degree of euphoria. MDA was the first of these compounds to be widely abused but in the 1990s, MDMA has taken over that distinction.

MDMA ("ecstasy," "rave," "XTC," "X," "Adam," "Eve," and others)

The compound MDMA, chemical name 3,4 methylenedioxymethamphetamine, is shorter acting than MDA (4–6 hours versus 10–12 hours) and can be swallowed or injected, much like amphetamines, though it is usually sold in capsule or tablet form. A capsule costs anywhere from $10 to $25 and has been manufactured illegally since it was banned in 1987 by the U.S. Federal Government.

Physical Effects. MDMA has many stimulant effects similar to amphetamines, such as increased heart rate, faster respiration, excess energy, and hyperactivity. Some claim that it has the opposite effect and calms these bodily functions. Part of this contradiction has to do with the amount ingested. The more that is used, the greater the physical effects. MDMA can trigger nausea, loss of appetite, and the clenching of jaw muscles. Since tolerance to its mental effects develops rapidly, increased doses can result in greater physical harm.

Mental Effects. Twenty minutes to one hour after ingestion, MDMA causes stimulation and mild distortions of perception but most often, according to some users, it has a calming effect and increases empathy with others. It doesn't give the visual illusions most often associated with psychedelics. Physical dependency is generally not a problem but as with amphetamines and cocaine, psychological dependence can cause compulsive use. If used daily, tolerance develops rather quickly, as with the amphetamines.

Toxicity. Major problems seen with MDMA abuse consist of a high body temperature resulting from the effects of the drug plus dehydration caused by physical exertion, the combination of which has caused death in some users. High-dose use also results in high blood pressure and seizure activity much like that seen in amphetamine overdose. Following an "ecstasy" experience, users have also been known to become extremely depressed and suicidal. Despite the claim that the drug does not produce major psychedelic reactions, high-dose use has resulted in an acute anxiety reaction ("bum trip"), prolonged reaction, and even flashbacks.

In recent experiments, it was found that MDMA damages serotonin neurons in the brain. Since it releases less adrenaline than most amphetamines, a user doesn't receive quite as much sympathetic nervous stimulation of heart rate and blood pressure.

"Rave" Clubs. One of the dangerous effects of MDMA, becoming overheated and dehydrated, has much to do with the way the drug is being used. Starting in 1990 in Europe, particularly in the Netherlands and England and quickly spreading to the United States, there has been an upsurge in "rave" clubs, dance and party clubs where drug taking is common. Anywhere from a few hundred to thousands of young people attend these gatherings. Some of the clubs are legal and some are nomadic. Flyers are handed out during the week for a party at an empty warehouse that weekend. "Rave" clubs have become so popular that they have become a big business enterprise.

These clubs hark back to the psychedelic ballrooms of the 1960s where not only

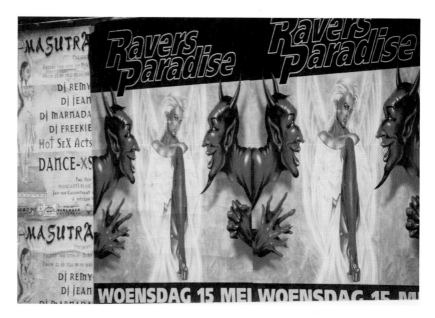

In Amsterdam in the Netherlands, "rave" clubs have fewer worries about being busted for drugs than do clubs in the United States since drug use in Amsterdam is quasi-legal.

light shows, the music of the times, and current hip fashions were on display but where marijuana, LSD, amphetamine, and almost any other abused drug were common. In the "rave" clubs of the '90s, the drugs of choice are MDMA, LSD, amphetamines, marijuana, volatile nitrites, and of course alcohol. Combinations of these drugs are also being used, e.g., "ecstasy" and LSD called "X's and L's," "flip flops," or "candy snaps"; "speedballs" of "ecstasy" and heroin; "ecstasy" and methamphetamine; "ecstasy" and the so-called "smart drugs" or "smart drinks," such as ephedrine, vasopressin, or amino acid. Further, there has been an increasing use of other psychedelic drugs at these "raves," including "euphoria," 2CB, CBR, GHB, and "illusion."

A recent variation of the nomadic "raves" are "desert raves." Invitations are passed out during the week, designating a location in the desert or some isolated piece of property. Hundreds of "ravers" show up to party and take drugs. There have been problems with environmental damage from so many people on an ecologically sensitive piece of land. Medically, "ravers" have suffered from overheating or hypothermia from the hot sun in the daytime and later, from the cold night desert air aggravated by the effects of certain drugs on body temperature (e.g., alcohol causes heat loss).

STP (DOM) (4 methyl 2,5 dimethoxy amphetamine)

STP, also called the "serenity," "tranquillity," and "peace pill," is similar to MDA. It causes a 12-hour intoxication characterized by intense stimulation and several mild psychedelic reactions. There are, however, reports that it is a "thicker" "duller" trip than those experienced from mescaline or LSD. The combination of STP and LSD, called "pinks" and "purple (or orange) wedges," was popular in the late 1960s but is rarely seen in the '90s because of the high incidence of bad trips in the '60s.

BELLADONNA AND OTHER ANTICHOLINERGIC PSYCHEDELICS

BELLADONNA, HENBANE, MANDRAKE, DATURA (jimsonweed, thornapple)

From ancient Greek times through the Middle Ages and the Renaissance, these plants, which contain scopolamine, hyoscyamine, and atropine, have been used in magic ceremonies, sorcery, witchcraft (Black Mass), and religious rituals. They've also been used as a poison, to mimic insanity, and even as a beauty aid by ancient Greek, Roman, and Egyptian women because they dilate pupils. In fact, *belladonna* in Latin means beautiful woman. Datura is more widely grown and references to it are found in Chinese, Indian, Greek, and Aztec history.

One of the effects of these plants is to block acetylcholine receptors in the central nervous system. Acetylcholine helps regulate reflexes, aggression, sleep, blood pressure, heart rate, sexual behavior, mental acuity, and attention. This disruptive effect can cause a form of delirium, make it hard to focus, speed up the heart, create an intense thirst, and raise the body temperature to dangerous levels. Anticholinergics also create some hallucinations, a separation from reality, and a deep sleep for up to 48

hours. They are still used today by some native tribes in Mexico and Africa. Synthetic anticholinergic prescription drugs, like Cogentin® and Artane®, which are used to treat the side effects of antipsychotic drugs and Parkinson's disease symptoms, are diverted from legal sources and abused for their psychedelic effects. Further, even belladonna cigarettes (Asmador®), used to treat asthma, are abused by young people in search of a cheap high.

PCP AND OTHER PSYCHEDELICS

PCP

Phencyclidine or PCP, also called "angel dust," "peep," "KJ," "Shermans," or "ozone," is usually misrepresented as THC or LSD. Two other names used for PCP are "ice" and "krystal," which are also the street names for methamphetamine. Many users end up with PCP instead of the methamphetamine they were looking for and the unexpected effects can be hazardous.

PCP was originally created as a general anesthetic for humans. However, the frequency and severity of toxic effects soon limited its use to veterinary medicine and use of PCP was later even discontinued in veterinary medicine. Now, the only supplies are illegal. PCP can be smoked in a joint, snorted, swallowed, or injected. It appears to distort sensory messages sent to the central nervous system. It stifles inhibitions, deadens pain, and results in an experience which has been described by users as a separation of the mind from the body.

"If you smoke it, depending on how strong the joint is, you just kind of get a floating sensation about one minute after you take

PCP ("angel dust") comes in liquid, crystal, or a powder. It is often smoked in a Sherman® cigarette or sprinkled on a marijuana joint. It can also be snorted, swallowed, or injected and is often misrepresented as THC, the active ingredient in marijuana.

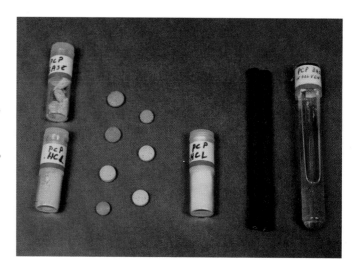

your first few tokes. And you just get a really numbed sensation. I mean, there are actual rooms I go in that don't exist."
Recovering PCP user

Since PCP is so strong, particularly for first-time users, the range between a dose that produces a pleasant sensory deprivation effect and one that induces catatonia, coma, or convulsions is very small. Low dosages (2–5 milligrams) produce first mild depression, then stimulation. Moderate doses (10–15 milligrams) can produce a desirable sensory-deprived state. They can also produce extremely high blood pressure and very combative behavior. Other adverse reactions to moderate doses include an inability to talk, rigid or robotic movements, tremors, confusion, agitation, and paranoid thinking. Dosages just a little higher, above 20 milligrams, can cause catatonia, coma, and convulsions. Large PCP doses have also produced seizures, respiratory depression, cardiovascular instability, and even kidney failure. PCP also induces amnesia in people under its influence.

"I've had seizures before on it and banged my head really hard—continually, on hard objects—and got lots of bumps and everything and felt them the next few days but never realized I was doing it and never felt hurt from it." Recovering PCP user

The effects of a small dose of PCP will last 1–2 hours but the effects of a large dose can last much longer (up to 48 hours), longer than effects produced by a similar dose of LSD. Further, current evidence shows that PCP is retained by the body for several months in fatty cells. The PCP stored in fat can be released during exercise or fasting, resulting in a true chemical PCP flashback. The flashback also results because of the drug's recirculation from the brain, to the blood, to the stomach, to the intestines, then back to the blood and brain. This is called enterogastric recirculation.

PCP is not widely used by the general drug-using population because of the frequency of bad trips associated with it. PCP is often sold as THC or mescaline to unsuspecting drug users. When the psychedelic effects kick in, surprised users can have a bad trip and not even remember what happened during the trip. Sometimes they even forget that they used the drug. However, PCP can cause an emotional addiction resulting in high levels of abuse in certain populations.

Some studies of patients handled by the Los Angeles County Psychiatric Emergency Unit found PCP in a large percentage of patient urine samples despite the fact that it was rarely reported as having been used by patients on admittance to the crisis center.

KETAMINE (Ketalar®, Ketajet®, "super-K")

A close relative of PCP, ketamine is still available by prescription. It is used as a surgical anesthetic to control severe pain and is not as closely watched as other restricted drugs. It is available by being easily diverted from medical and veterinary supplies. It is usually injected but can be evaporated to solid crystals, powdered and smoked, snorted, or swallowed. The liquid containing ketamine is heated which causes the chemical to form a crystalline structure. These crystals are then smoked like "crack" or PCP, making it easy to abuse. Users experience a disassociation effect which separates the mind from the body senses. They enter a dreamlike state, often filled with illusions and even hallucinations which last for about six hours. They are also impervious to pain, such as that caused by injuries sustained by rough activities like dancing in a "mosh pit" at rock concerts where people bang against each other. Because of these effects, ketamine has recently become popular as a "rave" club drug and is also often abused by veterinarians. Since its effects are similar to those of PCP, toxic reactions, such as coma, convulsions, and combative

or belligerent behavior, also result from its misuse.

AMANITA MUSHROOMS

Most members of this family of mushrooms, except the *Amanita muscaria* (fly agaric) and the *Amanita pantherina* (panther mushroom), are deadly. The *Amanita muscaria* can cause dreamy intoxication, hallucinations, and delirious excitement though there are also some dangerous physical toxic effects as well. The effects start a half an hour after ingestion and can last for four to eight hours. The active ingredients are ibotenic acid and the alkaloid muscimole.

The amanita mushroom is mentioned in sacred writings in India in 1500 B.C. where it is referred to as the god Soma. Statues of the mushroom found in Mexico and dating back to 100 A.D. indicate its early use in the Americas. Amanita has also been used by native tribes in Siberia but its use is limited in the modern age because of the unpredictability of its effects and because many deadly mushrooms can be mistaken for it. The use of *Amanita muscaria* in ancient ritual ceremonies is still practiced today by some Ojibway Indians in Michigan.

NUTMEG, MACE

At the low end of the "desirable" psychedelic drug spectrum, nutmeg and mace, both from the nutmeg tree, can cause varied effects from a mild floating sensation to a full-blown delirium. So much has to be consumed (about 20 grams) that the user is left with a bad hangover and a severely upset stomach. The active chemicals in nutmeg and mace are variants of MDA (methylenedioxyamphetamine). Since this dose exposes a user to the nauseating and toxic effects of other chemicals in nutmeg, its abuse is extremely rare outside of prisons where convicts are driven to use it since they have limited access to other psychedelics.

MARIJUANA AND OTHER CANNABINOLS

The Cannabis or hemp plant, also called marijuana, produces fibers used to make rope, cloth, roofing materials, and floor coverings. It grows edible seeds (akenes), an oil that is used as a fuel and lubricant, a number of other active ingredients that can treat various illnesses, and a psychedelic resin that can alter consciousness.

"The marijuana high—it's relaxing, it's pleasant. It opens the other side of the mind. It's like the left side saying 'Hi,' to the right and they're saying, 'Hey, we're together. We're having fun.'"
50-year-old marijuana smoker

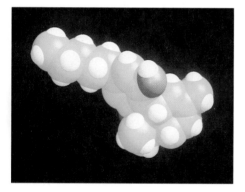

Computerized chemical model of Δ-9-tetrahydrocannabinol or THC, the main active psychedelic component in marijuana.
Courtesy of the Molecular Imaging Department, University of California Medical Center, San Francisco

Marijuana is also written about endlessly, researched in dozens of laboratories, smoked in hundreds of countries, and forbidden by thousands of laws. And, in spite of the fact that research has led to the discovery of neurotransmitters and receptor sites that are specific for marijuana, uncertainty is still prevalent in many medical, political, legal, and user circles as to the real benefits and dangers of the drug.

HISTORY OF USE

The relationship between Cannabis and humans has existed for at least 10,000 years. From its probable origin in China or central Asia in Neolithic times, hemp cultivation has spread to almost every country in the world. There are a variety of species. Some are better for fiber, some for food, and some for inducing psychedelic effects.

The first use of the plant was probably as a source of nutrition since Neolithic man (after 6500 B.C.) were always searching for food. When parts of the plant were eaten, our ancient ancestors doubtless experienced some psychedelic effects, particularly if the species had a high enough concentration of psychedelic chemicals. Next, Cannabis was most likely tried as a source of fiber. After that, various medicine men and women experimented with Cannabis for its medicinal benefits. Finally, different ways to extract and consume psychedelic parts of the plant were discovered.

The Indian *Vedas,* around 1500 B.C., described Cannabis as a divine nectar that could deter evil, bring luck, and cleanse a person of sin. Indian writings also described its medicinal use to relieve headaches, control mania, counteract insomnia, treat venereal disease, cure whooping cough, and even arrest tuberculosis.

Galen wrote in 200 A.D. that it was sometimes customary to give marijuana to guests to induce enjoyment and mirth.

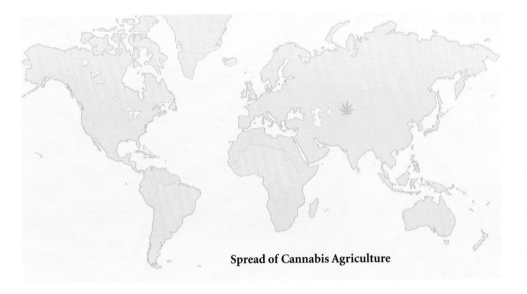

Spread of Cannabis Agriculture

Figure 6-2 •
From its origin in central Asia, Cannabis has spread to almost every country.

Ropes and sails were made from the fiber in third century Rome. Medieval physicians recommended weedy hemp to treat cancer and cultivated hemp for jaundice and coughs. Because Cannabis was not specifically banned in the Koran by the Prophet Mohammed, Islamic cultures spread its use to Africa and Europe. In Africa, it was used in social and religious rituals and in medicinal preparations to treat dysentery, fevers, and even the pain of childbirth.

Starting in the fifteenth century, the Age of Exploration increased the need for rope, sails, and paper, so many colonies were introduced to Cannabis and encouraged to grow and export the more fibrous variants. Even George Washington had large fields of it growing on his plantation to produce hemp. Cannabis was widely cultivated in the Americas until the nineteenth century when the end of slavery made it less profitable to grow.

Mexican laborers who worked in the United States introduced Americans to the habit of smoking marijuana for its psychedelic effects after World War I. Initially, its use was confined to poor and minority groups but in the 1920s, the use of Cannabis as a substitute for the prohibited alcohol spread its popularity. In the 1930s, the expanded use of marijuana alarmed prohibitionists who were left without a cause when the Eighteenth Amendment, which banned the sale of alcohol, was repealed. Marijuana, the Mexican word for Cannabis, was popularized by the Hearst newspapers in a series of crusading articles against use of the drug. The use of Cannabis (except for sterilized bird seed and medical treatment) was banned by the Marijuana Act of 1937. Although medical use was still permitted, any prescribing of the substance was actively discouraged.

The fear of an interruption in the importation of hemp fiber to America during

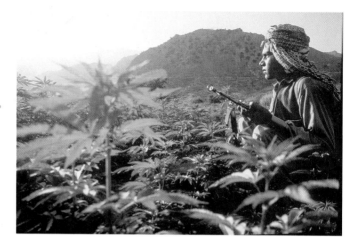

A young Uzbekistan tribesman guards his fields of marijuana.

Reprinted, by permission, Alain Labrousse, Observatoire Geopolitique Des Drogues.

World War II temporarily lifted the ban on growing the plant but since the end of the war, its use has been illegal in the United States as well as in most other countries worldwide. The level of prohibition varies widely from country to country. In spite of restrictions, marijuana is used in some form by 200–300 million people worldwide. In addition, several countries are cultivating a fibrous variant of the Cannabis plant to supply pulp and fiber to make paper, textiles, and rope. France, Italy, Yugoslavia, and to a lesser extent England and Canada now grow hemp.

EPIDEMIOLOGY

"My parents were hippies, so having drugs around wasn't like a bring down or anything and this was in the '70s when it was peace, love, and everything was happening on a cool, mellow level. So, you know, I enjoyed being the little kid around with a bunch of partying hippies in their 20s just having a good time. So, I was very much accustomed to having 'pot' and smoking it."
25-year-old marijuana smoker

In 1960, only 2% of people in the United States (3–4 million) had tried any illegal drug. By the mid-'60s, the growth of the counterculture, fueled by the baby boom, greatly increased the psychedelic use of marijuana and other illicit drugs. By 1979, 68 million people in the United States had tried marijuana and 23 million were using it on a monthly basis. The popularity of the drug led 10 states to decriminalize possession of small amounts of the drug for personal use but by the '90s, the resurgence of the concept of complete prohibition had recriminalized use of the drug in most states (and greatly increased the number of people in prison for marijuana possession). By 1992, the monthly rate of use had dropped to 1/3 of its 1979 peak level of use but recently, those levels have begun to climb, particularly among teenagers. By 1995, more than 10 million Americans were using marijuana on a monthly basis.

"Coming into high school there's a lot of pressures and stuff socially and academically and it's like a break for me. Me and my friends would run out of school Friday and smoke. It was like a little vacation for a night." *16-year-old smoker*

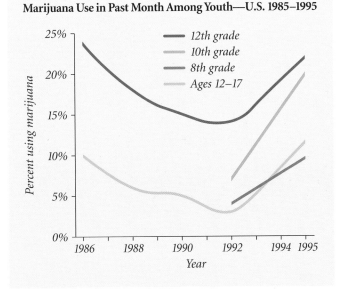

Marijuana Use in Past Month Among Youth—U.S. 1985–1995

- 12th grade
- 10th grade
- 8th grade
- Ages 12–17

BOTANY

There is much confusion over the various terms used to describe the Cannabis plant. *Cannabis* is the botanical genus of all these plants. Hemp is generally used to describe Cannabis plants that are high in fiber content, whereas marijuana is used to describe Cannabis plants that are high in psychoactive components.

"Back in the old days they had all the 'Michoacan,' 'Panama red,' 'Acapulco gold,' and all that stuff. I had no problem with that. But when all that faded out and the only thing left was like sinsemilla and Thai stick, that's when I started thinking about quitting. Number one, it became so expensive and number two, it caused that draining high where you would just sit around and just kind of not be there."

43-year-old recovering compulsive marijuana smoker

Species

Marijuana (the psychedelic Cannabis plant) has many street names: "pot," "buds," "herb," "chronic," "dank," "the kind," grass," "ganja," "charas," "sens," "weed," and "dope." There are also hundreds of strains that sound like brand names: "Maui wowie," "Humboldt green," "British Columbia bud," and "Buddha Thai." Constant experimentation by growers has resulted in variations in the size, concentration of psychoactive resin, and even shape of leaf. Some botanists say that *Cannabis sativa* is the only true species. Many other botanists think that there are three distinct species. Unfortunately, intensive hybridization and cultivation has made them hard to identify. In this book we will identify three species: *Cannabis sativa, Cannabis ruderalis,* and *Cannabis indica.*

The most common species is *Cannabis sativa,* grown throughout the world. Variations of *Cannabis sativa* have sufficient quantities of active resins to cause psychedelic phenomena while other variations have a high concentration of fiber and are used for hemp. It grows easily in tropical, subtropical, and temperate regions. The average plant will grow from 5–12 feet tall but can grow up to 20 feet. There are generally five thin serrated leaves on each stem. A typical plant will produce between one to five pounds of buds and smokable leaves, both of which contain the highest concentration of the psychedelic resin. *Cannabis ruderalis*, a small thin species, has few psychoactive components and is especially plentiful in Siberia and western Asia. The third species, *Cannabis indica*, is a shorter, bushier plant with fatter leaves and is generally not used for its fibers. It is especially

plentiful in the Middle East and India and is the source of most of the world's hashish. Modifications of *Cannabis indica* have resulted in a stronger, smellier variety of this plant nicknamed "skunk weed." Many illegal growers have come to prefer *Cannabis indica* as the base plant on which to use the sinsemilla-growing technique.

Sinsemilla

The sinsemilla-growing technique, used with both *Cannabis indica* and *Cannabis sativa* plants, increases the potency of the marijuana plant. The sinsemilla technique involves separating female plants from male plants before pollination. Female plants produce more

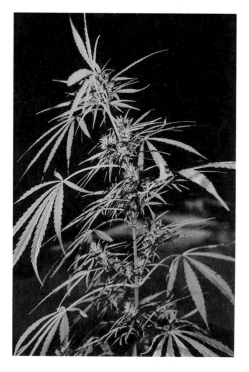

Female flowering top of Cannabis sativa *with relatively long slender leaf projections.*

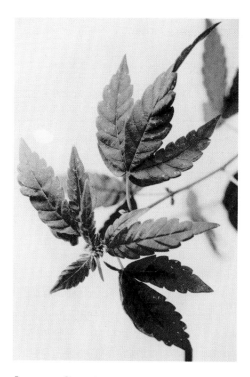

Immature Cannabis indica *with shorter stout leaves.*

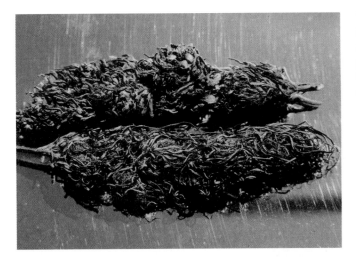

Two marijuana buds grown by the sinsemilla technique are saturated with THC, the psychedelic ingredient in marijuana.

psychoactive resin than male plants especially when they are unpollinated and therefore bear no seeds. *Sinsemilla* means without seeds in Spanish. (The term commercial grade refers to marijuana that is not grown by the sinsemilla technique.)

Marijuana buds, leaves, and flowers can be crushed and rolled into cigarettes. They can also be used in food or in drinks or the leaves can be chewed. In India, marijuana is divided into three different strengths, each one coming from a different part of the plant. Bhang is made from the stem and leaves and has the lowest potency. Ganja is made from the stronger leaves and flowering tops. Charas is the concentrated resin from the plant and is the most potent. The sticky resin which contains most of the psychoactive ingredients can be collected and pressed into cakes. This concentrated form, called hashish, is usually smoked in special pipes called bongs or hookahs or it can be added to a joint to enhance the potency of weaker leaves.

Hash oil can be extracted from the plant (using solvents) and added to foods. Most often it is smeared onto rolling paper or dripped onto crushed marijuana leaves to enhance the psychoactive effects of marijuana cigarettes called joints.

Growers

The majority of marijuana used in the United States comes from Mexico and Columbia, according to the U.S. Department of State. In addition, tens of thousands of Americans grow their own marijuana, either a few plants for their own use or hundreds, even thousands, for large-scale dealing. Because of stiffer penalties and greater surveillance by law enforcement agencies, more growers are moving their operations indoors.

PHARMACOLOGY

At last count, researchers had discovered some 360 chemicals in a single Cannabis plant. At least 30 of these chemicals have been studied for their psychoactive effects. The most potent psychoactive chemical is considered to be the cannabinoid called Δ9 tetrahydrocannabinol or THC. When smoked or ingested, this potent psychoactive chemical is converted by the liver

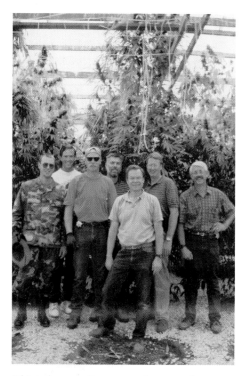

This indoor marijuana-growing operation was raided by JACNET, a drug task force run by the Sheriff's Department in Jackson County, Oregon. Growers can use grow lights or filtered sunlight to avoid detection by law enforcement agencies or passers-by.

into over 60 other metabolites, some of which are also psychoactive. In addition, the sinsemilla technique has increased the concentration of THC from 1% to 3% in the 1960s to 6% to 14% in the '80s and made potent marijuana more readily available on the streets. What this means is that a user would have to smoke 5 to 14 of the weak joints from the 1960s to equal just 1 of the stronger joints readily available in the 1990s. Unfor-tunately, many of the studies on marijuana and many of the attitudes of the counterculture about the effects of the drug were based on the weaker plants. There has been an increase in research over the last few years using a higher potency form of the drug (4–5% THC).

Recent Discoveries

In the last few years, three important discoveries were made that have greatly expanded knowledge of the way marijuana works. The first was the discovery in 1992 at John Hopkins University of receptor sites in the brain that were specifically reactive to the THC in marijuana. This discovery implied that the brain had its own natural neurotransmitters that fit into these receptor sites which affected the same areas of the brain as marijuana.

In 1995, the National Institute on Drug Abuse announced the discovery of anandamide, the natural neurotransmitter that fits into the receptor sites. Receptors for anandamide were found in several areas of the limbic system, including the reward-pleasure center. Other parts of the brain with anandamide receptor sites are those regulating the integration of sensory experiences with emotions as well as those controlling functions of learning, motor coordination, and some automatic body functions. The presence of anandamide receptors means that these are the areas of the brain most affected by marijuana. It is important that there are few anandamide receptors in the brain stem for marijuana compared to enkephalin receptors for opioids and norepinephrine receptors for cocaine. Since involvement of this area of the brain that controls heart rate, respiration, and other body functions is the reason dangerous overdoses can occur with cocaine and opioids, it helps explain why it is so difficult to physically overdose with marijuana.

The discovery by French scientists in 1994 of an antagonist that instantly blocks the effects of marijuana enables researchers to search for true signs of tolerance, tissue dependence, and withdrawal symptoms in long-term users. They can conduct their search by using the antagonist to precipitate withdrawal in a long-term marijuana user and by studying the symptoms.

SHORT-TERM EFFECTS

Physical Effects

The immediate physical effects of marijuana often include physical relaxation or sedation, bloodshot eyes, coughing from lung irritation, an increase in appetite, and a loss in muscular coordination. Other physical effects include an increased heart rate, decreased blood pressure, decreased pressure behind the eyes (Marinol® capsules or marijuana joints are used as a treatment for glaucoma), and decreased nausea (capsules and joints are also used for cancer patients undergoing chemotherapy).

Marijuana impairs tracking ability (the ability to follow a moving object, such as a baseball) and causes a trailing phenomenon where one sees an after-image of a moving object. Impaired tracking ability, the trailing phenomena, and sedating effects make it more difficult to perform tasks which require depth perception and good hand-eye coordination, such as flying an airplane or catching a football pass.

Marijuana can act as a stimulant as well as a depressant, depending on the variety and amount of chemical that is absorbed in the brain, the setting in which it is used, and the personality of the user.

"Marijuana is not a downer for me, it's a speed thing. I have plenty of friends who smoke marijuana and become quiet. They can't speak. They become immobile. They're total veggies, you know, sitting around and cannot move, whereas I become more active." Marijuana smoker

Marijuana also causes a small temporary disruption of the secretion of the male hormone testosterone. That might be important to a user with hormonal imbalance or somebody in the throes of puberty and sexual maturation.

Mental Effects

Within a few minutes of smoking marijuana, the user becomes a bit confused and mentally separated from the environment. It produces a feeling of deja vu where everything seems familiar but really isn't. Additional effects include detachment, an aloof feeling, drowsiness, and difficulty concentrating.

"It's kind of like life without a coherent thought. It's kind of like an escape. It's like when you go to sleep, you forget about things. It's like everything's dreamlike and there's no restraints on anything. You can have freedom to say what you want to say." 16-year-old marijuana smoker

Stronger varieties of marijuana can produce a giddiness, stimulation with increased alertness, and major distortions and perceptions of time, color, and sound. Very strong doses can even produce a sensation of movement under one's feet, visual illusions, and even hallucinations. One of the most frequently mentioned psychological problems with smoking marijuana is paranoia and a deeper depersonification (detachment from one's sense of self.)

"I'd keep smoking and keep smoking and keep smoking and I'd get paranoid. If you're not relaxed and having fun, it seems really insane to keep doing it and I did keep doing it for a long time after I had started developing fear." 35-year-old marijuana user

Like most psychedelics, the mental effects of marijuana are very dependent on the mood of the smoker and the surroundings. Marijuana acts somewhat like a mild hypnotic. Charles Baudelair, the nineteenth century French poet, referred to it as a "mirror that magnifies." It exaggerates mood and personality and makes smokers more empathetic to others' feelings but also makes them more suggestible.

"I mean, sometimes, in some relationships, it helps me to think about it and maybe I come up with a solution for my problem or whatever but sometimes it wouldn't, so it's a very back and forth type deal. It could go either way."
17-year-old recovering compulsive marijuana user

Marijuana disrupts short-term memory but not long-term memory.

"I'd be doing the job and all of a sudden I'd look up and freeze and not know what to do. I would have a handful of checks in my hand and just look at the machine for a while and just think to myself, 'What is this and what do I do with it?'"
Recovering marijuana addict

The loss of a sense of time is responsible for several of the perceived effects of marijuana. Dull repetitive jobs seem to go by faster. In Jamaica, some cane field workers smoke ganja (marijuana) to make their hard monotonous work pass by more quickly. On the other hand, students who smoke marijuana while studying get easily bored and often abandon their books.

The effects of mental confusion, distortion of the passage of time, impaired judgment, and short-term memory loss result in a user's inability to perform multiple and interactive tasks, like programming a VCR, while under the influence of marijuana.

LONG-TERM EFFECTS

Respiratory Problems

THC is a bronchodilator; it opens up the airways, at least initially. As smoking becomes chronic, so does irritation to the breathing passages. Since marijuana is unfiltered, harsh, crudely grown, and held in the lungs when inhaled, smoking four to five joints gives the same harmful exposure to the lungs and mucous membranes as smoking a full pack of cigarettes according to studies by Dr. Donald Tashkin at UCLA. For these and other reasons, a major concern of health professionals is the damaging effect that marijuana smoking has on the respiratory system. Marijuana smoking on a regular basis leads to symptoms of acute and chronic bronchitis. In microscopic studies of these mucous membranes, Dr. Tashkin has found that most damage occurs in the lungs of those who smoke both cigarettes and marijuana. This is significant because most marijuana smokers also smoke cigarettes.

"I'm sure I've done some damage to my lungs. I mean, you can't put that kind of tar down in your system, heated tar going into your system constantly for 23 years and sit here and say there's nothing wrong and nothing has happened."
Marijuana smoker

In the series of slides, the normal ciliated surface epithelial cells in the mucous membranes of a nonsmoker of either cigarettes or marijuana (Fig. 6-4A) show healthy densely packed cilia which clear the breathing passages of mucous, dust, and debris.

The breathing passage of a chronic smoker of only marijuana (Fig. 6-4B) shows increased numbers of mucous-secreting surface epithelial cells which do not have cilia, so phlegm production is increased but is not cleared as readily from the breathing passages. The result is increased coughing and chronic bronchitis. Some of the changes involve the nucleus,

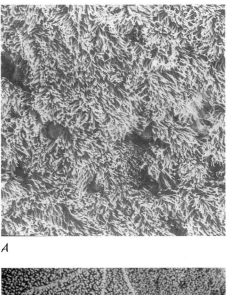

A

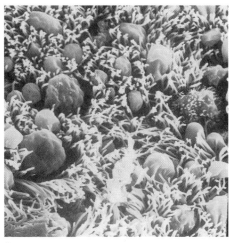

B

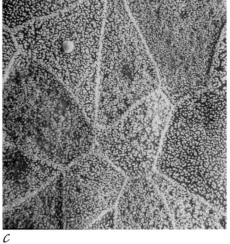

C

Figure 6-4 • (2,000 magnification)

A. Healthy mucous membrane of nonsmoker.

B. Mucous membrane of a marijuana smoker.

C. Mucous membrane of a marijuana and
   cigarette smoker.

Courtesy of Dr. Donald Tashkin, Chief, Pulmonary
Research Department, UCLA Medical Center, Los
Angeles

suggesting that malignancy may be a consequence of regular marijuana smoking since some of these changes are precursors of cancer.

Finally, the breathing passage of a chronic marijuana and cigarette smoker (Fig. 6-4C) shows that the normal surface cells have been completely replaced by nonciliated cells resembling skin, so the smoker has to cough to clear mucous from the lungs since the ciliated cells are gone. This leads to acute and chronic bronchitis.

Marijuana and cigarette smokers also have a greatly increased risk for developing cancer of the tongue, cancer of the larynx, and cancer of the lung.

Immune System

Some evidence suggests that heavy use can depress the immune system, making users more susceptible to a cold, the flu, and other viral infections. If such were the case, it would be a mistake for people who are already immune depressed, either as a result of AIDS or as a result of chemotherapy for cancer, to smoke marijuana for therapeutic purposes. The smoker is further suppressing an already depressed immune system and exposing the lungs to pathogens, such as fungi and bacteria, found in marijuana smoke.

Learning and Emotional Maturation

"If you go home and have homework to do that night and you say, 'O.K. I'm going to get stoned before I do my homework,' you're never going to get your homework done."
High school student

Marijuana has been shown to slow learning and disrupt concentration. Part of this influence comes from marijuana's effect on short-term memory. Short-term memory, in contrast to long-term memory, is a processing of information to be retained for only a short period of time, such as a grocery list, a proper assortment of tools for a certain job, or facts crammed into the head for an upcoming exam. Marijuana greatly impairs a person's ability to retain this information. However, it has very little effect on long-term memory which is the processing of information for a long period of time, such as a theory in physics that has been studied for several weeks. This explains why some students have been able to maintain good grades while using marijuana on a regular basis while others end up flunking out.

Although more research is needed into what some researchers call an amotivational syndrome, a number of chronic users do show a lack of motivation. They have a tendency to avoid problems.

"You know how they tell you go to school to get an education so you can get a good job?

They did tell me how to get a job, so that's eight hours a day. I knew how to sleep, that's eight hours a day. I had another eight hours a day that I didn't know how to fill and I used marijuana to fill those eight hours. Period."
38-year-old recovering compulsive marijuana smoker

The way this mechanism operates is similar to the effects of other psychoactive drugs. What happens is that a drug can be used as a shortcut to a pleasing physical sensation or as a way to counteract boredom or emotional pain. If users then come to depend on this method for gaining pleasure or avoiding pain rather than learning how to receive pleasure and satisfaction naturally or face up to and deal with painful situations directly, they will habituate their minds and bodies to this chemical solution.

"I liked to do it so much that, it's like, why not do it? I couldn't find a reason for not doing it. It was too enjoyable. It was like going and looking in your refrigerator and seeing a thing of ice cream and a thing of Hershey's chocolate syrup and going, 'No, I'm going to have a bran muffin instead.' Why? You can have ice cream and the chocolate syrup, man. That's what you want. Why don't you have it?"
17-year-old marijuana smoker

Since marijuana can be "the mirror that magnifies," smoking often exaggerates natural tendencies in the user. Thus, if a person really isn't interested in working, studying, having a relationship, or reading a book and smokes marijuana, his or her primitive brain is given the edge over the new brain and says, "You don't have to do those things." So rather than the new brain, the neocortex, giving guidance and saying, "These are necessary things that you're going to have to do," the primitive brain takes over and says, "Forget it, let's not do this."

"When I got high, I thought I was the smartest person in the world. I knew I had the answer to everything and one day, I sat down with the tape recorder and I started rattling off all this brilliance that I had and the next day when I woke up in the morning and I played it back, it was almost like I wasn't even speaking English."
Recovering user in Marijuana Anonymous 12-step program

With marijuana, many thoughts and feelings are internalized. Long-term marijuana smokers feel that they're thinking, feeling, and communicating better but often they're not.

"When I have worked with couples where one of the principal partners in the relationship has been using marijuana for a long period of time, the biggest complaint is that 'He never says anything' or 'She never says anything.' 'We don't talk. We don't communicate.' But for the marijuana user, that person feels when they're under the influence that they are trying to communicate. So the intentions are there, the feelings are there, and the emotions are there but it's all internal. It never gets out to the other person." *Counselor, Haight-Ashbury Detox Clinic*

Acute Mental Effects

Lasting mental problems from short-term use are unusual but in someone with preexisting mental problems or with latent emotional problems, particularly if marijuana with high THC levels is smoked, acute anxiety or temporary psychotic reactions can occur. Individuals believe that

they have lost control of their mental state. There's often paranoia or a belief that they have severely damaged themselves or that their underlying insecurities are insurmountable. These acute problems are usually treatable but what is problematic is when the symptoms persist. In medicine, this is called a post-hallucinogenic drug perceptual disorder where people who, after experiencing a bad trip, don't come all the way down and may have problems going on with their lives.

"I'm working with a 13-year-old client who had no premorbid symptoms that could be identified prior to his 13th birthday when his friends turned him on to a 'honey blunt,' which is a cigar packed with marijuana. It happened to be very strong sinsemilla and he experienced an acute anxiety reaction followed by a post-hallucinogenic drug perceptual disorder, including a profound depression and an inability to concentrate. We don't know how long these problems will last."
Counselor, Haight-Ashbury Detox Clinic

Even seasoned veteran smokers who've been smoking some low-grade "pot" and then get some strong "Buddha Thai" sinsemilla may feel that somebody has slipped them a psychedelic, like PCP or LSD. They begin to experience anxiety and paranoia which then create more anxiety than what they were feeling. Eventually, they could have an acute psychotic break.

TOLERANCE, WITHDRAWAL, AND ADDICTION

Tolerance

Tolerance to marijuana occurs in a rapid and dramatic fashion. Although high-dose chronic users can recognize the effects of low levels of THC in their systems, they are able to tolerate much higher levels without some of the more severe emotional and psychic effects experienced by a first-time user.

"When you smoke a certain type of marijuana all the time, I think you get used to it. It takes more to get high. And that's why a lot of times I switch what I'm smoking— different types of 'pot'—because I get used to it so quickly." 22-year-old musician

One great concern about marijuana is that it persists in the body of a chronic user for up to 6 months though the major effects last only 4–6 hours after smoking. These residual amounts in the body can disrupt some physiological, mental, and emotional functions for a longer period.

Casual use of marijuana may result in positive urine tests for about 5–7 days, daily use for about 10–15 days, and chronic heavy use for about 12 months. However, some users try to stretch the truth too much when they have a positive result in a preemployment drug screening test by claiming they had one joint 6 months ago. Urine drug testing is nowhere near that sensitive (Fig. 6-5).

Withdrawal

Because there is not the rapid onset of withdrawal from marijuana as with alcohol or heroin, many people deny that withdrawal occurs. The withdrawal from marijuana is more drawn out because most of the THC has been retained in the fat cells and only after a period of abstinence will the withdrawal effects appear.

"Sometimes people who've been smoking for five years decide to quit. They stop one, two, three days, even a week, and they say (especially those who think marijuana is be-

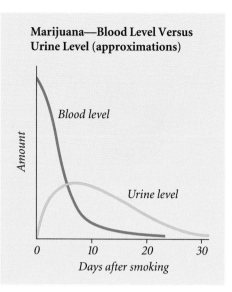

Marijuana—Blood Level Versus Urine Level (approximations)

Figure 6–5 •

This chart shows the blood and urine levels of marijuana over time. The marijuana persists in the urine longer than in the blood. Most drug testing only measures marijuana in the urine.

nign), 'Wow, I feel great. Marijuana's no problem. I have no withdrawal. It's nothing at all.' Then they start up again. They never experience withdrawal. We see that withdrawal symptoms to marijuana are delayed sometimes for several weeks to a month after a person stops."
Counselor, Haight-Ashbury Detox Clinic

The delayed withdrawal effects of marijuana include

- anger or irritability;
- aches, pains, chills;
- depression;
- inability to concentrate;
- slight tremors;
- sleep disturbances;
- decreased appetite;

- sweating;
- craving.

Not everyone will experience all of these effects but everyone will experience some of them, especially craving.

"I could break into a sweat in the shower. I could not maintain my concentration for the first month or two. To really treasure my sobriety it took me about three or four months before I really came out of the fog and really started getting a grasp of what was going on around me."
42-year-old recovering marijuana addict

Recent experiments have demonstrated that cessation of marijuana use can cause true physical withdrawal symptoms. Dr. Billy Martin of the Medical College of Virginia gave the THC antagonist SR14176A to rats who had been exposed to marijuana for 4 days in a row. The antagonist negated the influence of the marijuana. Within 10 minutes, the rats exhibited immediate physical withdrawal behaviors that included "wet dog shakes" and facial rubbing which is the rat equivalent of withdrawal. These experiments indicated that marijuana dependence occurs more rapidly than previously suspected. This experiment, which compressed the withdrawal to minutes instead of weeks, allowed the addictive potential of cannabinoids to be more clearly understood. Further, human studies have demonstrated rapid eye movement (REM) sleep changes, similar to those seen in other drug addictions: decreased REM while smoking marijuana and increased REM during withdrawal.

Addiction

"I thought I could control it because when I woke up in the morning, I didn't get high for the first hour or hour and a half. I figured an hour and a half, that proves that I'm not hooked on this stuff because I don't really need it."
Recovering user in Marijuana Anonymous 12-step program

The 1990s has made us take a different view of the addiction potential of this substance. Today, many people smoke the drug in a chronic compulsive way and have difficulty discontinuing their use. Like cocaine, heroin, alcohol, nicotine, and other addictive drugs, marijuana does have the ability to induce compulsive use in spite of the negative consequences it may be causing in the user's life.

"Why am I doing this? What's wrong with me? Why do I have to keep doing this? And I did this for a good 8 to 10 years. I used to buy it by the pound and then I found after awhile that I wanted to make it harder on myself to smoke. So I started buying dime bags, figuring it would cost a lot more and then eventually, I got to the point where it didn't work. I just kept on buying. But yeah, with me, I just could not stop."
39-year-old recovering marijuana addict

Finally, all available research on marijuana was based on a THC calculation of 20 milligrams per marijuana cigarette (considered in the 1960s to be a high-dose exposure). Current marijuana joints used for research contain 40 milligrams of THC, still below most good quality street joints but closer than in the past. (The marijuana for these experimental joints are grown at a government farm in Mississippi.)

"The main problem we're dealing with today is that today's potent form of marijuana is causing a lot more problems than we saw in

the 1960s. I never treated a single self-admitted marijuana addict in the Clinic throughout the '60s nor the '70s and pretty much through the '80s but by the late '80s, we started seeing people coming in, everyone of them on their own volition saying, 'Help me. I want to stop smoking 'pot.' It is causing me these problems, causing me to have memory problems, causing me to be too spaced out, not to function in my work. I can't complete tasks. It's causing me to be sick in the morning and cough. I have withdrawal symptoms. I want to stop and I can't stop.' At our program in San Francisco, we now have about 100 patients every month who are in treatment specifically for marijuana addiction. So people who claim that marijuana is harmless have to sit down and listen to those people who are the wounded, what we call the walking wounded or the casualties from marijuana use. For them, marijuana has caused some problems—not propaganda or other people telling them it's causing problems but they themselves saying it's so."

Darryl Inaba, Director, Haight-Ashbury Detox Clinic

Is Marijuana a Gateway Drug?

In antidrug movies like "Reefer Madness" and "Marijuana, Assassin of Youth," the claim was that marijuana physically and mentally changed users, so they started using heroin and cocaine and became helpless addicts. The exaggeration of this idea led to an undermining of drug education because people who smoked marijuana didn't becoming raving lunatics or depraved dope fiends. The experimenters who had tried marijuana said, "I tried marijuana and that didn't happen, so I guess they're lying about all the drugs."

This exaggeration and resultant ridicule, particularly by the younger generation, of propagandistic or scare films and books probably caused more drug abuse than it prevented. Scare tactics also obscured an important idea, that is, the real role marijuana use plays in future drug use and abuse.

"I've been in a 12-step program [Narcotics Anonymous] for a little over six years and I'm not going to say like one and one equal two but just about everybody I meet in the 12-step program started out with either marijuana or alcohol."
Recovering marijuana addict

Marijuana is a gateway drug in the sense that if people smoke it, they will probably hang around others who smoke marijuana or use other drugs, so the opportunities and pressure to experiment with other drugs are greater. Incidentally, the history of most addicts clearly demonstrates that the first drug they ever used or abused was either tobacco or alcohol.

No two people will have the exact same reaction to marijuana but what has been observed is that those who continue to use it regularly establish a pattern of use and begin to find opportunities where drugs other than marijuana are available.

"The majority of people that I know that I hang around with, if they ain't smoking weed, they're smoking 'crack,' or drinking. I'm not saying that they are bad people but that's just how it is."
38-year-old polydrug user who started smoking marijuana at the age of 13

The Medical Use of Marijuana

Controversy has always existed around marijuana. One major area of contention is whether it should be legalized, decriminal-

Agents raid marijuana club
Operation sells drug to AIDS, cancer patients

By **MARK EVANS**
The Associated Press

SAN FRANCISCO — State drug agents on Sunday burst into the headquarters of a controversial group that sells marijuana to AIDS, cancer and other terminally ill patients and shut the operation down.

Armed with a search warrant, the agents raided the Cannabis Buyers' Club headquarters at about 7:45 a.m. and spent four hours hauling away computers, marijuana and a cabinet full of customer information.

In addition, volunteers involved

ple who were not using it for medical reasons."

Officials later said at a news conference that they suspected the club was being used as a focal point for the distribution of large quantities of marijuana under the guise of medical treatment.

Calvin Martin, a 46-year-old AIDS patient who is a member of the club, said he was sleeping near the club's back entrance to guard against burglaries when the agents swarmed in.

The Cannabis Buyers' Club has operated for at least four years, and

fact they sold the illegal drug. About a year ago, the club moved its office from a relatively obscure site to a storefront shop.

Organizers maintain that marijuana is sold only to members who furnish a photo identification and a doctor's letter certifying a condition that could be alleviated by the drug.

AIDS patients use the drug because it enhances their appetite, helping them fight weight loss and weakness. Cancer patients say it counters the waves of nausea that result from chemotherapy. Glaucoma patients use it to relieve the

The police raided the Cannabis Buyers' Club in San Francisco which had been established to make marijuana available to ill patients. The police claimed a number of the smokers weren't using it medicinally.

ized, or kept illegal. A second major area is whether it should be available for medical use.

Historically, marijuana has been used to treat insomnia, anxiety, venereal disease, whooping cough, headaches, jaundice, cancer, and dozens of other illnesses. Recently, it has been recommended for some types of glaucoma, nausea control, asthma, and to help a patient who has lost too much weight (wasting disease) to gain it back.

There is evidence that marijuana does reduce intraocular pressure, does calm nausea, and does encourage people to eat though there are other drugs that are as effective or better. Many people smoke marijuana therapeutically for their glaucoma, cancer, AIDS or other illness even though it is illegal. There are also people and places, such as the Cannabis Buyers' Club in San Francisco, that procure marijuana for those who are ill. In addition, Marinol®, a synthesized form of THC, is theoretically available for treatment of these and other health problems but in practice is hard to have

prescribed. People say they prefer marijuana in its smokable form because it works faster than Marinol®. In addition, if they smoke, they can smoke just as much or as little as they need to relieve symptoms, whereas if they take a premeasured Marinol® capsule, it may not be enough or may be too much for their condition. A major obstacle with smoking or eating marijuana for medical purposes is the great variation in the marijuana plant. Variations in THC potency, the relative concentration of other active cannabinoids, and the inconsistency of other botanical factors make it difficult to rely on this substance to treat medical problems. For example, some forms of marijuana have been shown to increase intraocular pressure, making someone's glaucoma worse although normally, most forms of marijuana will lower intraocular pressure.

But beyond the physiological effects, there are the mental effects of marijuana that are the real issue. Like opium cure-alls, such as theriac and laudanum, it is the mental effects of calming, anxiety relief, or mild euphoria that make people feel good and think they are getting better even if the drug isn't actually helping the illness.

There is, however, a reluctance in the medical community to prescribe or even approve of marijuana for medical use for several reasons, including those already stated.

- There are a number of drugs on the market which physiologically have the same therapeutic effects or even better effects than marijuana or Marinol®.

- The THC content and even the potency of all the other chemicals vary from one joint to the next, so even if a few puffs worked a certain way one time, there's no guarantee the reaction would be the same the next time.

- Marijuana smoke contains a number of irritants, carcinogens, pathogens, and other chemicals, most of which have not been studied. If marijuana is baked in brownies or otherwise eaten, the respiratory effects are avoided but the 360 drugs contained in marijuana remain, along with all their side effects.

- Marijuana does somewhat impair the immune system, making the user more vulnerable to other illnesses.

- Marijuana is a psychoactive drug with abuse and addictive potential, particularly dangerous for those who are recovering from abuse or addiction.

Contrary to popular belief, medical research about marijuana continues in many countries. Since the 1970s, there have been more than 10,500 scientific studies conducted on marijuana. Yet, results continue to be conflicting, making it difficult to substantiate appropriate medical use of marijuana.

CHAPTER   SUMMARY

Classification

1. The most commonly used psychedelics are marijuana, LSD, PCP, peyote, psilocybin ("magic mushrooms"), and MDMA (or other variations of the amphetamine molecule).

General Effects

2. A major physical effect of psychedelics, other than marijuana, PCP, or anticholinergics, is stimulation.

3. The most frequent mental effects of psychedelics are intensified sensations (particularly visual ones, illusions, and delusions), mixed up sensations (synesthesia), suppressed memory centers, and impaired judgment and reasoning.

4. The effects of all arounders are particularly dependent on the size of the dose, the emotional makeup of the user, the mood at the time of use, and the user's surroundings.

LSD, Mushrooms, and Other Indole Psychedelics

5. LSD is extremely potent. Doses as low as 25 micrograms (25 millionths of a gram) can cause some psychedelic effects.

6. Like many other psychedelics, LSD overloads the brain stem, the sensory switchboard for the mind, and creates illusions and delusions.

7. Psilocybin is the active ingredient in "magic mushrooms."

8. After initial nausea or vomiting, visual illusions and a certain altered state of consciousness are the most common effects of mushrooms.

9. Mushrooms and peyote buttons have been used in religious ceremonies by many Native American and Mexican Indian tribes.

Peyote, MDMA, and Other Phenylalkylamine Psychedelics

10. Mescaline is the active ingredient of the peyote cactus.

11. Eating peyote buttons or drinking them in a prepared tea causes vivid hallucinations after an initial nausea and physical stimulation.

Belladonna and Other Anticholinergic Psychedelics

12. Belladonna and other nightshade plants contain scopolamine and atropine. In low doses, these substances cause a mild stupor but as the dose increases, delirium, hallucinations, and a separation from reality are common.

PCP and Other Psychedelics

13. PCP ("angel dust") is an anesthetic, now illegal, which besides deadening sensation, disassociates users from their surroundings and senses.

14. Effects of the drug PCP include amnesia, extremely high blood pressure, and combativeness. Higher doses can produce tremors, seizures, catatonia, coma, and even kidney failure.

15. Ketamine, another anesthetic, has become a popular drug in the "rave" club scene.

Marijuana and Other Cannabinols

16. Historically, the Cannabis plant has been grown to produce fibers for rope and cloth, seeds for food, various chemicals for medicinal effects, and a psychoactive resin for psychedelic effects.

17. Marijuana is the most widely used illicit psychoactive drug. Use has increased, particularly by high school students, since 1991 after a decade of decline.

18. Recent discoveries in the 1990s of a marijuana receptor site, a neurotransmitter (anandamide) that fits into that receptor site, and a marijuana antagonist all have accelerated research into the effects of marijuana.

19. The two most widely used marijuana species are *Cannabis sativa* and *Cannabis indica*. *Cannabis sativa* can be used for hemp or psychedelic effects. *Cannabis indica* is only used for its psychedelic effects.

20. The sinsemilla technique of growing *Cannabis sativa* or *Cannabis indica* greatly increases the concentration of THC, the main psychoactive ingredient in marijuana.

21. Street marijuana that is readily available in the 1990s is 5–14 times stronger than the marijuana of the 1960s and '70s. Much growing is done indoors to avoid detection.

22. Short-term effects of smoking marijuana include a dreamlike effect, sedation, and a mild self-hypnosis, making users more likely to exaggerate their mood and react to the surroundings.

23. Some of the negative effects of short-term marijuana use are lowered testosterone levels, a decrease in the ability to do complicated tasks, a temporary disruption of short-term memory, decreased tracking ability (an impairment of hand-eye coordination), a trailing phenomenom, and a loss of the sense of time.

24. Large amounts of marijuana or prolonged use can cause anxiety reactions, paranoia, and some illusions.

25. Respiratory effects include a decrease in the cilia lining the mucous membranes in the breathing passages which makes the smoker more susceptible to coughs, chronic bronchitis, emphysema, and possible cancer. A smoker of both marijuana and cigarettes does much more damage to the air passages and lungs than smoking only one of the drugs.

26. Chronic marijuana use can make some smokers less likely to do anything they don't want to do, leading to a tendency to neglect life's problems or to think about problems rather than do something about them.

27. Tolerance develops fairly rapidly with chronic marijuana use.

28. When stopping chronic marijuana use, a person can suffer delayed withdrawal symptoms which include headache, anxiety, depression, restlessness, tremors, sleep disturbances, and continued craving for the drug.

29. Medical use of marijuana is the controversial new battleground. Proponents say it should be available as a medicine, whereas opponents say there are better medicines that are more reliable and don't have all the other chemicals with unresearched side effects.

Other Drugs,
Other Addictions

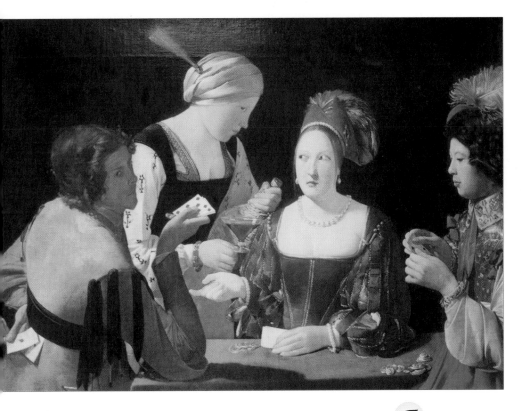

T *he Cheat with*
the Ace of Diamonds
by Georges de La Tour,
c. 1647, Louvre Museum,
Paris.

Photo reprinted, by permission,
Simone Garlaund.

OTHER DRUGS

- **Inhalants:** Volatile solvents, volatile nitrites, and anesthetics, the major inhalants, can cause CNS depression, disorientation, and inebriation. Dangerous effects include nerve damage, lack of coordination, and even learning disabilities.

- **Sports and Drugs:** Athletes have used therapeutic drugs, performance-enhancing drugs (especially steroids), and recreational street drugs. Steroids can build muscles and increase weight but they can also cause aggression, abuse, and addiction.

- **Miscellaneous Drugs:** Toad secretions, embalming fluid, hairspray, and even C-4 explosive have been used to get high. Amino acids, herbal preparations, vitamins, and nutrients are used to improve health and brain power and slow aging.

OTHER ADDICTIONS

- **Compulsive Behaviors:** People get into compulsive behaviors to change their moods, forget problems, get a rush, or self-medicate in much the same way they begin to use psychoactive drugs.

- **Heredity, Environment, and Compulsive Behaviors:** These influences make compulsive behaviors progressive diseases just like substance addictions.

- **Compulsive Gambling:** Gambling has grown dramatically over the past 20 years. One to three percent of adults are compulsive gamblers.

- **Eating Disorders:** Compulsive overeating, bulimia (eating and purging), and anorexia (starving oneself) are the three most common eating disorders. They combine behavior and a substance (food) to create compulsive behaviors.

- **Other Compulsive Behaviors:** Other addictions include workaholism, shoplifting, hair pulling, and many other impulse control disorders. Sexual compulsivity, particularly pornography and masturbation, are often used to cope with personal problems and childhood trauma or stress. Cyberaddiction involves compulsive use of the Internet, other online services, chat rooms, list servers, and e-mail.

- **Conclusion:** Because the roots of many compulsions are so similar, one has to treat the basic emotional causes of addiction as well as the specific substances or behaviors.

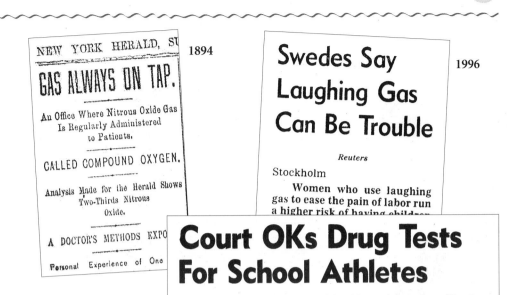

NEW YORK HERALD, SU 1894

GAS ALWAYS ON TAP.

An Office Where Nitrous Oxide Gas Is Regularly Administered to Patients.

CALLED COMPOUND OXYGEN.

Analysis Made for the Herald Shows Two-Thirds Nitrous Oxide.

A DOCTOR'S METHODS EXPO

Personal Experience of One

Swedes Say Laughing Gas Can Be Trouble

1996

Reuters

Stockholm

Women who use laughing gas to ease the pain of labor run a higher risk of having childr

Court OKs Drug Tests For School Athletes

By Reynolds Holding
Chronicle Legal Affairs Writer

The U.S. Supreme Court yesterday allowed public schools to randomly test their athletes for drugs, ruling that the importance of deterring schoolchildren from taking drugs outweighs the students' right to privacy

subject to drug testing without suspicion, but yesterday's ruling makes clear that even people in more mundane pursuits may not

More Supreme Court News
SEE PAGE A2

be immune from the drug war's intrusions.

"Deterring drug use by our nation's schoolchildren is at least as

1996

Alzado Dies of Brain Cancer At 43 — He Blamed Steroids

Chronicle Wire Services

Portland
Lyle Alzado, once among the most feared players in professional football, died yesterday of brain cancer, a disease he blamed on his prolonged use of body-building steroids. He was 43.

The two-time, all-pro defensive lineman died peacefully in his sleep at home

book at the tumor. He wanted us to go in with both guns blazing. I never knew him to believe that he wasn't going to beat it."

Alzado played 15 seasons in the NFL, including eight with the Denver Broncos and four for the Los Angeles Raiders before retiring in 1985 and beginning an acting career. He failed in a comeback attempt with the Raiders in 1990.

1991

OVERVIEW

One reason to use psychoactive drugs is to change one's state of consciousness. In fact, the definition of psychoactive drugs is any substance that will alter one's nervous system. Users, whether through curiosity or desperation, have found many substances which alter their mood and perception in much the same way that psychoactive drugs do. When certain behaviors are practiced over a long period of time, they too can become compulsive and addictive in the same way that cocaine or heroin use becomes compulsive and addictive.

OTHER DRUGS

In addition to stimulants, depressants, and psychedelics, many other drugs are used for their psychoactive effects. Inhalants have been around for millennia. Drugs used in sports to heal, increase performance, or to reward performance have been used for several thousand years. "Smart drugs" and herbal preparations have also been available since Neolithic times. Herbals have been discovered, forgotten, and discovered again while some have been synthesized in laboratories.

INHALANTS

Inhalants, sometimes classified as deliriants, comprise a wide variety of volatile substances, including certain gases, liquids that give off fumes, and aerosol sprays. The volatile substances are often present in commercial products. Inhalants are used for their stupefying, intoxicating, and less often, slight psychedelic effects. Inhalants which are sniffed are different from those substances like tobacco which are heated or burned and then smoked, or powders like cocaine hydrochloride which are sniffed.

Inhalants have some distinct differences from other psychoactive drugs.

- They are quick-acting and have intense effects. Inhalants are absorbed through the lungs into the bloodstream which carries them rapidly to the brain. Their intoxicating effects occur within 7–10 seconds and last no more than 30 minutes to 1 hour after exposure has ceased. People who abuse inhalants can very quickly become intoxicated and can display strange, erratic, and unpredictable behavior and poor judgment. They can become violent, even suicidal.

- They are cheap, readily available, and widespread. Thousands of chemical products can be inhaled for their psychoactive effects. Because psychoactive gasses and liquids are present in a wide variety of substances in the home, garage, and workplace, they are readily accessible to children and adolescents.

The three groups of inhalants are volatile solvents, volatile nitrites, and anesthetics.

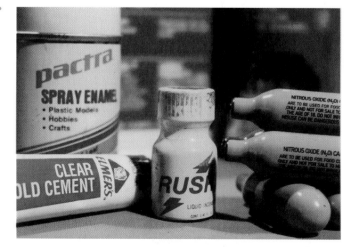

TABLE 7–1   INHALANTS

Products	Chemicals
VOLATILE SOLVENTS AND SPRAYS	
Airplane glue	Toluene, ethyl acetate
Rubber cement	Toluene, hexane, methyl chloride, acetone, methyl ethyl ketone, methyl butyl ketone
PVC cement	Trichloroethylene
Paint sprays (especially gold and silver metallic paints)	Toluene, butane, propane, fluorocarbons, hydrocarbons
Hairsprays and deodorants	Butane, propane, fluorocarbons
Lighter fluid	Butane, isopropane
Fuel gas	Butane
Dry cleaning fluid, spot removers, correction fluid, degreasers	Tetrachloroethylene, trichloroethane, trichloroethylene
Nail polish remover	Acetone
Paint remover/thinners	Toluene, methylene chloride, methanol
Local anesthetic	Ethyl chloride
Analgesic/asthma sprays	Fluorocarbons
VOLATILE NITRITES	
Room odorizers, Locker Room®, Rush®, Climax®, Quicksilver®, Bolt®, Bullet®, ("poppers")	(Iso)amyl nitrite, (iso)butyl nitrite, isopropyl nitrite
ANESTHETICS	
Nitrous oxide Whipped cream propellant, Whippets, laughing gas, ("blue nun," "nitrous")	Nitrous oxide
Chloroform	Chloroform
Ether	Ether

- They have serious effects. Short-term effects include disorientation, hallucinations, and an intoxication resembling drunkenness. Long-term inhalant abuse can damage muscles, vital organs, and the brain. Neurologic damage can include hearing and visual impairment, loss of coordination and memory, and learning disabilities.

- They get inadequate attention from parents, educators, the media, and law enforcement personnel because of the low status of inhalant abuse as a drug problem. Derogatory and dismissive attitudes towards solvent abusers compound the difficulty of getting warnings and treatment to them.

The three major classes of inhalants are volatile solvents, volatile nitrites, and anesthetics. Volatile solvents are used in glue, gasoline, plastic cement, varnish remover, paint, paint thinner, lighter fluid, and nail polish remover. The nitrites used to be sold over-the-counter as room fresheners. Nitrous oxide is still used as an anesthetic or aerosol propellant. Some aerosols, which can be sprayed to produce a foggy mist, are inhaled for their gaseous propellants rather than for their primary contents.

HISTORY

The practice of inhaling gaseous substances to get high goes back to ancient times. The Greek Oracle at Delphi was said to breathe in vapors from the earth before uttering her prophecies. In the Judaic world, burnt spices, gums, herbs, and incense were inhaled during religious ceremonies, a practice shared by other Mediterranean, African, and Native American peoples.

Our modern version of inhalant abuse began in the late 1700s with the discovery of nitrous oxide (laughing gas), chloroform, and ether. Later, at the turn of the twentieth century, when petroleum began to be refined and manufactured into new products, such as solvents, thinners, and glues, many more substances began to be inhaled for their intoxicating or euphoric effects. Shortly after World War II, the abuse of glue and metallic paints rose dramatically, particularly in the midwestern United States and in Japan. The phrase glue sniffing is still used to include inhalation of many substances besides glue. The practice has persisted as a drug abuse problem into the 1990s where inhalants are responsible for up to 1,200 deaths each year in the United States. (The actual number of deaths is thought to be underreported since medical examiners probably mistake death from inhalant abuse for suicide, suffocation, or an accident.)

EPIDEMIOLOGY

Since inhalants, especially volatile solvents, are readily available and inexpensive, they provide a cheap quick high, especially for those who are young and/or poor. Inhalant abuse often has an episodic pattern with brief outbreaks or fads in particular schools or regions. Abuse is most prevalent among young adolescents. However, adults also abuse inhalants, including painters, chemical company workers, health care professionals (especially in dentistry and anesthesiology), and others who have access to inhalants at work.

"In college, we'd have 'Whippet' parties where someone would go and get six or seven of those small nitrous oxide cylinders and we'd pass them around. By the time it came around again, you'd be down from the giddy, stupid feeling." 25-year-old ex-student

In a recent survey asking respondents whether they had ever used an inhalant, the most frequently abused substances were typewriter correction fluid, glue, gasoline, and spray paints. When a mixture of substances is involved, the solvents toluene and trichloroethylene are the most frequent ingredients.

"We got a 911 call about a kid in a coma. It seems that three of them were inhaling a waterproofing spray and this one kid did too much. Basically, he starved his head of oxygen because the spray temporarily replaced the oxygen. It took him three months to recover."
Emergency medical technician, Kansas City

Inhalant abuse continues to be a worldwide problem, according to a World Health Organization report. It afflicts primarily the young, the poor, especially street children, recent migrants to cities, and children exposed to chemicals daily, such as children of cleaners or shoemakers. The inhalant of choice in many countries is gasoline because of its wide availability, low price, and the rapid onset of psychoactive effects.

Use by Sex and Age

Generally, more young people than adults abuse inhalants in the 1990s and among 12 to 17 year olds, more young women than young men. About 17% of the adolescents in the United States have sniffed inhalants at least once. In older populations, more men abuse inhalants than women but the numbers of overall abusers decline by 2/3 or more after the age of 25.

Ethnically, earliest use is highest among Hispanics and lowest among Whites. Besides low price and easy availability, people abuse inhalants because the packaging is convenient, the substances themselves are generally legal, the high comes on quickly, and they are cheaper than marijuana, LSD, or even alcohol. Inhalants are also widely abused in Asia, Africa, and Latin America.

METHODS OF INHALATION

Although there have been reports of people spraying aerosols onto bread and eating the bread or inserting small bottles of inhalants, such as typewriter correction fluid, into the nostrils, the more common forms of inhalation are listed below.

- "Sniffing" is breathing in the inhalant directly from the container. Sniffing puts the vapor into the lungs in contrast with snorting which puts solids, like cocaine, in contact with the mucosal lining of the nose.

- "Huffing" is soaking a rag with a dissolved inhalant, putting the rag in the mouth, and inhaling; also, inhaling from a solvent-soaked rag, sock, tissue, or glove. Generally, huffing puts more vapors into the lungs.

- "Bagging" means placing the inhalant in a plastic bag and inhaling. Rebreathing the exhaled air intensifies the effect.

- "Spraying" means spraying the inhalant directly into the nose or mouth.

TABLE 7–2	NUMBER OF AMERICANS WHO HAVE USED INHALANTS		
Age	Ever Used	Last Year	Last Month
12–17	1,639,000	930,000	380,000
18–25	3,110,000	870,000	260,000
26–34	3,132,000	310,000	131,000
35 & up	4,135,000	198,000	125,000
Total	12,016,000	2,308,000	896,000

(NIDA Household Survey on Drug Use, 1995)

- "Balloon and cracker" means the cracker punctures a container with a pin, releasing the inhalant which inflates a balloon and then is inhaled.

Other methods include

- putting a bag over one's head, spraying an aerosol into the bag, and inhaling;

- pouring or spraying inhalants onto cuffs, sleeves, or collars and then sniffing over a period of time;

- heating the solvent to make it more volatile, a particularly dangerous practice that has resulted in explosions, burns, and deaths.

Directly ingesting and spraying inhalants are particularly toxic methods. These methods expose an abuser's fragile membranes to the caustic effects of these substances, put a harmful amount of pressure into the lungs, and even freeze respiratory membranes as the substances vaporize quickly, taking heat from everything around them. "Bagging," because it limits oxygen, concentrates the effects. The choices of inhalant and method of inhalation allow great control over the intensity and duration of the effects.

"In the classes I take care of, we have a problem with kids soaking their collars with this waterproofing spray and then getting loaded in class by sniffing them. It is a cheap high for 4th graders who can't afford other drugs." Oklahoma elementary school nurse

VOLATILE SOLVENTS

These solvents are often carbon- and -hydrocarbon-based compounds. Refined from petroleum oil, they are used as fuels, aerosols, and solvents. They include such common materials as gasoline and kero-

sene, paints, paint thinners (especially metallic paints), nail polish and spot removers, glues and plastic cements, lighter fluid, and a variety of aerosols, and even STP®, a gasoline additive. Some are inhaled, not for the primary substance but for the effects of the solvents they are dissolved in or the propellant gasses used.

These volatile solvents are quick acting because they are absorbed into the blood almost immediately after being inhaled and then they move to the liver, brain, and other tissues. Solvents are exhaled by the lungs (in which case a telltale odor from the inhalant remains on the breath) or are excreted by the kidneys.

Inhaling these substances produces a temporary stimulation, mood elevation, and reduced inhibitions before the central nervous system (CNS) depressive effects begin. Dizziness, slurred speech, unsteady gait, and drowsiness are seen early on. Impulsiveness, excitement, and irritability may also occur. Because judgment is impaired with abuse of these substances, there is substantial danger of accident and injury.

"I asked this kid who came into the office if he sniffed gas and he got indignant and said, 'I don't sniff it, I huff it.' This kid reeked of gas fumes, answered in words of one syllable, and had dropped out of school at the age of 14 and wanted to return. He was really unkempt and dirty. If he doesn't accept treatment, I don't think he'll make it to the age of 18." High school drug counselor

If, because of high dosage or individual susceptibility, the CNS becomes more deeply affected, illusions, hallucinations, and delusions may develop. The abuser may experience a dreamy stupor, culminating in a short period of sleep. The effects resemble alcohol or sedative intoxication (inhalant abuse has been called a "quick drunk"), though psychedelic effects may also occur, depending on the inhalant.

The intoxicated state may last from minutes to an hour or more, depending on the kind, quantity, and length of exposure to the substance inhaled. Headaches and nausea may follow as part of an inhalant hangover. After prolonged inhalation, delirium with confusion, psychomotor clumsiness, emotional instability, impaired thinking, and coma have been reported. Both low-level and high-level (acute) exposure to volatile solvents usually involve reversible brain and neurologic effects.

Chronic abuse (abuse that continues over a period of time) is characterized by lack of coordination, inability to concentrate, weakness, disorientation, and loss of weight. Since chronic abuse can involve extremely high concentrations of fumes, sometimes thousands of times higher than industrial exposure, mental and neurologic effects may be irreversible, though not usually progressive, after abuse ceases. For example, chronic abuse of toluene can result in dementia, spasticity, and other CNS dysfunctions, whereas occupational exposure to toluene has not produced similar effects.

Complications may result from the effects of the solvent or other toxic ingredients, such as lead in gasoline. Injuries to the brain, liver, kidney, bone marrow, and particularly the lungs may result either from heavy exposure or from individual hypersensitivity. Blood irregularities and chromosome damage can result, as well as respiratory arrest, cardiac arrhythmias, or asphyxia due to occlusion of the airway. Some of these substances produce ulcers around the nose and mouth and cancerous growths when abused chronically. Body injuries result from falling, fainting, or other accidents experienced while under the influence of these substances.

Toluene

Probably the most abused solvent, toluene is a component of many substances—glues, drying agents, solvents, thinners, paints, inks, and cleaning agents. Chronic abuse can affect balance, hearing, eyesight, and most often, neurological functions and cognitive abilities. In one study of chronic abusers of toluene in spray paint, 65% had neurologic damage. Heavy abuse results in deafness, trembling, and dementia.

Trichloroethylene

This is the most common solvent used in typewriter correction fluids, paints, and spot removers. Like the other volatile solvents, toluene and acetone, this substance causes overall depression effects and moderate hallucinations. The toxic effects are similar to those of toluene.

Gasoline

Gasoline sniffing, especially common among solvent abusers on Native American reservations, introduces various components of gasoline into the system, including solvents, metals, and chemicals. Symptoms include insomnia, tremors, anorexia, and sometimes paralysis. When leaded gas is inhaled, symptoms can also include hallucinations, convulsions, and the chronic, irreversible effects of lead poisoning.

Warning Signs

Though inhalant abuse is difficult to spot, there are still various warning signs. They are

- chemical odor on body and clothes or in a room;
- red, glassy, or watery eyes and dilated pupils;
- slow, thick, or slurred speech;

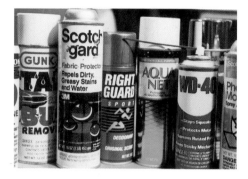

Many common household sprays have been huffed.

● ●

- staggering gait, disorientation, and lack of coordination;
- inflamed nose, nosebleeds, and rashes around nose and mouth;
- pains in chest and stomach, headaches, fatigue, nausea;
- shortness of breath, loss of appetite;
- intoxication, irritability, aggression;
- seizure, coma.

Drug Enforcement Administration bulletin, 1995

VOLATILE NITRITES

Amyl nitrite as well as butyl and isobutyl nitrite dilate blood vessels so the heart receives more blood. Medically, they are used for heart-related chest pains or for cyanide poisoning. Other effects include a rush of blood to the brain and the relaxation of smooth muscles in the body. Effects start in 7–10 seconds and last for about 30 seconds. Blood pressure reaches its lowest point in 30 seconds and returns to normal at 90 seconds.

"My roommate uses 'poppers' at 'raves' because he feels it helps his dancing and makes him more lively. It works for him some of the time but a couple of times he got

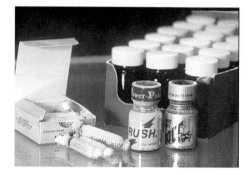

Isobutyl, butyl, or amyl nitrite, sold under various trade names from the 1970s, were some of the first successful designer drugs. For example, a prescription drug, amyl nitrite, was chemically rearranged to create a nonprescription derivative and sold as a room odorizer to circumvent drug laws.

● ●

dizzy and fell over. The last time he fell over and broke his nose." 17-year-old "raver"

On inhalation, there is a feeling of a fullness in the head, a rush, and mild euphoria. (First-time abusers have reported feeling panic attacks.) This may be followed by severe headaches, dizziness, and giddiness. A tolerance develops rapidly to the gas, though excessive prolonged abuse may cause oxygen deprivation, nitrite asphyxiation, and possible death. An extreme increase in heart rate and palpitations makes nitrite inhalation unpleasant. First aid for the headaches includes abstinence. Overdose treatment requires removing the abuser from exposure and insuring that respiration and blood flow are maintained. Occasionally CPR is used.

Nitrites, thought to enhance sexual activity, are sought after especially by male homosexuals for both their euphoric and physiological effects, which include relaxation of smooth muscles such as the sphincter muscle. Repeated abuse may alter blood cells and impair the immune system, thus increasing susceptibility to HIV infection. There is some evidence that nitrites inhibit the functioning of the white blood cells and that the activity of these killer cells is suppressed.

ANESTHETICS

In 1772, Joseph Priestly discovered nitrous oxide. Inhalant parties were given featuring the euphoric effects of the gas. At one of these parties, Humphrey Davy, a noted physician of his day, observed that the gas had pain-killing ability and recommended it be used as an anesthetic during surgery. The euphoric effects of this and other gases, such as chloroform, ether, and pure oxygen, were sought starting in the 1800s. Abuse of nitrous oxide was even reported among Harvard University medical students in the nineteenth century.

Abuse continues today by young experimenters as well as among middle class and affluent groups, including dentists, doctors, anesthesiologists, hospital workers and health-care professionals. They abuse nitrous oxide, halothane, and other anesthetics like ether, ethylene, ethyl chloride, and cyclopropane.

Nitrous Oxide

Currently, nitrous oxide (laughing gas) is available in large blue painted gas tanks for dental offices where it is used as an anesthetic and in bakeries where it is used as a propellant in whipping cream aerosol cans and small metal cylinders. Nitrous oxide is abused for its mood-altering effects. Within 8–10 seconds of inhalation, the gas produces a giddiness and stimulation often accompanied by silly laughter. The maximum effect lasts only 2 or 3 minutes. There is a buzzing or ringing in the ears along with a sense that one is about to collapse or

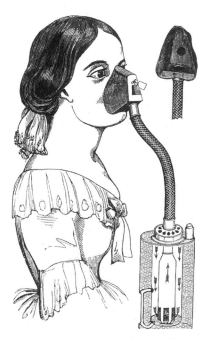

This mask was used not only by early day anesthesiologists but by genteel inhalers at oxygen or nitrous oxide parties in the 1800s.

pass out. These feelings quickly cease when the gas leaves the body.

"This one kid's dad was a dentist, so he'd rigged some deal where he got this 'blue nun,' this four foot tank of nitrous oxide, from the office. He filled a bunch of balloons with the gas and we'd pass them around and breath it in." 20-year-old

Dangers from the abuse of nitrous oxide, especially if inhaled directly from a pressurized tank, include exploded or frozen lung tissue and frostbite of the tips of the nose and vocal cords. This risk is minimized when the gas is inhaled from a balloon inflated with the gas. Inhalation can deplete the body's supply of oxygen and cause death.

Long-term exposure can cause central and peripheral nerve cell and brain cell damage due to lack of sufficient oxygen in the blood since nitrous oxide replaces oxygen in the blood. Symptoms of long-term exposure include numbness, loss of balance and dexterity, weakness and numbness in the arms and legs, and passing out and getting hurt from the fall. Further, nitrous oxide abuse can lead to physical dependence.

Halothane

Halothane is a prescription surgical anesthetic gas sold under the trade name Fluothane®. Its effects are therefore extremely rapid and powerful enough to induce a coma for surgery. Because of its limited availability, it has been most often abused by anesthesiologists and hospital personnel.

PREVENTION

Inhalants present a special challenge to prevention efforts. The dangers of inhalant abuse have not been publicized as widely as the dangers of alcohol, tobacco, and other drugs. Young people may be unaware that they risk sudden death or brain damage from inhaling volatile substances. Inhalants are plentiful, cheap, and easily accessible even to young people. Law enforcement officers, health workers, and teachers may not be trained to recognize signs and symptoms of inhalant abuse and the youth who are particularly at risk are often far from the usual prevention resources.

SPORTS AND DRUGS

"I was so wild about winning. Winning, winning, winning. I never thought about anything else." Lyle Alzado, former NFL star

BACKGROUND

Years ago, several hundred superior athletes were asked, "If you could take a drug that would guarantee a world record or an Olympic gold medal in your sport but afterwards the drug would kill you within the year, would you take it?" More than half the athletes said, "Yes," meaning that they were willing to die just so they could be the best in their chosen sport.

Some athletes perceive drugs as the quick way to put on pounds, to increase stamina, to get up for a game, to relieve pain, or to keep up with other athletes suspected of using drugs. Since many drugs used in sports create feelings of confidence and excitement, drugs themselves can motivate athletes to abuse them.

"What you have to understand is that a young man doesn't think past tomorrow. All he is interested in is winning the neighborhood game and having the best looking girl on his arm and looking the best that he possibly can. And these are technically the motivations for him taking the drug. And then he goes to college where peer pressure and the desire not to disappoint the home town folks put further pressure on him. Then if he's lucky enough to make it to the pro ranks, it becomes a matter of money."
High school football coach giving testimony to a congressional panel on drugs and sports

History

The use of drugs in sports is not new. Greek Olympic athletes in the third century B.C. ate mushrooms or meat to improve their performance. If they were caught, they were expelled from the games. About the same time, athletes in Macedonia prepared for their events by

Athletes probably use drugs at the same rate as the general public but since they are in the spotlight, their problems get banner headlines.

John Daly to Enter Rehab Facility

Associated Press

John Daly's career hit bottom yesterday, almost as quickly as it took off.

One of pro golf's most popular and controversial figures, the 28-year-old Daly withdrew from the PGA Tour to seek help for an alcohol-related problem.

"I will check into an alcohol rehabilitation facility and will return to tournament play only when I am comfortable my life is

decision over Mercer in ¦ City, N.J., and earned a ti against Evander Holyfield a unanimous decision to F on June 19 in Las Vegas. into the hospital immedia the Mercer fight and had tion," Holmes said.

"I don't know anythi it, I don't recall anythi Larry Hazzard Sr., athl missioner for New Jers der for a fighter to fi

Drug-related cases put Irvin, Morris back in spotlight

By Jarrett Bell
USA TODAY

NFL notes

Two months ago, Pittsburgh
Steelers tailbacl sive captain ¦ ecause of ees. New ty Myron

▪ TENNIS

Capriati Checks Into Rehab Center

Associated Press

Jennifer Capriati ....

Capriati's arrest prompted team of Patrick McEnroe and Richie Reneberg also lost as France upset the United States, 2-1, in the World Team Cup in Duesseldorf, Germany. The only U.S. victory came from Pete Sampras in singles, his 29th straight win.

▪ BASEBALL NOTES

Gooden: I Came Close To Commiting Suicide

Associated Press

Dwight Gooden pointed a gun at his head and thought about pulling the trigger nearly two years ago during his drug suspension, the New York Yankees pitcher has revealed

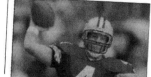

NFL MVP in drug treatment

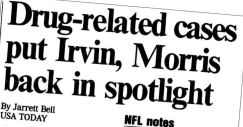

Brett Favre, who led Green Bay to NFC title game, says he has a dependency on painkillers, 1,8C

By Robert Hanashiro, USA TODAY

Favre: Seeks help after seizure.

---

drinking ground donkey hooves boiled in oil and garnished with rose petals. Roman gladiators took stimulants (betel nuts or ephedrine) to give them endurance.

By the 1800s, cyclists, swimmers, and other athletes used opium, morphine, cocaine, caffeine, nitroglycerin, sugar cubes soaked in ether, and even strychnine. Boxers drank water laced with cocaine between rounds. Long-distance runners were followed on bicycles by doctors who gave

them a mixture of brandy and strychnine.

New versions of amphetamines which initially increase alertness and energy also appeared. In World War II, amphetamines had been used by various countries to delay fatigue and increase endurance of their troops. When veterans returned home to the playing fields, some continued to rely on the drugs to try to give themselves a competitive edge or increase their athletic endurance.

International Politics

The male hormone testosterone had been isolated in the 1930s and was used in its pure form or in compounds to help injury victims and survivors of World War II concentration camps gain weight. During the Cold War era, the Soviet weightlifting team used steroids in the 1952 Olympics to garner medals. The Soviets were rumored to be using anabolic steroids at the 1956 Olympics, as were many of the Communist Bloc countries, especially East Germany, in succeeding Olympics.

The argument was made that the United States team should also have access to steroids. America wanted its athletes to stay ahead of the Soviets and the rest of the Communist Bloc. The use of performance-enhancing drugs was thought to be the only way that Americans could maintain their competitiveness in international athletics. By 1958, steroids were available and abuse by athletes had become widespread, even in face of growing evidence of negative side effects. At first, they were abused by bodybuilders and weightlifters who wanted to increase weight and strength, and later by many athletes to try to accelerate their training and development. Typical dosages have been greatly increased from 30–40 milligrams per day in the 1970s up to 300 milligrams per day in the '90s. In the 1994 World Championships, winning swimmers from The People's Republic of China were accused of using performance-enhancing drugs and subsequently, a number of them tested positive.

Commercialization of Sports

Beginning in the 1950s, the excellence of an athlete's performance began to matter less and less. With televised sports events, the explosive growth of professional sports, larger and larger salaries, purses, prizes, and big money for commercial endorsements of products, the public's attitude changed from respect for athletic excellence to envy of athletes' salaries and an expectation that for that kind of money, they had better be a winner. This attitude of "win at any cost" was echoed by many coaches.

"Winning is not the most important thing, it's the only thing."
Vince Lombardi, Green Bay Packers coach, 1956–1964

Over the past 30 years, the financial and social pressures to win have encouraged athletes to try drugs as a way to gain an advantage. "Do what you have to, but just win, baby, win" became our society's best advice to athletes. Many athletes earn more from endorsements than from salary, making winning even more crucial in their minds.

Extent of Abuse

In the 1990s, some athletes continue to abuse substances that cover a very large diverse group of drugs, chemicals, and other substances, many of which are not psychoactive but most of which are being misused in the context that they are taken. A special problem in sports comes with performance-enhancing or strength-enhancing drugs. In the '70s, over half of the NFL football players admitted to using amphetamines on a regular basis. One study in 1982 suggested that 70% to 80% of anabolic steroids prescribed in the United States were being diverted from medical uses.

A 15-year study published in 1985 reported that 20% of college athletes said they used anabolic steroids compared with 1% of nonathlete students, though anecdotal evidence in football and other strength sports suggests the numbers are much higher.

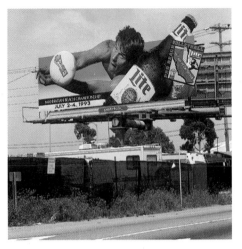

Advertisements that combine sports and alcohol are as plentiful as advertisements that combine sex and alcohol. Reprinted, by permission, Jason Moss.

Athletes in certain sports use more of one drug than another. For example, football players in one survey reported 10% use anabolic steroids. In 1990, steroids were designated a controlled substance so the use has been declining in collegiate and professional sports. The National Collegiate Athletic Association (NCAA) has an off-season anabolic steroid random testing program. Of 2,000 student athletes tested under this program, 3.5% tested positive. Unfortunately, the NCAA neither requires nor assists its member schools in drug testing. National sports federations frequently have been lax in enforcing rules against athletes found in violation of drug rules.

Currently, it is estimated that at least 350,000 junior high and high school students have used or are using anabolic steroids. Another report indicates that as collegiate testing for steroids becomes more stringent, young athletes are encouraged to bulk up on steroids during high school and then go clean when they get to college. This is particularly disturbing because an effect of anabolic steroids is to stunt hormonal and bone development in young people.

To understand the physical, mental, legal, and moral consequences of drug use in sports, it is necessary to examine the drugs themselves. Although there are literally hundreds of drugs and techniques that are used in connection with sports, we have focused on the most used and abused. The following three categories of drugs used in sports are based on athletes' motives and the context in which use occurs rather than pharmacological properties of the substances:

- therapeutic drugs;
- performance-enhancing (ergogenic) or appearance-enhancing drugs;
- recreational/street drugs.

THERAPEUTIC DRUGS

Therapeutic drugs are used for specific medical problems, usually in accordance with standards of good medical practice.

Analgesics (painkillers)

Analgesics are normally used to deaden pain. They include both topical analgesics which desensitize nerve endings on the skin (alcohol and menthol or local anesthetics such as procaine and lidocaine), and systemic analgesics, such as aspirin and Tylenol® for mild to moderate pain, or narcotic (opioid) analgesics for moderate to severe pain. The most common opioids used in sports are meperidine (Demerol®, the most widely prescribed), morphine, codeine, and propoxyphene (Darvon®). These drugs are either ingested or injected. Besides the pain-killing effects, opioids can cause sedation, drowsiness, dulling of the senses, mood changes, nausea, and euphoria. Opioids allow users to play through the pain and perform at or near their previous levels.

The biggest danger from these drugs results from their ability to block pain without repairing the damage. Normally, pain is the body's warning signal that some muscle, organ, or tissue is damaged and that it should be protected. If those signals are constantly short-circuited, the user becomes confused about what the body is saying. In addition, since tolerance develops so rapidly with opioids, increasing amounts become necessary to achieve pain relief. The problem is that tissue dependence can develop along with the analgesic effects, making it easier for the user to slip into compulsive use of the drug.

Muscle Relaxants

Muscle relaxants are drugs that are used to treat muscle strains, ligament sprains and the resultant severe spasms, and to control tremors or shaking. Some athletes also use them to control performance anxiety. The classes of muscle relaxants include skeletal muscle relaxants, such as Soma® and Robaxin®, and benzodiazepines, such as Valium® or Klonopin®.

As with analgesics, the performance enhancement of these drugs is minimal because the drugs are depressants and can also cause sedation, blurred vision, decreased concentration, impaired memory, respiratory depression, and mild euphoria. Skeletal muscle relaxants are only occasionally abused for their mental effects. Benzodiazepines and barbiturates have a higher dependence liability since accelerating use causes tolerance and tissue dependence. The benzodiazepines also stay in the body for a long period of time, causing delayed effects when they're not wanted.

"I couldn't imagine anyone performing under the influence of alcohol or a barbiturate. If they got to that point they would probably hurt themselves. Occasionally, some competed with a stimulant." Former college diving champion

Anti-inflammatory Drugs

These drugs control inflammation and lessen pain. Anti-inflammatory drugs come in two classes: NSAIDs or nonsteroidal anti-inflammatory drugs (typically Motrin® or Advil®, Indocin®, Butazoliden®, or Clinoril®) and corticosteroids, such as cortisone and Prednisone® (corticosteroids are different than androgenic-anabolic steroids described below).

With the corticosteroids, side effects are a significant consideration. Prolonged use can cause water retention, bone thinning, muscle and tendon weakness, skin problems such as delayed wound healing, vertigo, headaches, and glaucoma. Psychoactive effects are minimal at low doses but severe psychosis results from excessive high-dose use.

As with analgesics and skeletal muscle relaxants, when athletes are using anti-inflammatory drugs, a careful examination must be done to insure that the injury is not serious and that practice or play can continue without risk of aggravating the injury. There is the risk that these drugs will be used as a cure for the injury. They should not be used solely to enable the athlete to resume activity but should be part of the overall healing process. Ice, elevation, rest, physical therapy, and other treatment measures must accompany pharmacological relief of pain and inflammation.

STEROIDS AND OTHER PERFORMANCE-ENHANCING (ergogenic) OR APPEARANCE-ENHANCING DRUGS

To this very broad general category of drugs we will add other substances and even techniques used to enhance performance. Anabolic steroids are used by physicians to treat osteoporosis, anemia, some breast cancers, and other conditions. But many of the drugs are illegal without a prescription. Most of the drugs, substances, and techniques are banned by various sports-governing bodies such as the International Olympic Committee and the NCAA.

The goals that motivate users make these drugs different from alcohol and other psychoactive drugs. These ergogenic or energy-producing drugs, substances, and techniques are thought to possess various capabilities for boosting an athlete's performance by giving a temporary competitive edge. They are also abused to enhance self-image by adding muscle mass (bulking up) and shaping physique. Young adolescents might want them to hasten maturity or to develop the look of others using them. Unfortunately, one of the side effects in young adolescents is to limit growth. Steroid use in junior high and high school will limit increases in height.

Anabolic-Androgenic Steroids (AASs or "rhoids")

The most abused performance-enhancing drugs today, anabolic-androgenic steroids are derived from the male hormone testosterone or synthesized versions of it. Androgenic means producing masculine characteristics, anabolic means muscle building, and steroid is the chemical classification of the natural and synthetic compounds resembling bodily hormones like testosterone. Rapid weight gain is one of the most apparent effects but other less desirable effects occur such as bone weakness, tendon injury, cancer, sexual problems, and even feminization in males or masculinization in women. So far no pharmacological process has been able to separate the desirable muscle-building proper-

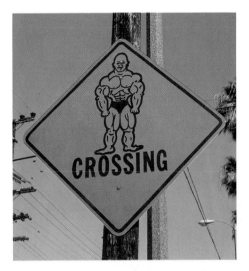

The use of steroids by bodybuilding competitors is so common that "natural" bodybuilding competitions are now being held where competitors are tested for the presence of these drugs.
Reprinted, by permission, Jason Moss.

ties of AASs from their dangerous hormonal side effects. These drugs have marked benefits that include increases in body weight, lean muscle mass, and increased muscular strength. The drugs can also increase aggressiveness and confidence, traits that are of value in many sports. Many students use AASs strictly to enhance personal appearance.

"The men I knew who used steroids the most were 5'8" and under and they talked about how they were the runts of the class and the 98 pound weakling at the beach. Steroid use is one way they felt they could overcome that." Ex-weightlifter

Patterns of Use—Cycling and Stacking. Anabolic steroid users may take from 20–200 times the usually prescribed daily dosage. Some athletes practice steroid stacking by using three or more kinds of oral or injectable steroids and by alternating between cycles of use and nonuse.

Cycling means taking the drugs for a 4- to 18-week period during intensive training and then stopping the drugs for a period of several weeks to several months to give the body a pharmacological rest and then beginning another cycle. Some athletes cycle to escape detection. Studies have reported that 82% of those using "rhoids" during a training cycle combined three or more different anabolic steroids in that time and 30% used seven or more. Of special concern is the fact that up to 99% of "rhoid" users have injected the drug and most increase their dosage during the course of their training.

Physical Side Effects. In men, these drugs can result in an initial masculinization effect which includes an increase in muscle mass and muscle tone. Most users also report an initial bloated appearance. However, long-term use results in suppression of the body's own natural production of testosterone. As a consequence, men who are long-term steroid users develop more feminine characteristics (e.g., swelling breasts, nipple changes), decreased size of sexual organs, and an impairment of sexual functioning.

In women, similar gains in muscular development may be considered beautiful to some but long-term use results in masculinizing effects, such as increased facial hair, decreased breast size, lowered voice, and clitoral enlargement.

"This woman friend of mine walked into the gym after being gone for three weeks. Her face was square and had unusual amounts of blond hair all over it. Her voice was really deep and her back had cystic acne on it which she never had before. I found out later that she had shot up straight testosterone. That was just one

more reason for me to stop competing. She went from beauty to freak in three weeks."
Former bodybuilder

If injections of steroids are taken to supplement oral doses and the large-gauge reusable needles purchased on the black market are shared, users are liable to contract or transmit infection, including HIV (AIDS).

Mental and Emotional Effects. Anabolic steroids can make users feel more confident and aggressive while using these substances. Some researchers think that the confidence that "rhoids" can induce is as sought after as the physical effects. As use continues, emotional balance starts to swing, from confidence, to aggressiveness, to emotional instability, to rage, and back to depression or to psychosis. This "rhoid rage" can lead to irrational behavior.

"After a dinner date, this one guy attacked me in my apartment. He was in the middle of a "rhoid" cycle. I put up a great fight and he gave up but if he was determined, there was no way I could have overpowered him. I don't know if it was the drugs or he was just crazy."
Female college student

The "rhoid rage" is more likely to occur in people who already have a tendency to anger or who take excessive amounts of steroids.

Compulsive Use and Addiction. About 1/3 of the users experience a sense of euphoria or well-being (at least initially) which contributes to their continued and compulsive abuse of "rhoids." In a survey of hard-core AAS users in their senior year in high school, 25% said they wouldn't stop using even if it were proven beyond a doubt that AASs cause permanent sterility, liver cancer, or heart attacks.

Yale University researchers have discovered that long-term steroid users have addictive cravings, difficulty in ceasing use, and withdrawal symptoms. In a college survey of 45 weightlifters who were regular AAS users, half reported three or more symptoms of addiction, particularly withdrawal symptoms. Withdrawal symptoms include fatigue, depressed mood, restlessness, insomnia, lack of appetite, and diminished sexual desire. Even between cycles, users will continue with low doses to avoid withdrawal. As with other drugs, compulsive use of steroids makes the user more likely to take other psychoactive drugs to enhance performance, as a reward, or in social situations.

"It was addicting, mentally addicting. I just didn't feel strong unless I was taking something. When I retired, I kept taking the stuff. I couldn't stand the thought of being weak." Lyle Alzado, former NFL star

Do Steroids Work? In 1984, the American College of Sports Medicine stated that steroids could increase mass and muscle strength when combined with diet and exercise. A 1996 study by Dr. Shalender Bhasin of Charles R. Drew University in Los Angeles showed large measurable increases in strength and weight due to steroids in research involving 43 male volunteers. What the study didn't cover was the use of multiple steroids and the use of excessive amounts of steroids over long periods of time.

"I took steroids from 1976 to 1983. In the middle of 1979, my body began turning a yellowish color. I was very aggressive and combative, had high blood pressure and

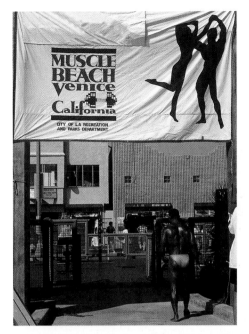

At Muscle Beach in Venice, California where the latest bodybuilding techniques are discussed, the topic turns occasionally to anabolic-androgenic steroids.
Reprinted, by permission, Jason Moss.

testicular atrophy. I was hospitalized twice with near kidney failure, liver tumors, and severe personality disorders. During my second hospital stay, the doctors found I had become sterile. Two years after I quit using and started training without drugs, I set six new world records in power lifting, something I thought was impossible without the steroids."
Richard L. Sandlin, former assistant coach, University of Alabama, before the U.S. House of Representatives Subcommittee on Crime, 1990

Supply and Cost

"We all knew who was using. We exchanged information on any new drugs

TABLE 7–3   ANABOLIC-ANDROGENIC STEROIDS

Chemical Name	Trade Name
U.S. APPROVED	
Danazol	Danocrin®
Fluoxymesterone	Halotestin®
Methyltestosterone	Android®, Metandren®, Testred®, Virilon®
Nandrolone phenpropionate	Durabolin®
Nandrolone decanoate	Deca-Durabolin®
Oxymetholon	Anadrol-50®
Stanozolol	Winstrol®
Testolactone	Teslac®
Testosterone cypionate	Depo-Testosterone®, Vioilon IM®
Testosterone enanthate	Delatestryl®
Testosterone propionate	Testex®, Oreton Propionate®
NOT U.S. APPROVED	
Ethylestrenol	Maxibolan®
Mesterolone	
Methandrostenolone	Dianabol®
Methenolone enanthate	Primobolan Depot®
Morethandrolone	
Nethenolone	Primobolan®
Norethandrolong	Nilexor®
Oxandrolone	Anavar®
Oxymesterone	Oranabol®
Trebelone	Finajet®
Trebolone acetate	Parabolin®
VETERINARY	
Bolasterone	Finiject 30®
Boldenone	Equipoise®
Mibolerone	

that were on the market. We got our steroids through the gym owner. In fact, he would inject them for us, in the rear."
Weightlifter

Athletes obtain steroids in different ways: from the black market, at gyms, from mail order companies, from friends or from unscrupulous doctors, veterinarians, or pharmacists. Serious users spend $200 to $400 per week on anabolic steroids and other strength drugs, so a single cycle can cost thousands of dollars. Some professional athletes spend $20,000 to $30,000 a year. At a conservative estimate, the black market for steroids grosses up to $500 million a year. Most of the product comes from up to 20 underground laboratories in the United States and foreign countries.

Beta Blockers (propranolol [Inderol®]and atenolol [Tenormin®])

Beta blockers constitute a class of drugs banned by the International Olympic Committee which block nerve cell activity at the heart, kidney, and blood vessels. They block adrenaline from binding onto beta receptors on the heart. They also block nerve cell activity in the brain and are used to calm and steady the body. Beta blockers are also used to control the symptoms of a panic attack or performance fright. Because of their ability to calm the brain and tremors, they are sought by some athletes involved in riflery, archery, diving, ski-jumping, and biathlon and pentathlon.

Beta blockers can cause fatigue, lethargy, dreams, occasional nausea, vomiting, and temporary impotence. Another negative effect of these drugs is interference with production of the liver enzyme needed to eliminate wastes. A great danger in the use of these drugs is their potential to intensify some forms of asthma and heart problems which can be fatal to the user.

Diuretics

Diuretics are drugs that increase the rate of urine formation, thus speeding the elimination of water from the body. Athletes use these drugs for two reasons:

- to lose weight rapidly which is important in sports where people compete in certain weight classes;

- to avoid detection of illegal drugs during testing by increasing urination.

"I was given a diuretic a week before I was to compete with instructions not to drink more than a half cup of water per day. I probably lost 12 pounds of water that week. I left the dorm the morning of my competition and my neighbor across the hall didn't recognize me because my face was so drawn. Competitive wrestler

Athletes trying to make their weight will use diuretics, laxatives, exercise, fasting, self-induced vomiting, and excess sweating in a sauna. This is done in spite of the evidence that dehydration significantly diminishes performance. Some athletes will lose three to five percent of their weight in a couple of days.

Blood Doping

While not involving a drug, the practice of injecting extra blood, either one's own or someone else's, is used to increase endurance by increasing the number of red blood cells available to carry oxygen. Blood doping is used by athletes in such sports as cycling, long-distance running, cross-country skiing, and other events that require endurance. Because doping involves blood transfusion, dangers include damaged blood due to poor storage, viral or bacterial infections, and even fatal reactions due to mislabeling. No test yet exists to accurately detect blood doping, so athletes have a clear-cut decision to make: to cheat or not to cheat.

Erythropoietin (EPO)

EPO is a synthetic version of the human hormone that stimulates the production of oxygen-laden red blood cells. It is used as a substitute for blood doping and there is evidence that it increases performance in endurance sports.

The dangers from unsupervised EPO administration result from the thickening of the blood which can lead to clots that might cause stroke or heart attack. Sweating and the accompanying increase in blood viscosity magnifies this potential danger of blood clots even more. A number of deaths among European cyclists from this kind of blood doping have been reported.

Miscellaneous Drugs

- **Bee pollen:** used in sports to increase endurance; can cause severe allergic reaction.

- **Calcium pangamate:** (also called B-15 or pengamic acid) keeps muscle tissue better oxidated; high rate of liver cancer.

- **Ephedrine:** found in hundreds of legal, over-the-counter cold and asthma medications as well as in some herbal teas; is used to supposedly increase strength and endurance.

- **Ornithine:** amino acid used in sports to increase growth and performance; high doses can lead to kidney damage.

- **Primagen:** increases steroid production; used by European athletes.

- **Vitamin B-12:** injected supposedly to ward off illness and provide extra energy; also used to mitigate the effects of heavy drinking.

- **HCG or human chorionic gonadotropin:** this drug and clomiphene or tamoxifen occasionally used after anabolic steroid treatment to restart the body's own testosterone production; toxic effects on the liver and reproductive system have been reported.

- **Periactin:** used for colds and allergic reactions; believed to increase strength

and cause weight gain; side effects include decreased performance, sweating, and sedation.

- **Adrenaline and amyl or isobutyl nitrite:** taken by weightlifters just prior to their performance to increase strength; the downside includes dizziness (a dangerous side effect with a 400 pound barbell over one's head), rapid heart beat, and hypertension.

STREET DRUGS AND ALCOHOL

Some athletes take drugs to adjust their moods, to fit into social situations where drug use is encouraged as they comply with peer pressure, to imitate the behavior of older role models, or to conform to their own image of an athlete. Athletes may also turn to drugs to help cope with the demands of a heavy schedule (practice, course work), to reduce stress, to compensate for loneliness, or to fill up time on long road trips.

Uppers

Some athletes use stimulants such as amphetamines ("crank," "whites," "black beauties") as a way of getting up for competition. The user feels energetic, alert, and confident. Athletes take (or are given) amphetamines to make themselves more aggressive and alert and to reduce fatigue. Athletes take them before an athletic event: football players to become more aggressive, runners to increase speed and energy, and tennis players to improve concentration and reaction time. Some take them after an event to sustain the competitive high.

"When you have played before 70,000 people and come off the field, you're back down to normal, so to speak. You want to get back up there with cocaine. It replaces that high

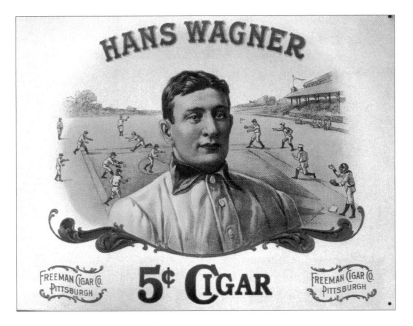

The use of sports celebrities to advertise alcohol and tobacco products is nothing new. It started in the late 1800s. Hans (Honus) Wagner objected to the use of his name and likeness on tobacco trading cards and had the manufacturer destroy them.

with an artificial stimulation. But the comedown from cocaine is very, very draining, emotionally, physically, and nutritionally. It's totally different than coming down from the natural high."
Former NFL running back

The nicotine in cigarettes is a mild stimulant but does very little for performance and in fact, reduces lung capacity. Like other stimulants, it also constricts blood vessels, thus raising blood pressure. Smokeless tobacco has many of the same effects as cigarettes except for a reduction in lung capacity. The image of the baseball player with a large wad of chewing tobacco in his cheek, spitting in the dugout was common but fortunately, it is becoming less popular. One of the reasons is that ball players such as Brett Butler who underwent surgery for throat cancer which he feels was caused by chewing tobacco are speaking out.

Downers

Some athletes will use drugs, such as alcohol, Xanax®, Valium®, barbiturates, opioids, and even marijuana, as self-rewards for enduring the stress they experience while performing before so many people. They also use these drugs as a tranquilizer to calm down after the excitement of competition or to counteract the effects of stimulants used to enhance their performance.

In general, alcohol consumption negatively affects reaction time, coordination, and balance, although studies suggest that low-dose alcohol consumption does not produce impaired performance in all people. The NFL Drug Policy statement calls alcohol "without question the most abused drug in our sport." The problem is how to alert athletes to the health and performance consequences of a drug that has general social, legal, and moral acceptance in society.

Marijuana

This all arounder can either stimulate or depress the user depending on the strength of the drug and the mood of the smoker. Marijuana lowers blood pressure which has caused fainting spells in football linemen who have to go quickly from a down position to a standing one often during a game. It inhibits sweating which has caused heat prostration and strokes in athletes and it impairs the ability of users to follow a moving object like a ball in play (decreased tracking ability). It also diminishes hand-eye coordination.

In a study at a major university, athletes admitted who was using marijuana and who wasn't. All of the athletes thought they were doing well and performing well but when an objective study was made of their performance, those who smoked marijuana did much more poorly: they dropped more passes, committed more errors, and suffered more injuries during their college careers.

ETHICAL ISSUES

Using illegal drugs or abusing legal drugs to improve athletic performance is against the rules in all sports and is illegal in most states. Drugs undermine the assumption of fair competition on which all sports rest. It is a kind of cheating that goes on before a game as well as during a game. Drugs violate the very nature of sport which, since the time of the Greeks, was a measure of personal excellence, the result of a sound mind in a healthy body. The outcome of athletic contests was to be determined by discipline, training, and effort.

There is a real threat today that the public will walk away from sports if they perceive that winning is based on access to the latest pharmacology and schemes to evade drug testing. Drugs also rob the athlete of feelings of self-accomplishment and tarnish the pride of winning. Because our society treats sports figures as heroes and role models, drug-abusing athletes diminish all of us.

MISCELLANEOUS DRUGS

UNUSUAL SUBSTANCES

It's amazing what substances and methods some people will use to get high: inhaling typewriter correction fluid, drinking rubbing alcohol, ingesting C-4 (a plastic explosive), smoking toad secretions, and swallowing antihistamines. Steroids, cough suppressants, over-the-counter diet pills, and even ginseng root are also abused.

Other psychoactive substances are provided by street chemists who either synthesize drugs that were once legally available, such as Quaaludes®, PCP, and fentanyl, or produce illegal drugs, such as MDMA, MDE, and cathinone (synthetic khat). The danger is that street drugs have not been tested and are not made under any kind of control. Irregular doses, unexpected effects, or contaminants in the manufacturing process can have disastrous effects on an unsuspecting user.

For example, in the 1980s, a group of heroin users who had been sold a supposedly synthetic Demerol® derivative, MPPP, were later found to have an 80% incidence of Parkinson's disease symptoms (rigid muscles, loss of voluntary body control) caused by contamination of the drug with MPTP. Street drugs can be dozens of times stronger than the expected dose. Overdoses

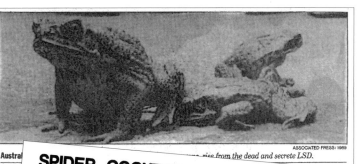

Aussies can't lick cane toads

The poisonous pests are taking over

By Uli Schmetzer
CHICAGO TRIBUNE

BRISBANE, Australia — Yuk lives on the third floor of the Museum of Queensland. He has become a permanent warning against man's folly in tampering with nature and a reminder that his ravenous family advances another 17 miles across the country every

...rise from the dead and secrete LSD.

ASSOCIATED PRESS/1989

SPIDER COCKTAIL: Doctors at a California emergency department report they successfully treated a 37-year-old woman who had crushed a black widow spider, mixed it with distilled water and injected it to get high. "One hour later she (complained) of severe cramping ... headache and anxiety," say Drs. Sean Bush, John Naftel and David Farstad in the April *Annals of Emergency Medicine.* She had an extremely fast heart rate and trouble breathing, but three days of hospital treatment returned her to normal. The heart and lung problems could have been from an allergy to the spider protein or a direct result of the spider venom. The woman was referred to a psychiatrist.

Some substances such as the secretion of certain frogs do produce psychoactive effects but others can be deadly.

occur such as those in Baltimore where in 1993, street fentanyl killed 30 people.

Camel Dung

Some Arab countries produce hashish by force feeding ripe marijuana plants to camels. Their four-chambered stomachs compact the marijuana into hashish camel dung.

C-4 Explosive

Soldiers have been known to ingest C-4 or cyclonite plastic explosives for their psychedelic effects. Tremors and seizure activity can result but usually not an explosion since it takes a blasting cap to set off the chemical.

Toad Secretions (bufotenine)

The *Bufo* genus of toads (Colorado River, Sonoran Desert, Cane, and others) secrete a psychedelic substance from pores located on the back of their necks. This substance, bufotenine, is milked and harvested onto cigarettes which are then smoked to induce a psychedelic experience.

Embalming Fluid (formaldehyde)

Mortuaries have been broken into and robbed of their embalming fluid. It can either be directly abused (inhaled for its depressant and psychedelic effects) or it can be used in the manufacture of other illicit drugs. Some abusers soak marijuana joints or cigarettes in the fluid and smoke it.

Called "clickers," "clickems," or "Sherms," the mixture gives a PCP-like effect. Formaldehyde, the main ingredient of embalming fluid, is a known carcinogen. Recently, formaldehyde, has also been used in the illicit manufacture of "crank" or "crystal" methamphetamine.

Gasoline

In spite of the toxicity of leaded or unleaded gasoline, a few people have been known to mix it with orange juice and drink it; they call it "Montana Gin," a particularly lethal beverage. Most often, gasoline fumes are inhaled for their effects.

Ginseng Root

Ginseng has been used for thousands of years as an herbal tonic or health aid. Today, the plant extract is also used to help develop muscles rapidly. The root does contain small amounts of anabolic steroids and can cause blood problems in massive doses.

Kava Kava

The roots of the South American *Piper methysticum* plant are chewed or crushed into a soapy liquid and drunk. The milky exudate of the root contains at least six chemicals that produce a drunken state, similar to that of alcohol, to the observer but users claim that the effects are more pleasurable, relaxing, and psychic than the effects of alcohol, and without the hangover. Since human saliva is an important ingredient in the preparation of this drug, its use has not found popularity.

Raid®, Hairspray, and Lysol®

Abusers puncture the aerosol cans, draining out the liquid which they swallow mainly for its alcohol content. These items are rarely abused in the general population but find more use in isolated rural areas where access to alcohol is limited.

M-99

M-99, a powerful injectable opioid which is 400–1,000 times stronger than morphine, is sold under the trade names of M-99® or Immobilion®. This drug is used in veterinary practices to immobilize large animals. Its abuse seems limited to the veterinary professionals who know how to deal with its high toxicity. In fact, when it is abused, the user will also have a needle into a vein, ready to administer the antidote Narcan®.

Dextromethorphan (Robitussin D.M.®, Romilar®, and other cough syrups)

Dextromethorphan has been known to be a psychedelic compound for 25 years. A full six ounces of the liquid is ingested to get a proper dose of dextromethorphan. This also provides the abuser with six ounces of up to 20% alcohol, so the effects are that of a drunken deliriant.

Coriciden®, Benedryl®, and Sudafed®

Decongestants and antihistamine tablets or capsules, sold over-the-counter to relieve cold symptoms, are taken in excessive doses (6–10 pills at a time) to produce sedation or psychic effects.

"SMART DRUGS"

"Smart drugs" ("SDs") are the drugs, nutrients, drinks, vitamins, extracts, and herbal potions that manufacturers, distributors, and proponents think will boost intelligence, improve memory, sharpen attention, increase concentration, detoxify the body, especially after alcohol or other drug abuse, and energize the user. Popular drugs include Cloud 9®, Herbal Ecstasy®, Brain Tonix®, Brain Booster®, Nirvana®, and many others. Proponents range from AIDS activists to health faddists, New Agers, anti-aging questors, and members of the technoculture who feel they are on the edge of a new field of mental development. Consumers of "smart drugs" are estimated to number 100,000.

For some consumers, "smart drinks" are nonalcoholic, usually a mixture of vitamins or powdered nutrients and amino acids in a fruit drink purchased in a "smart bar" for $4 to $6 or at a health food store. More recently, "smart drinks" and drugs have contained combinations of medications usually prescribed for Parkinsonism, Alz-heimer's disease, or dementia. It is felt that these drugs more effectively rebalance the brain after abusing drugs, for instance, MDMA during a "rave." It is also claimed that they will slow or reverse the aging process. The consumers are typically young (17–25) urban students or professionals looking for an intellectual edge or more stamina to work or party harder.

Vitamin supplements and nutrient products, once purchased through ads in New Age magazines, are now sold through health food stores. Critics of these supplements and products attribute their success to either a placebo effect (only the expectation, not the product, produces the effect) or to the caffeine or sugar that is part of the ingredients. "Smart drugs" with stimulant effects could lead to problems if someone with high blood pressure, for example, were to take too high a dose.

Americans have begun to import powerful pharmaceuticals called nootropic drugs (nootropic means acting on the mind) from Europe where many can be purchased that are not yet approved by the Food and Drug Administration (FDA) for sale in the United States. Critics of these

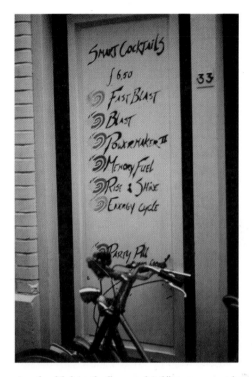

At a health bar, the "smart drink" names are advertisements for their supposed effects.
Reprinted, by permission, Simone Garlaund.

and other prescription drugs, including researchers, doctors, and the FDA, point out that, at the very least, claims for the efficacy of the drugs have not been substantiated. Advocates argue that these and other smart drugs improve mental ability for people suffering from debilitating mental disorders and that they can enhance mental capacity in normal people too. Drugs commonly called nootropic include those prescribed for debilitating mental disorders (but not FDA approved for other uses) such as ergoloid mesylates, selegiline hydrochloride, phenytoin (Dilantin®), and vasopressin. Other nootropics are prescription drugs not approved in the United States for any use, such as pracetam, aniracetam, fipexide, vinpocetine, and lucidril.

OTHER ADDICTIONS

COMPULSIVE BEHAVIORS

Compulsive sexual behavior, cyberaddiction on the Internet, compulsive shopping, pathological lying, shoplifting, hair pulling, fire setting, and compulsive TV watching or video game playing, all offer opportunities for repetitive, compulsive behaviors. Because of the similarities among these disorders, they are sometimes referred to as impulse control disorders. Two British psychologists compared children who play continuous computer games with heavy smokers and drinkers, noting the same euphoric responses and the same withdrawal symptoms.

The reasons that people engage in compulsive behavior are the same reasons that they engage in compulsive drug use: to get an instant rush, to forget problems, to control anxiety, to oblige friends, to alter consciousness, and so forth. But to understand how similar they are, it is instructive to look at the hallmarks of addiction to psychoactive substances and compare them to compulsive behaviors. They are

- using and thinking about using most of the time;
- continued use despite adverse medical, social, family, and legal consequences;
- denial that use is a problem;
- a strong tendency to relapse after stopping use.

If one takes these definitions of drug addiction and replaces the word use or using with the words eating, gambling, surfing the Internet, shopping, watching TV, or having sex, then it is easier to see that compulsion isn't limited to psychoactive substances (although many regard certain foods as psychoactive drugs). For example, compulsive gamblers would say

- they are always figuring odds, buying lottery tickets, trying to raise money, or making trips to Las Vegas in order to gamble;
- even though they lose most of their paycheck each month through bad bets, they continue gambling;
- they can control their gambling but are enjoying it too much to stop;
- when they can't gamble, they become restless, irritable, and discontent and have to find some action, almost as if they are going through withdrawal.

Compulsive eaters would say

- they are always eating, thinking about where they are going to eat next, or in the case of anorexics, figuring out how they are going to avoid eating;
- they continue overeating despite diabetes, increased risk of heart disease, impaired relationships, and a decreased ability to function physically;
- they could stop eating but why give up something that gives instant pleasure, blocks out worries, and is as easy to find as the next fast-food restaurant;
- even when they lose large amounts of weight dieting, they are extremely likely to gain all that back and more.

Another example of the relationship between compulsive drug use and compulsive behaviors is that in 12-step groups which help people with compulsive behaviors, such as gambling, overeating, or obsessions with sex, the members use literature taken directly from Alcoholics Anonymous. Even

Researchers Say Cause of Obesity Is a Flawed Gene

Associated Press

Boston

[...] weight people that [...]

metabolic rates and get diabetes at younger ages."

Three reports on the discovery, [...] and Johns Hop-

kins colleagues, were published in today's issue of the New England Journal of Medicine.

Experts estimate that from

eight to 30 genes may contribute to obesity. Although no single gene probably causes obesity by itself, those who inherit several are more likely to have weight problems.

A Shameless Addiction to TV

By Tenley Harrison

MY FRIENDS, "20-somethings," talk about television an awful lot. That's nothing new. But it came to my attention recently because I have spent the past two years in Asia, where I lived blissfully without knowing the comings and goings of TV characters, safe from syndicated reruns and somewhat protected from the "Friends" and "Seinfeld" mania.

The absurdity of many of my conversations with friends, jammed with refer-

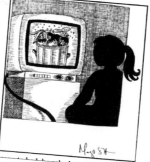

friends, who live in Japan, explained that Americans there received taped copies of the hit shows and then pass them around. While living in Japan, I too had been pathetically excited when the next episode arrived.

This concentration on television is disturbing because I do not want to be sucked back into that scene. After leaving Japan in December, I traveled around Southeast Asia for 2½ months and didn't have the choice to watch TV. At night, I would sit around with other travelers and talk, play cards, go for a walk, or go swimming under the moon. I never sped up a meal because I felt anxious about missing a show, nor did I turned down an invitation because it [...]

Addicted teenage gamblers

Washington

ASK ED LOONEY about gambling, and he starts telling horror stories. Looney serves as executive director of [...]

the N[...]
sive [...]
hotli[...]
and r[...]

Lo[...]
slit hi[...]
the lo[...]
sente[...]
livery [...]

casinos alone. Lotteries contributed $10 billion.

Nationwide, it is estimated that about 10 million Americans have a [...]ling habit that is out of control. [...]indt, a professor of commerce [...]gal policy at the University of [...], says when gamb[...]ng activities [...]alized and made [...]risdictions, the [...] gamblers increa[...])0 percent to 55([...] Grinols, an ec[...]

Judge William L. Stewart, who has served on chancery court along Mississippi's Gulf Coast for 17 years, says he knows gambling to be a factor in about a third of the divorce cases he now oversees.

Meanwhile, data from communities where gambling is legal point to [...] legal[...]
[...]ctivity.
[...]f casi-
[...]0th to
[...]ties in

Criminals Drawn to Cardrooms

Police leery of expansion efforts

By David Dietz
Chronicle Staff Writer

To someone crossing his path, Khiem Pham was just a struggling businessman who ran a small Vietnamese cafe, drove an aging Hyundai hatchback and lived modestly with family and friends on a leafy street in south San Jose.

But Pham was anything but run-of-the-mill in 1993 to authorities. They tapped his phone, spied on him with un-

Net overuse called 'true addiction'

By Marilyn Elias
USA TODAY

Obsessive Internet users have a true addiction that can hurt their relationships and leave them hung over or disabled at work, suggests the largest mental health study so far of heavy Net participants.

The study of 396 men and women on line for an average of 38 hours a week was prethe structure of the meetings is similar as is the philosophy which tries to get people to understand that addiction involves lack of control over the behavior and tries to make them see the necessity of changing their life style and beliefs.

HEREDITY, ENVIRONMENT, AND COMPULSIVE BEHAVIORS

Apparently, like substance abuse, these behaviors can be triggered by genetic predisposition, by environmental stresses, and by the comfort, reassurance, or escape provided by the repetitive behavior itself. Increased dopamine levels in those involved in the behaviors suggests a common biochemical thread.

It is fairly easy to understand how environment could intensify certain compulsive behaviors. Compulsive overeating is magnified by all the fast-food restaurants, by the abundance of fat and refined carbohydrates which can induce a certain euphoria, by parents who overfeed their children, by the endless ads for junk foods, such as ice cream, by chaotic childhoods which make people search for an instant escape, by the lack of daily physical activity which allows fat rather than muscle to form, and by the endless media examples of how important it is to look thin.

Compulsive gambling is influenced environmentally by the abundance of state lotteries, the growth of gambling casinos in states outside of New Jersey and Nevada, along with the growth of legal off-track-betting. Compulsive shopping is influenced by the ease of obtaining credit, the endless barrage of advertisements and shopping networks urging people to buy, and a materialistic view of how life should be lived.

The presence of physical and sexual abuse and other childhood traumas in many who practice these compulsive behaviors also suggests the importance of environmental conditioning and reinforcement.

It is also easy to understand how engaging in the activity itself could lead to compulsive behaviors. Straining the digestive system with excessive food, particularly fats and sugars, or eating too many reward foods rather than life-enhancing foods changes the body's chemistry, so the person eats to change mood rather than sustain life. Compulsive shopping imprints the brain so it can anticipate buying a coveted item, thereby kindling a surge of pleasure from the act of buying something with no regard for financial responsibility or even the need for such an item. The repeated use of pornography and participation in other compulsive sexual behaviors can make the participant avoid normal relationships.

HEREDITY AND COMPULSIVE BEHAVIOR

Twin studies have already identified a genetic connection to alcoholism and other drug addictions. Other twin studies have shown a connection between heredity and other compulsive behaviors which don't involve psychoactive drugs.

"I never was a very good alcoholic though my dad and granddad were quite successful at it. Now eating—that I excelled in. I could put down five or six meals a day without a second thought. I got pretty good at cards and slots. I can play poker for 20 hours straight without a thought for going home. And work—I can get lost in that too. In truth, I don't do anything halfway. Check that. I can't do anything halfway."
37-year-old recovering compulsive overeater

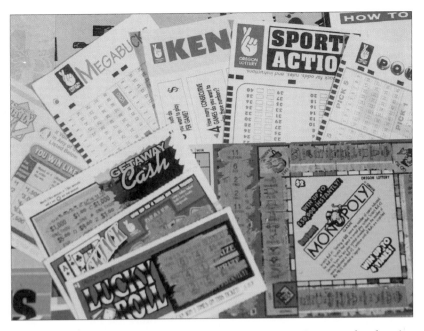

States started with scratch-off tickets and lotteries as a way to raise money for education and other state services. They have expanded the action to Keno, sports betting, and poker machines.

Compulsive eating was the first behavioral addiction shown to be partly hereditary. A recent study by the *National Institutes of Health* of 400 twins over a period of 43 years found that "cumulative genetic effects explain most of the tracking in obesity over time." This means that a much higher than normal percentage of twins born to obese parents but subsequently raised in totally different households ended up obese. The researchers also found that "shared environmental effects were not significant" in affecting the twins' weight gain. Five studies of adopted children bolstered this finding by discovering that the family environment, such as the size and frequency of meals, the amount of food in the house, and the level of exercise of the family, plays very little or no role in determining the obesity of children. They found that only dramatic environmental differences could mitigate the influence of a genetic profile that made one susceptible to obesity.

Twin studies of risk takers have also found a genetic component which resulted in a higher percentage of children of risk takers being risk takers themselves.

By the mid-1990s, genetic connections between alcohol abuse, compulsive drug use, and other compulsive behaviors were starting to be confirmed by research efforts. Kenneth Blum, John Cull, Eric Braverman, David Comings, researchers at various universities, and others have postulated a genetic basis not only for alcoholism but for people with other addictive, compulsive, and impulsive disorders, such as compulsive overeating, pathological gambling, attention deficit disorder, and Tourette's syndrome. They call this genetic predisposition the **reward deficiency syndrome.**

Specifically, their studies indicate that a marker gene associated with the most severe forms of alcoholism also has a strong association with several addictive-compulsive behaviors. This is only one of several, yet to be discovered marker genes that indicate a deficiency of certain neurotransmitters in the reward/pleasure center. They found that, whereas this marker gene (DRD_2 A_1 allele gene) appears in only 19–21% of nonalcoholic, nonaddicted, and noncompulsive subjects, it exists in

- 69% of alcoholic subjects;
- 45% of compulsive overeaters;
- 48% of smokers;
- 52% of cocaine addicts;
- 51% of pathological gamblers;
- 76% of pathological gamblers with drug problems;
- and in 45% of the people with Tourette's syndrome (compulsive verbal outbursts or strong tics).

In addition, a study of children with attention deficit disorder found that 49% had the marker gene compared to only 27% of the control group.

These findings suggest that a biochemical deficiency or anomaly draws some people to compulsive behaviors. The researchers postulate that carriers of this A_1 allele gene have a deficiency of dopamine receptors in the reward/pleasure center. What the dopamine receptor site deficiency means is that activities which will normally give people a surge of satisfaction, pleasure, and satiation by releasing dopamine do not give that same level of satisfaction to people with a lack of dopamine receptor sites. Such people are more likely to seek out substances and activities that release additional dopamine (e.g., alcohol, drugs, and repetitive compulsive behaviors). The release of extra amounts of dopamine caused by compulsive repetitive behaviors stimulates the reward/pleasure center to a greater degree than normal. People with this lack of receptors all of a sudden feel pleasure that they normally don't experience.

It is important to note that there isn't just one marker gene for compulsive drug use and behaviors. There are several neurotransmitters involved in the reward cascade chain and several that can alter the reward reinforcement sites in the brain (see Chapter 2). For example, in the urine and spinal fluid of pathological gamblers, researchers have discovered higher than normal levels of norepinephrine, the neurotransmitter that produces stimulation, alertness, and confidence. Scientists funded by the National Institute of Mental Health discovered abnormal functioning in serotonin and norepinephrine in acutely ill, bulimic, and anorexic patients, further suggesting a link between these disorders at the level of neurotransmitters.

It is instructive to look at specific compulsive behaviors to better appreciate the similarities among most addictions.

COMPULSIVE GAMBLING

HISTORY

The record of human gambling predates recorded history. Archeologists have unearthed prehistoric gambling bones. The casting of lots is recorded in the *Bible* and crusading knights gambled at dice. Lotteries, popular for centuries in both Asia and Europe, were imported to the American colonies in the 1700s where, among other things, their proceeds were used to support roads, schools, hospitals, and other public works. Betting on horse races, cock fights and dogs fights was popular. Gambling financed some of the

Revolutionary War, though some antigambling laws were later passed by the original 13 States.

For much of the nineteenth and twentieth centuries, gambling continued to be popular, though it was considered immoral, either because it encouraged greed and was sinful or because it preyed on human weakness and was criminal. Gambling has also been considered decadent, irresponsible, or insane. But in the last 30 years, gambling has become a respectable pastime or hobby and its legalization has increased. By the mid-1990s, all states except Hawaii and Utah had established some kind of gambling. In addition, the Indian Gaming Regulatory Act of 1988 gave Native American tribes the right to operate on their reservations any form of gambling that legally exists in a state. By 1995, 65 of the 550 Native American tribes in the United States had gambling operations.

State-supported lotteries were established through the 1980s and '90s to replace dwindling tax dollars and generate jobs. From 1974 to 1993, the public increased its wagers on legal gambling from $17 billion to $394 billion per year, generating profits in 1993 of over $35 billion. Some argue that legalized gambling imposes a very regressive tax on low-income gamblers. The poor devote two and a half times more of their income on gambling than the middle class.

Unfortunately, many states have not adequately studied compulsive gambling nor have they established prevention or treatment programs. Critics contend that government encourages gambling and legitimizes it but does not address the problem of gambling addiction (The gambling industry sees concern over compulsive gambling as an impediment to its growth.)

The media directly or indirectly supports gambling by publishing odds, sports' scores, players' injury reports, winning lottery numbers, stories of big winners, and ads for gambling excursions. CNN Headline News offers a sports ticker, listing running scores across the bottom of the screen. There is also simultaneous picture-in-picture coverage of multiple games. It is possible to gamble in airports, gas stations, bars, and supermarkets.

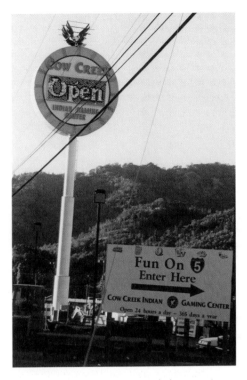

Gambling establishments on tribal reservations have increased the prevalence of gambling in communities surrounding the reservation as well.

EPIDEMIOLOGY

For most people who gamble, gambling is an occasional, recreational pastime. But for approximately 1–3% of adults, gambling is compulsive and pathological. Male compulsive gamblers outnumber female

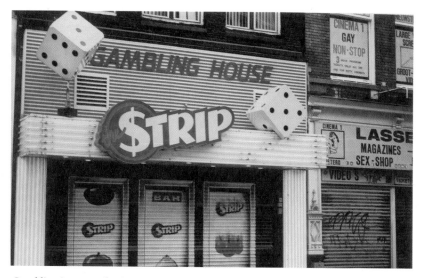

Gambling is as popular in most countries as it is in the United States. Lotteries, betting parlors, and casinos were popular in many other countries before they became legal in the United States.

Reprinted, by permission, Simone Garlaund.

compulsive gamblers 2 to 1 but probably because of the greater stigma put on women gamblers, only about 2–4% of women belong to Gamblers Anonymous. Women more than men seem to use gambling as a means of escape from depression, traumas, or relationship problems.

"I won $2,000 once and I spent it all back on Keno and a trip to Reno. The money's not important to me. What I like is the excitement of playing and seeing my numbers come up on the board. Keno takes my mind off everyday problems and gives me something to look forward to."
30-year-old recovering compulsive gambler

College students have a higher rate of pathological gambling than the general population: 5 1/2%, with 15% reporting at least some problems associated with gambling. College male pathological gamblers outnumbered their female counterparts approximately 4 to 1, suggesting that problem gambling surfaces at an older age for women. Among college students, pathological gamblers were absent more often and got lower grades than other students.

CHARACTERISTICS

Like other addictions, pathological gambling seems to be a progressive disorder, requiring more episodes and larger amounts of money bet to relieve anxiety and tension. Other behavioral and substance addictions occur in 30–50% of pathological gamblers. Alcoholism occurs in half of all compulsive gamblers.

"I discovered pretty quickly that I might be a compulsive gambler as well as an alcoholic. I had been sober for two years before I drank again. While I was sober, I had more money

and my gambling escalated. I was losing my whole paycheck some weeks. Eventually, I resumed drinking. I lost my job because of my drinking but still I kept betting on baseball and football."

Recovering compulsive gambler (From <u>Deadly Odds</u>, by Estes and Brubaker)

Symptoms of persistent recurrent pathological gambling (positive diagnosis with five or more of the following) are

1. preoccupation with gambling (reliving past experiences, planning future ones);

2. gambling with increased amounts of money;

3. repeated, unsuccessful efforts to control, cut back, or stop gambling;

4. restlessness and irritability when attempting to control, cut back or stop;

5. gambling as escape;

6. attempts to recoup previous losses;

7. lies to others to conceal gambling;

8. illegal acts to finance gambling;

9. jeopardization or loss of job, relationship, or educational or career opportunity;

10. reliance on others to bail gambler out of pressing debts.

Adapted from Diagnostic and Statistical Manual of Mental Disorders, Fourth Edition (DSM-IV™)

A pathological male gambler often began gambling as an early adolescent. Female pathological gamblers typically began in later life. They both are more likely to have a parent who was a problem gambler than the general population. Initially, gambling is recreative and pleasurable. Then a gambler begins to devote more time and wager more money. He or she develops an uncontrollable passion for gambling. Compulsive gamblers report feeling a high, the euphoria and excitement they get from the action of the risks and thrills involved in gambling. Money is often only a way to be part of the "action." Another part of the compulsion involves "chasing", that is, the attempt to recover losses, to get even by increasing either the money bet or the risks.

As losses multiply, the gambler tries to recover them by gambling more, tries unsuccessfully to cut back, and then maxes out credit cards, borrows from friends and family, and even turns to illegal activities like theft, embezzlement, and drug dealing in order to finance gambling episodes. A sports gambler may listen to three or four games simultaneously, a compulsive stock or commodities speculator may call for quotes frequently or be glued to a quote screen. Social, job, and family tensions multiply. Gamblers may deny there is a problem or lie to conceal the amount of money involved or the frequency of the gambling. Law enforcement officials point to problems associated with gambling such as illegal loans, extortion, threats and beatings to collect debts, and the embezzlement and theft to pay them off.

In the end stages, which may take decades to develop, a compulsive gambler often loses a job because of absenteeism or poor work performance. The gambler bankrupts his or her family with second mortgages, credit card debt, or personal loans or suffers divorce or separation because of deteriorating family relations, long absences from home, arguments over money and gambling, and indifference to the welfare of family members and others. Gamblers can experience insomnia attacks, health problems, and elated moods when they win and mania, depression, panic attacks, and suicidal thoughts or attempts when they lose. Often, the problems become so overwhelming that they can precipitate the final crisis that leads the compulsive gambler into treatment.

TREATMENT

Compulsive gambling is treatable. The standard assessment test of this condition is the South Oaks Gambling Screen (SOGS) and The Gamblers Anonymous 20 Questions usually accompanied with an in-depth assessment and formal diagnosis. Treatment options developed over the last 30 years include self-help groups, such as Gamblers Anonymous, for the compulsive gambler, inpatient and outpatient treatment programs, and private therapy. The recovery process relies on a 12-step process that parallels the one used by Alcoholics Anonymous. It also employs sponsors, mandatory group meetings, commitment to complete abstinence, and contact numbers and support to help the gambler. Additional support groups include Gam-Anon for the families of compulsive gamblers and also a group for children of pathological gamblers called Gam-A-Teen.

Inpatient or residential treatment programs are also available, though insurance companies rarely pay for a primary diagnosis of compulsive gambling. It usually takes a diagnosis of a mood disorder or other coexisting condition to get insurance coverage for treatment. Frequently, however, compulsive gamblers have already lost their jobs and insurance coverage before they seek help for their addiction.

EATING DISORDERS

There is a central paradox in contemporary society surrounding body images and food. Being thin is a culturally established sign of youth, beauty, and health. Being greatly overweight may subject a person to social and job discrimination or ridicule which create a feeling of inferiority and guilt. A common compliment in our

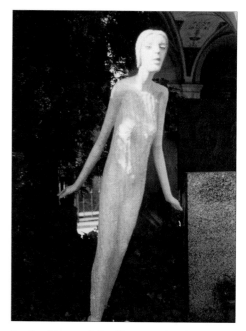

Reprinted, by permission, Simone Garlaund.

society is, "You've lost weight. You look good." Yet our supermarkets are filled with an astonishing variety of foods that are fattening, most of which are advertised insistently. People are given mixed messages— look thin, stay slim, but eat up, eat up.

Fashion, media, and entertainment industries perpetuate a thin ideal, especially for females. The average height and weight of women in the United States is 5'4" and 142 lbs. The average height and weight of fashion models is 5'9" and 110 lbs. Diet and exercise industries capitalize on this disparity and persistently urge us to maintain a slim look. At the same time, food and advertising industries take the bulk of their profits from convincing people that to eat prepared foods, often high in calories and fats, is a sign of the good life. That a number of chronic eating disorders have sprung from these conflicting messages is no great surprise.

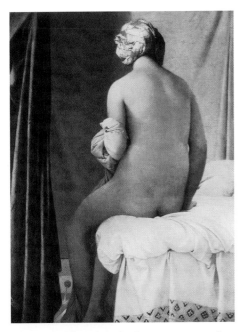

The ideal of femininity in the 1700s was much different than the ideal in the 1990s.
Louvre Museum, Paris. Photo, reprinted, by permission, Simone Garlaund.

•••••••••••••••••••••••••••••••••••

The three main eating disorders are anorexia nervosa, bulimia nervosa, and compulsive overeating. **Anorexia** is an addiction to weight loss, fasting, and control of body size. **Bulimia** is an addiction to binge eating of large amounts of food often followed by purges using self-induced vomiting, laxatives, or fasting. **Compulsive overeating** is an obsessive consumption of food.

Like other addictions, eating disorders involve a sense of powerlessness when dealing with food or eating. They also involve obsession with thoughts of food, use of food to escape from undesirable feelings, secretive behavior, guilt, denial, and dysfunctional reliance on eating or not eating such that the behavior is continued regardless of the harm done.

Some regard eating disorders as learned behaviors that can be unlearned in treatment. Others believe they are physiological and psychological addictions. Recent evidence suggests that part of eating disorders is rooted in biochemical imbalances. Some bulimics, for instance, report feeling a rush while purging or a peacefulness afterwards. Anorexic women describe feelings of powerfulness, blissfulness, and even a floating sensation. Preliminary studies indicate that there is an addiction to the neurotransmitters produced during both bingeing and purging. Clearly, eating often involves control of moods through compulsive eating and the process can be addicting. Eating disorders are complex syndromes with multiple causes.

EPIDEMIOLOGY

Anorexia and Bulimia

Anorexia and bulimia are overwhelmingly female disorders. An estimated 90–95% of anorexics and bulimics are women. Women have been socialized to regard their self-worth as closely tied up with their physical appearance, especially their size and weight. In *The Beauty Myth*, Naomi Wolf points out that, whereas a generation ago models weighed 8% less than average, today they weigh 23% less. Secondly, both bulimia and anorexia involve collateral elements of low self-esteem, depression, and secrecy. Often illness is provoked by a stressful event like the breakup of a relationship or going off to college.

Historically, anorexia appeared in the "holy anorexia" of the Middle Ages, during which monks and nuns piously starved themselves to achieve a control over the desires of the flesh and an ideal of holiness. Today, anorexia seems more common in developed nations with an abundance of food and media promotion of thin-body beauty ideals for women. But recent studies of school girls in Cairo, Egypt found rates for anorexia and bulimia about the same as those in England. The globalization of culture seems to have spread these disorders.

Certainly, in the United States, anorexia and bulimia are quickly reaching epidemic proportions. From the mid-1950s to the mid-'70s, cases of anorexia grew by 300%. During the early 1980s, the estimates of these two disorders among women were 5–6%. By the late '80s, the estimates had grown to 9–12%. Currently, it is estimated that 5% of college women are bulimic to some degree. In some colleges, the figure is as high as 20%.

These illnesses are most frequent in young women from 14–18 years old, afflicting an estimated 0.5–1.0% of women in their late teens and early adulthood.

Women over 40 seldom develop anorexia. The illnesses do however strike all age groups from children to the elderly. In one study of elderly men, 11% had some form of eating disorder. A high incidence of anorexia in males is found in high school and college wrestlers who must maintain a certain weight to stay in a category. There is also a high incidence among rowers.

"It was our coach who taught us how to throw up to maintain our weight in high school on the wrestling team. We'd go to smorgasbords, eat a bunch, throw up in the bathroom, eat again, throw up again. Most of the team did it. Of course we weren't supposed to tell anybody but about a year and a half later, word got out and he was fired." College senior

Magazines give mixed messages. One week they extol the "most beautiful people" and the next week they write about eating disorders.

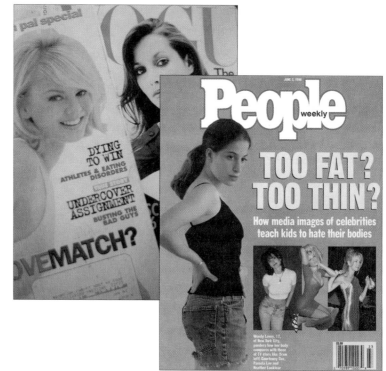

Females involved in sports who are at risk include gymnasts, runners, swimmers, dancers, cheerleaders, and figure skaters, many of whom are prodded or compelled by teachers, coaches, and trainers to maintain a certain weight, no matter what.

A complex of disorders afflicting women athletes has been called the female athlete triad. It consists of

1. an eating disorder, such as anorexia and bulimia, but also includes elimination of certain food groups and abuse of weight control methods, such as dieting, fasting, and use of diet aids and laxatives;

2. irregular menstruation, e.g., missing more than one period;

3. osteoporosis or irreversible loss of bone density which can result in pain or fractures.

It is not clear whether eating disorders precede or follow women's participation in sports.

"I went to this eating disorder clinic for my bulimia. There were also anorexics and overeaters there. At the meal table, the staff kept an eye on everyone. They made sure the anorexics ate something and didn't give it to the overeaters or bulimics or go to the bathroom immediately after to throw up or start exercising to incredible excess. They also checked under the table for thrown away food. Us bulimics, they just had to keep away from the bathroom, so everyone had to stay in the meal room for at least a half-hour after eating. A year after I stopped throwing up because of health reasons, I ballooned up to 360 pounds. Now I'm just a plain old compulsive overeater."
35-year-old recovering bulimic (male, ex-college wrestler)

ANOREXIA NERVOSA

Definition

Although anorexia means without appetite, the condition has less to do with loss of appetite than with what one expert calls weight phobia. Some anorexics, the so-called anorexia restrictors, will maintain weight by limiting their food intake through fasts and diets. Others, anorexic bulimics, limit weight by purging through the use of diuretics, laxatives, or enemas. Additional ways of controlling weight include excessive exercise and liposuction or surgical removal of fat.

"Bingeing and purging is the choice of my best friend and it's easy to see the signs: the skin on a finger eaten away and yellow from the acids in the vomit. You feel guilt for eating even a salad with no dressing. If you eat only once a day, your mind screams at you to not eat, to say no. The guilt of eating anything almost consumes you. I used to do it too." College student

People afflicted with anorexia nervosa are afraid of weight gain and eventually may lose from 15–60% of their weight. They will not maintain a normal body weight and they have a distorted perception of their body's shape and size, often feeling, even when emaciated, that their body or parts of it are overweight. Their emotional state is tied to their weight. They let the scale dictate how they feel about themselves. Often there is ignorance or denial of the seriousness of low body weight. Peer approval may aggravate the condition by praising the anorexic and encouraging "the look" which confers high status among adolescents.

"Our whole culture promotes a thin look. I never realized how bad I looked. I wore

baggy clothes so no one could tell. Even when I wore a bathing suit, my friends told me how good I looked, not how sick I was."
Recovering anorexic

Causes

Some psychologists see anorexia as a compensatory behavior for people who are too concerned with following directions and pleasing others. Young females may be considered good girls and be model students, academically talented, good athletes, and may have a tendency to perfectionism. But they may lack self-esteem and a sense of separate, individual self. A refusal to eat gives them a measure of control in their lives and continuous loss of weight can be an index of their discipline, achievement, self-esteem, and status among their peers.

"I didn't have a sense of myself or my body growing up but I tried to be so perfect. But whenever I do anything, I feel I'm going to be criticized for it, especially by my mother. I mean, even when she's not around, I still hear her. And she's not a bad person. So the only thing I could control was my eating. And the more they tried to get me to eat, the more I could say no. I thought that if I could control my eating, I could control the rest of my life."
19-year-old recovering from anorexia

Additional factors that either contribute or predispose one to anorexia include delusions (persistent, unshakable ideas that one is unattractive or overweight) and compulsions (rigid, self-imposed rituals, such as weighing food, dividing it into small pieces, or eating in a prescribed order).

Family studies, including twin studies, indicate a higher prevalence of anorexia among first-degree relatives. A current theory suggests that what initially may begin as a strict diet, in about three months begins to change brain chemistry, so that more of the body's natural opioids (endorphins) are produced and the person becomes addicted to those brain chemicals.

Effects

The results of semistarvation can put strains on almost all the body systems, including the heart, liver, and brain. Dehydration from vomiting depletes electrolytes, a dangerous condition that can lead to cardiac arrest. In addition, mild anemia, swollen joints, constipation, and light-headedness can also occur. Females can decrease their estrogen levels, and males, their testosterone levels. Other disturbances include stomach cramps, dry skin, and lanugo (a downy body hair that develops on the trunk).

When vomiting is practiced, the tooth enamel can be permanently eaten away by acid, high incidence of cavities can occur, and front teeth can appear ragged, chipped, and mottled. (Dental professionals often are the first to spot bulimia.) The back of the fingers and hands can become scarred from abrading the skin on the teeth while pushing the hand down the throat to induce vomiting. With anorexic nervosa, osteoporosis, sterility, miscarriage, and birth defects are additional dangers. Death rates among anorexic patients have been estimated at 4–20%, with risks increasing as weight loss approaches 60% of normal. The most frequent cause of death is heart disease, especially congestive heart failure.

Treatment

Many hospitals and clinics (available through associations such as the National Anorexic Aid Society) treat this eating disorder. A first priority in treatment is to prevent death by starvation. Severely ill patients are hospitalized where body weight, serum electrolytes, and diet are monitored as the patient is returned to normal nutrition. Fluoxetine (Prozac®) has helped some patients improve eating behavior and reduce anxiety, depression, and obsessive actions. Generally though, antidepressants and antipsychotic drugs have had marginal effects on aiding recovery. For an adolescent, a weight gain of 4 oz. (0.1 kg.) per day is aimed for. The patient is generally monitored by staff for 2–3 hours after eating to prevent self-induced vomiting. In one study, the recovery rate among 84 anorexic women after 12 years was 54% based on the restarting of menstruation (41% based on the criterion of general well-being). The mortality rate was 11% (*Psychology Today*, Mar/Apr. 1995).

One of the first problems in treatment is convincing the patient that anorexia is a potentially fatal problem. Often, it is a parent who brings a young woman to treatment. She herself will think that her body weight is normal or that she is overweight. Programs involve stabilizing the patient and psychological counseling to alert the anorexic to the problem and its causes; to devalue an overemphasis on thinness, weight, dieting, and food; to build self-esteem; and to promote healthy behaviors. They also involve family therapy to provide the family with understanding, support, and the ability to cope.

BULIMIA NERVOSA

Definition

Although bulimia means ox hunger ("I'm so hungry I could eat an ox"), the term generally is used to designate the eating disorder characterized by eating large amounts of food in one sitting, bingeing, followed by inappropriate methods of ridding oneself of the food or purging. These methods may include self-induced vomit-

ing (used by 80–90% of those with this disorder), use of diuretics or laxatives, fasting, and excessive exercise. These methods of eliminating food are used primarily to keep from gaining weight. People with bulimia often are ashamed of their behavior, do it secretly, and consume food rapidly. Although a slightly overweight condition may precede bulimia, those suffering from the disorder often are within normal weight ranges. People with bulimia may feel loss of control during binges and guilt after them.

Generally, a binge means an abnormally large amount of food on the order of a holiday meal, eaten in two hours or less but definitely more than other people would eat in the same time. Continuous snacking during the day does not constitute a binge. Diagnosis of bulimia requires that bingeing and purging average at least twice a week for three months. Although many binge eaters prefer sweet high-caloric foods like ice cream, soft drinks, and cookies, bulimia has more to do with the large amount of food consumed than the types of food. During binge episodes, there may be a feeling of frenzy, of not being in control, and a sense of being disconnected from one's surroundings. Between binges, typically low calorie foods and drinks are consumed.

In the United States, most people with bulimia are White and 90% or more are female, although the disorder is found in a number of ethnic groups from a variety of classes, with only Blacks under-represented. From 1–3% of adolescent females have the disorder, ten times the rate for males.

Causes

As with anorexia, the causes of bulimia are multiple. Because bulimia spans different races and classes, it is clear that all American women are subject to the social pressures to be slim. Except for a few notable exceptions, most television personalities are slender, a look promoted by fashion and entertainment industries.

Some claim that the socialization of women to an ideal of excessive thinness begins with the Barbie® dolls young girls are given, dolls which if extrapolated into an adult female's measurements, would produce a woman with a 36 inch bust, an emaciated 18 inch waist, and 33 inch hips. The contemporary starved look became popular in the 1960s, partly influenced by the 92 pound, 5'6" inch model named Twiggy and the child-like waif called the "flower child" of the late '60s and early '70s. One study that examined *Playboy* centerfold models and Miss America contestants found average weights declined from 1959–1978. Another study found that between 1979 and 1988, weights of the models and contestants averaged 13–19% below the average weights of women in relevant age groups. The number of articles on dieting and exercising has also been increasing through the mid-1990s and social historians say the feminine ideal is the most emaciated since the pencil-thin figure of the flapper (ballroom dancer) in the 1920s.

The biochemical changes involved with bulimia can make the disorder self-perpetuating. A severe diet can precipitate a bulimic cycle. Some studies indicate that 50% or more of bulimics have also been involved in self-starvation. Like other addictions, the process of bingeing and purging may encourage and continue the condition. There is evidence that metabolism adapts to the cycle and slows down, so that more weight is gained with the same intake of food. This increased weight gain is then seen as even more reason to continue to binge and purge. There is also evidence that purging through vomiting or laxatives produces higher levels of natural opioids (endorphins), so that people suffering from bulimia become addicted to the body's own natural drugs.

"It was like depression, you know. I'd just keep eating all day and so I got to the point where I was gaining weight too fast and I spoke with a friend about it and she said, 'Do like I do, throw it up.' I went into this mad trip of eating everything I could shove down my throat and then if I felt bad about it or if I felt any guilt at all, I could throw it back up and all the guilt would go away. And so to me, it was like stuffing down all my problems—the drinking, the smoking—and all of that stuff was replaced with the food and then throwing it back up."

28-year-old recovering bulimic

Effects

Effects and health consequences are less severe with bulimia that does not progress into anorexia. Problems include dental problems and a greater liability for alcohol and drug abuse than other people, including those suffering from anorexia. Dependency on laxatives for normal bowel movements can result. There is a high rate of depression associated with bulimia, as well as a greater risks of suicide.

Because of the frequency of vomiting, bulimia puts people at risk for stomach acid burns to the esophagus and throat, resulting in chronic sore throat and greater risk of cancer. As with anorexia, heart problems, such as arrhythmias, can develop as can electrolyte imbalances and irregular menstrual periods or no periods at all.

Psychological effects include loneliness and self-imposed isolation, difficulty in dealing with any activities involved with food, irritability, mood changes, and depression.

Treatment

Bulimia presents special problems. As with other eating disorders, bulimia is best treated in its early stages. But because people with bulimia often are in a normal weight range, their problem may escape detection for years. After diagnosis is made, a decision is made to treat an individual in hospital or on a outpatient basis.

Because of the multiple problems involved, a multidisciplined integrated treatment is generally used. An internist advises on medical problems. A nutritionist provides help with diet and eating patterns. A psychopharmacologist may counsel on which psychoactive medications might be effective. (In recent years, antidepressants have been used, especially selective serotonin reuptake inhibitors. One scientist combined naltrexone, usually prescribed to help people get off heroin or alcohol, in combination with psychotherapy for 19 women with bulimia or anorexia with good results.) A psychotherapist provides emotional support and counseling and may begin therapy which involves changing attitudes and behaviors.

Family and group therapies also are useful to provide understanding and emotional support to the patient. Group therapy may provide great relief for a person who doesn't need to keep the disorder secret any longer. Family, friends, and colleagues can help an ill person start and complete treatment and then provide the encouragement to make sure the disorder does not reoccur. There are also self-help and peer support groups organized specifically for bulimia but these are currently less effective than groups for compulsive overeating.

COMPULSIVE OVEREATING

Definition

When people regularly binge eat but do not purge themselves afterward, the disorder is called compulsive overeating or binge-eating disorder. With this disorder, people eat in response to emotional states rather than to hunger signals. Symptoms of a serious binge-eating disorder include the following:

- frequent episodes of eating what other people consider large quantities;
- eating rapidly, swallowing food without chewing;
- eating when not hungry;
- a preference for high-fat and high-sugar junk food;
- a feeling of not being able to control eating;
- feelings of depression or guilt after a binge-eating episode.

A pattern of frequent eating and snacking over periods of several hours is also a symptom of compulsive eating. As with those with bulimia, people with a binge-eating disorder feel that they cannot control the amount eaten, the pace of eating, or the kind of food eaten. They will only stop when it becomes painfully uncomfortable. Most who suffer from this disorder are obese but those with normal weight suffer this disorder as well. A newly recognized disorder, binge-eating disorder is estimated to afflict about two percent of the adult population in the United States. Although more women than men compulsively overeat, men constitute from 1/4 to 1/3 of those who have this disorder, a much higher proportion than for anorexia and bulimia.

Causes

Food is used to modify emotions, especially anxiety, solitude, and stress. Depression is found in about half of those with the disorder, though it is not clear whether depression is in fact a contributing cause. Food has a calming and sedating effect on some people. Dieting may trigger binge-eating disorder in some cases but in one study, nearly 50% of all cases had the disorder before starting to diet. Some report that solitude, boredom, anger, or other negative feelings can initiate binge eating. Unfortunately, weight gain may increase stress, guilt, and depression, perpetuating the overeating cycle.

"I couldn't at first tell what that hunger was that had me eating all the time. Now I know that it was my problems popping up again. When they come up, I get the nervousness that I need to eat. Now I know what time I should feel hungry. When I get that craving between meals, I ask myself, 'What's wrong with you? What are you worried about?' I know what my eating's about now."

Recovering 34-year-old compulsive eater

Effects

People who compulsively overeat are generally overweight and may suffer from those conditions associated with obesity, including high cholesterol, diabetes, high blood pressure, gall bladder disease, and heart disease. They are at greater risk for cancer, stroke, gout, and arthritis. They also have higher rates of depression than the population at large.

Psychological problems often develop. People who binge eat become distressed, develop a negative body image, and avoid going out in public or gathering socially.

Treatment

Many people with this disorder have unsuccessfully attempted to control it. Professional treatment generally recognizes that either physiological or psychological causes underlie the disorder and address those issues before initiating a weight-loss program. Treatment often concentrates on accomplishing positive life style changes, not just focusing on the narrower issues of eating behavior or the emotional states associated with the disorder itself. Common treatment methods include

- psychotherapy which focuses on changing attitudes and ideals;
- psychiatric counseling that addresses underlying traumas;
- behavioral therapy to help monitor and control responses to stress and to change eating habits;
- pharmacological treatment with antidepressants, for example, Zoloft® or Paxil®; or with newly approved combination therapies (e.g., fenfluramine and phentermine);
- self-help groups, such as Overeaters Anonymous, to reassure people who overeat that they are not alone and to provide the examples and support for positive changes.

As with all eating disorders, because people must eat to live, abstinence from all food is impossible, unlike alcohol and other drug dependencies where total abstinence is possible. A current saying among those recovering from eating disorders is, "You must walk the tiger three times a day and hope it doesn't eat you." The treatment goal is to learn to manage one's intake and to avoid foods such as refined sugars, chocolate, or carbohydrates that trigger binges. Binge foods are substances that give a much greater emotional reaction than

TABLE 7–4   COMPULSIVE OVEREATING SELF-DIAGNOSTIC TEST

The following questions are used by Overeaters Anonymous (OA) to help someone determine whether he or she is involved in compulsive overeating. Members of OA typically answer "yes" to many of the questions.

1. Do you eat when you're not hungry?
2. Do you go on eating binges for no apparent reason?
3. Do you have feelings of guilt and remorse after overeating?
4. Do you give too much time and thought to food?
5. Do you look forward with pleasure and anticipation to the time when you can eat alone?
6. Do you plan these secret binges ahead of time?
7. Do you eat sensibly before others and make up for it alone?
8. Is your weight affecting the way you live your life?
9. Have you tried to diet for a week (or longer) only to fall short of your goal?
10. Do you resent others telling you to "use a little willpower" to stop overeating?
11. Despite evidence to the contrary, have you continued to assert that you can diet on your own whenever you wish?
12. Do you crave to eat at a definite time, day or night, other than mealtimes?
13. Do you eat to escape from worries or troubles?
14. Have you ever been treated for obesity or a food-related condition?
15. Does your eating behavior make you or others unhappy?

other foods and they vary from person to person. The goal in treating eating disorders is to teach people to solve underlying problems without resorting to destructive eating behaviors.

OTHER COMPULSIVE BEHAVIORS

SEXUAL COMPULSIVITY

Sexual addiction is marked by sexual behavior over which the addict has no control and no choice. Compulsive sexual behavior is practiced by males and females, young and old, gay and straight. It can include masturbation, pornography, serial affairs, phone sex, and visits to topless bars and strip shows. Some sexual activity that can be compulsive has legal penalties, such as prostitution, sexual harassment, sexual abuse, voyeurism, exhibitionism or flashing, child molestation, rape, and incest. Pornography and masturbation are the most frequent combination. Collateral addictions include love addictions, such as romance addiction, the compulsion to fall in love and be in love, and relationship addiction, either a compulsive relationship with one person or with relationships in general.

Compulsive sexual behavior is practiced as a way to cope with anxiety, stress, solitude, or low self-worth. The body becomes conditioned to release pleasure-giving neurotransmitters, especially dopamine, enkephalins, and endorphins, with the repetitive practice of the sexual activity. But compulsive sex is not an effective way of solving problems. Often, progressively more time must be spent in the sexual activity to reduce the stressor. Damage is done to careers, relationships, self-image, and peace of mind but the activity continues despite all negative consequences.

With sexual addiction, sex becomes the person's most important, all-consuming activity. Part of the elevated mood generated by the activity may involve risk. The pursuit of the addiction has been described as trance-like. A special routine or pattern may be followed that increases the excitement. Usually there is a culminating sexual event (orgasm, exposure, rape, molestation) over which the addict feels no control. It is often followed by remorse, guilt, fear of being discovered, and resolutions to stop the behavior. Throughout, the sexual behavior is pursued with a sense of desperation and the person is demoralized and may suffer from low self-image, self-hatred, and despair at the time and money wasted on the danger or injury involved. Sexaholics Anonymous (SA) and other affiliated groups see compulsive sex as a progressive disease that can be treated.

CYBERADDICTION

America Online® established a chat group (room) for those suffering from cyberaddiction, an AOL-Anon group that deals with the addictive relationship with the Internet. Also called Internet compulsion disorder, cyberaddiction is marked by compulsive involvement in chat groups, interactive games, stock or commodities market watching, and sexual relationships, all on the Internet. Participation in virtual communities, sexual fantasy and role-playing games, and data hunts have also been noted in people who become addicted to surfing the Web.

Symptoms of Internet addiction are

1. logging on every chance you get at home, work, or school;

2. thinking about the Net constantly;

3. losing track of time while logged on so that hours go by like minutes;

4. neglecting your responsibilities because you are online;

5. allowing your relationships with spouse, family, co-workers, and friends to deteriorate;

6. getting involved in intense, obsessive, and damaging online relationships;

7. increasing the time you spend online;

8. posting more and more messages, downloading more and more data;

9. eating in front of your monitor;

10. checking your e-mail a soon as you get up in the morning and before you go to bed at night; getting up in the middle of the night to check it just in case.

Some people experience a stimulant-like rush when online while others speak of being tranquilized by their quiet isolated online time. Repetitive compulsive use of the Net induces tolerance and changes in mental states. Other symptoms of Internet (and computer game) addiction include blurred vision, lack of sleep, twitching mouse fingers, and relationship problems. People who spend hours of free time every day on the Internet or log on during work or school despite negative consequences may have a compulsive dependency problem.

CONCLUSION

As useful as seeing the similarities among substance abuse and other all-consuming behavior is, the danger in generalizing the concept of addictions is obscuring the distinctive characteristics of a specific addiction that need to be addressed in treatment. For example, in eating disorders and sex addiction, returning to normal levels of behavior is the preferred option, unlike alcohol and other drug abuse which stress abstinence. Fortunately, pharmacology, psychotherapy, and behavioral therapies tailored to specific compulsive disorders offer hope for treatment and recovery.

C H A P T E R   S U M M A R Y

OTHER DRUGS

Inhalants

1. The three main types of inhalants are volatile solvents, volatile nitrites, and anesthetics.

2. Volatile solvents consist of fluids such as gasoline, kerosene, airplane glue, nail polish remover, lighter fluid, carbon tetrachloride, and even embalming fluid.

3. The effects of volatile solvents, mostly depressant effects, include a dreaminess, dizziness, stupor, and slurred speech. Impulsiveness and irritability occasionally give way to hallucinations. Eventually, delirium, clumsiness, and impaired thinking occur.

4. Prolonged use of volatile solvents, especially leaded gasoline, can cause brain, liver, kidney, bone marrow, and especially lung damage. Death can occur from respiratory arrest, asphyxiation, or cardiac irregularities.

5. Volatile nitrites, "poppers" such as butyl or isobutyl nitrite, are sold as Bolt®, Rush®, and Locker Room®. The major effects are muscle relaxation, blood vessel dilation, and increased heart rate, causing a blood rush to the head. Dizziness and giddiness also occur. Too much can lead to vomiting, shock, unconsciousness, and blood problems.

6. Nitrous oxide, usually used as an anesthetic in the dentist's office, produces a temporary giddiness that lasts for just a couple of minutes. If not done very carefully, inhaling directly from the tank can cause frozen and exploded lung tissue.

Sports and Drugs

7. Athletes use drugs to lessen pain, improve performance, socialize, and as a reward.

8. Drug use among athletes dates from the time of the early Greeks. Drug use continues through the present because of increased availability of drugs, new drugs, a "win at any cost" attitude, and increased financial incentives to succeed.

9. Although use among collegiate and professional athletes is decreasing (possibly because of increased testing), use continues, especially among high school athletes.

10. Three classes of drugs available to athletes are therapeutic drugs, performance- or appearance-enhancing drugs, and recreational drugs.

11. A danger of various pain-killing drugs is that athletes will aggravate injuries while playing injured. Other undesirable effects of analgesics, such as opioids, include mood changes, nausea, and tissue dependence.

12. The two kinds of anti-inflammatory drugs are NSAIDs and corticosteroids. Side effects of the latter are more serious than those of the former.

13. Anabolic-androgenic steroids are derived from or imitate the male hormone testosterone. Athletes use them to increase weight, strength, muscle mass, and definition. Some use them to boost aggressiveness or confidence.

14. The side effects of anabolic steroid abuse are acne, lowered sex drive, shrinking of testicles in men, breast reduction in women, bloated appearance, anger, and aggressiveness.

15. Amphetamines, including methamphetamines, are used to boost the athlete's confidence and to increase energy, alertness, aggression, and reaction time. The negative effects from occasional use of amphetamines include irritability, restlessness, anxiety, and heart or blood pressure problems.

16. Blood doping involves injecting extra blood into an athlete to increase the oxygen content of the blood. Because of the risk of infection, it is considered dangerous.

17. Marijuana acts either as a stimulant or depressant and it is the most widely abused illegal drug. Athletes turn to marijuana to relax or calm down.

18. Cocaine may be used by athletes for its stimulant effects and as a reward or recreational drug. Psychological addiction is more usual than physical dependence.

19. Drug use in sports risks loss of fan support. It imperils the notion of fair competition and it robs athletes who abuse drugs of a sense of self-worth and personal achievement.

Miscellaneous Drugs

20. Other substances used to get high have included embalming fluid, toad secretions, gasoline, hairspray, C-4 explosive, and even camel dung.

21. "Smart drugs" are a mixture of vitamins, powdered nutrients, and amino acids. Some prescription drugs used to treat diseases of aging, such as Parkinson's disease or Alzheimer's disease, are also used as health drugs.

OTHER ADDICTIONS

Compulsive Behaviors

22. Compulsive behaviors are practiced for the same reasons that compulsive drug use occurs.

23. Many of the symptoms of compulsive behavior are the same as the symptoms of compulsive drug use, such as doing the behavior or thinking about doing it most of the time and continuing the behavior despite adverse consequences.

Heredity, Environment, and Compulsive Behaviors

24. Besides emotional needs created by chaotic childhoods, environmental influences that make users more susceptible to compulsive behaviors include bad diets, a glut of fast-food restaurants, state-sponsored lotteries, and easy to get credit cards.

25. Heredity plays a role in compulsive behaviors, making some people more susceptible.

26. A hereditary susceptibility to compulsive behavior involves many of the same areas of the brain and neurotransmitters that are involved in drug abuse.

27. A number of researchers postulate that a lack of arousal in the reward/pleasure centers causes people to engage in compulsive and repetitive behaviors to raise the level of arousal.

Compulsive Gambling

28. Historically, gambling has been used by governments to raise funds although at times, it was looked on as a vice.

29. One to three percent of American adults are compulsive gamblers. Male compulsive gamblers outnumber female compulsive gamblers two to one but only a fraction of women, compared to men, seek help.

30. More than 5% of college students are compulsive gamblers with another 10% experiencing some problems.

31. Other behavioral and substance addictions, such as alcoholism, occur in 30% to 50% of compulsive gamblers.

32. Some characteristics include preoccupation with gambling, betting progressive amounts of money, risky attempts to recoup losses, restlessness and irritability when trying to stop, and jeopardization of family, relationships, and job.

33. Compulsive gambling is treatable through Gamblers Anonymous, individual therapy, and abstinence from all gambling.

Eating Disorders

34. Society's promotion of underweight models has set up a false ideal of how we should look.

35. The three main eating disorders are bulimia, anorexia, and compulsive overeating.

36. Up to 95% of anorexics and bulimics are female.

37. Anorexia is similar to a weight phobia. It occurs mostly in women who are too concerned with pleasing others. They lack self-esteem and a sense of self.

38. Anorexic individuals lose up to 60% of their body weight. The health risks are enormous.

39. Treatment is difficult because anorexics think their weight is normal or even too high even though to others, they look emaciated.

40. Bulimics usually look normal but they stay that way by bingeing and then purging (throwing up) the large amounts of food they eat. The also use excessive exercise, laxatives, and fasting to keep control of their weight.

41. One to three percent of adolescent females have bulimia.

42. Low self-esteem, biochemical changes induced by constant dieting, and society's pursuit of thinness trigger and perpetuate bulimia.

43. Bulimia is best treated in its early stages through psychotherapy, emotional support by family and friends, and self-help groups.

44. With compulsive overeating, the desire to eat is triggered more by emotional states than by true hunger, e.g., to calm, to satisfy, to control pain, and to combat depression.

45. About 300,000 people die prematurely due to eating disorders, especially from heart disease, diabetes, stroke, gout, cancer, and arthritis.

46. Treatment includes psychotherapy, self-help groups, such as Overeaters Anonymous, pharmacological treatment with antidepressants or amphetamine congeners, and behavioral therapy to change eating habits and life style.

Other Compulsive Behaviors

47. Compulsive sexual behaviors, such as pornography, masturbation, phone sex, voyeurism, and "flashing" are practiced as a way to control anxiety, stress, solitude, and low self-worth.

48. The sexual activity is usually followed by guilt, remorse, fear of being caught, and resolutions to stop the behavior.

49. Cyberaddiction means using the Internet or the computer to the exclusion of a socially interactive life style.

50. Cyberaddiction can be stimulating or sedating to people while they are online.

Conclusion

51. Because the roots of any compulsion are so similar, one has to treat the basic emotional causes of addiction as well as the specific substance or behavior.

Drug Use and Prevention:
From Cradle to Grave

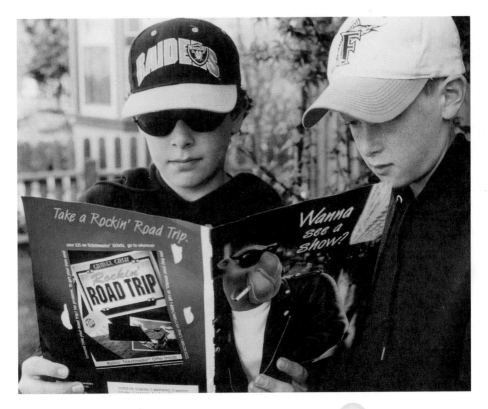

M uch controversy has surrounded advertisements or promotions of cigarettes or alcohol that could appeal to children. In some countries, all cigarette advertising is banned while in others, it is severely limited.

- **Introduction:** Drug use affects people from cradle to grave, so prevention should be taught from cradle to grave.

PREVENTION

- **Concepts of Prevention:** Historically, substance abuse prevention has included a vast array of interventions from total prohibition, to temperance, to harm reduction. Scare tactics, drug information programs, skill-building training, and resiliency programs have been some of the methods used over the years.

- **Prevention Methods:** The three main prevention methods are supply reduction (enforce legal penalties and interdict supplies), demand reduction (reduce craving for drugs), and harm reduction (try to minimize harm without demanding abstinence).

- **Challenges to Prevention:** The abundance of legal drugs and the availability of illegal drugs, the slow attainment of success of prevention programs, the inability to properly evaluate these efforts, and the lack of adequate funding hamper prevention efforts.

FROM CRADLE TO GRAVE

- **Patterns of Use:** The lowering of the age of first use and a recent increase in overall use are worrisome. Drug abuse is not limited by age, race, intelligence, or sex.

- **Pregnancy and Birth:** Drugs cross the placental barrier and affect the fetus more strongly than the mother. Drug effects continue long after birth.

- **Youth and School:** Alcohol is the number one problem in schools. Increased alcohol abuse is being countered by recognizing risk factors, bolstering resiliency, and using normative assessment. Prevention is needed throughout all grades.

- **Love, Sex, and Drugs:** Psychoactive drugs are used to lower inhibitions in order to enhance sexual activity. Initially, some drugs may increase sensation but with continued use, they can diminish sexual performance and pleasure. Sexual violence, such as date rape, is strongly associated with drug use. High-risk sex practices brought on by lowered inhibitions and contaminated needles spread sexually transmitted diseases, HIV (AIDS), and other infections.

- **Drugs at Work:** Employee assistance programs (EAPs) help control substance abuse in the workplace which costs businesses $140 billion a year.

- **Drug Testing:** Preemployment testing, testing of people in treatment, military testing, sports testing, and random testing of workers in positions potentially harmful to public safety (e.g., pilots, nuclear technicians) are the most widely used kinds of drug testing.

- **Drugs and the Elderly:** The elderly are more susceptible to drugs. Alcohol abuse and prescription drug abuse are the biggest problems.

- **Conclusion:** Prevention programs must be specific to each age, ethnic, and cultural group and the message must be consistent.

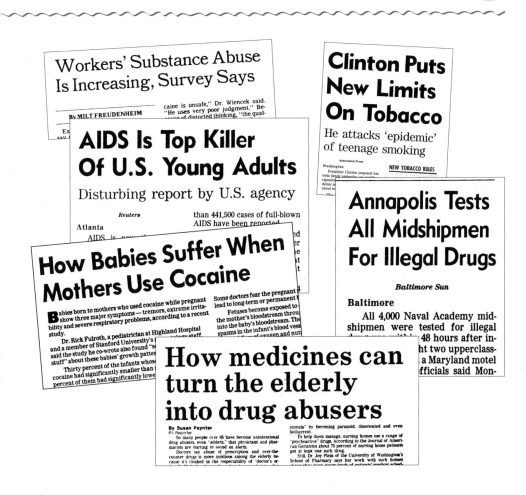

Workers' Substance Abuse Is Increasing, Survey Says

By MILT FREUDENHEIM

caine is unsafe," Dr. Wiencek said. "He uses very poor judgment." Be-

AIDS Is Top Killer Of U.S. Young Adults

Disturbing report by U.S. agency

Reuters

Atlanta

AIDS is

than 441,500 cases of full-blown AIDS have been reported

Clinton Puts New Limits On Tobacco

He attacks 'epidemic' of teenage smoking

Associated Press

Washington

President Clinton imposed his-

NEW TOBACCO RULES

Annapolis Tests All Midshipmen For Illegal Drugs

Baltimore Sun

Baltimore

All 4,000 Naval Academy midshipmen were tested for illegal 48 hours after in- two upperclass- a Maryland motel fficials said Mon-

How Babies Suffer When Mothers Use Cocaine

Babies born to mothers who used cocaine while pregnant show three major symptoms — tremors, extreme irritability and severe respiratory problems, according to a recent study.

Dr. Rick Fulroth, a pediatrician at Highland Hospital and a member of Stanford University's said the study he co-wrote also found "s stuff" about these babies' growth patte

Thirty percent of the infants whos cocaine had significantly smaller than percent of them had significantly lowe

Some doctors fear the pregnant lead to long-term or permanent
Fetuses become exposed to the mother's bloodstream throu into the baby's bloodstream. The spasms in the infant's blood vess of oxygen and nut

How medicines can turn the elderly into drug abusers

By Susan Paynter
P-I Reporter

So many people over 65 have become unintentional drug abusers, even "addicts," that physicians and pharmacists are starting to sound an alarm.

Doctors say abuse of prescription and over-the-counter drugs is more insidious among the elderly because it's cloaked in the respectability of "doctor's or-

stimula" by becoming paranoid, disoriented and even belligerent.

To help them manage, nursing homes use a range of "psychoactive" drugs. According to the Journal of American Geriatrics about 75 percent of nursing home patients get at least one such drug.

Still, Dr. Joy Plein of the University of Washington's School of Pharmacy says her work with such homes

INTRODUCTION

"Ours is not the first society to be concerned with drug problems. Throughout history, psychoactive drugs have had powerful and sometimes highly undesirable effects on individuals and society. Drugs have been banned, taxed, limited to certain classes, and otherwise regulated. We now understand that drug addiction is a primary, progressive, chronic, relapsing, and fatal disease that threatens our generation as it has threatened every past generation.

Happily, we now also understand that it is both preventable and treatable."
Darryl Inaba, Director, Haight-Ashbury Detox Clinic

Psychoactive drugs affect people's lives from conception to death. For example:

- a fetus absorbs the mother's heroin through the umbilical cord;

- an 8 year old samples some scotch at the household bar;

- a 14 year old is offered marijuana after school;

- a college student uses "speed" to stay awake for an exam;

- a young mother with three children hides in her room to smoke "crack";

- a 28-year-old IV amphetamine user infects his girlfriend with the HIV virus he got through a contaminated needle;

- an office worker takes a Xanax® to cope with job stress;

- a 50-year-old salesman on the road smokes and drinks to cope with boredom;

- a 74 year old borrows a prescription painkiller from a neighbor to relieve arthritic pain.

Since drug use and abuse affect all ages, prevention and treatment programs should also be continued throughout people's lifetimes. For example:

- teaching pregnant mothers not to use;

- showing 14 year olds how marijuana affects their studying;

- educating a college athlete on the health effects of amphetamines or steroids;

- letting the Xanax® abuser know about withdrawal convulsions;

- encouraging safe sex to prevent HIV infection;

- getting a heavily drinking salesman to use an employee assistance program;

- enlightening senior citizens about the dangers of borrowing medications;

- teaching all ages about resilience, support services, and healthy alternatives to using psychoactive drugs.

If the basic premise of practicing prevention at every age is accepted, then the questions that need be answered are: "What are the different theories and methods of prevention?" "Which prevention methods work?" and "How should they be implemented throughout people's lives?"

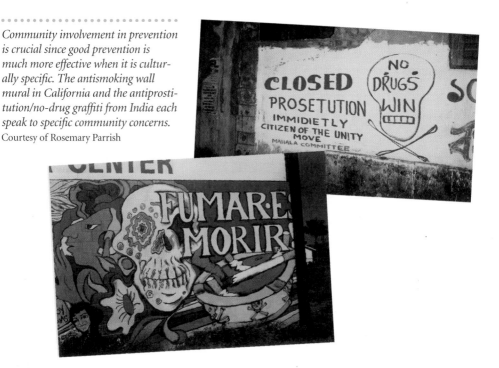

Community involvement in prevention is crucial since good prevention is much more effective when it is culturally specific. The antismoking wall mural in California and the antiprostitution/no-drug graffiti from India each speak to specific community concerns.
Courtesy of Rosemary Parrish

PREVENTION

CONCEPTS OF PREVENTION

PREVENTION GOALS

The first decision to make is about what we as a society are trying to prevent. Are we trying to prevent any use of any psychoactive drug or just illicit drugs or are we just trying to limit the damage caused by abuse and addiction? The consensus seems to be that we want to do both and therefore prevention needs to have several goals. Prevention is usually designed to

- keep the drug abuse from ever having a chance to develop;
- stop it as soon as possible where it has begun;
- in more advanced stages, reverse the progression and restore people to health;
- empower individuals with resistance, decision-making, and conflict resolution skills aimed at instilling resiliency and alternatives to drug use.

Traditionally, there have been three methods used to achieve the above goals. The first is to reduce the supply of illegal drugs available in society. This is usually done through interdiction, legislation, and legal penalties. The second method has been to reduce the demand for all psychoactive drugs, legal and illegal. This is done through treatment of drug abuse, education, emotional development, moral growth, and individual and community activities.

The third method, which is the most controversial, is to reduce the harm that drugs do to users, relatives and friends of users, and society as a whole. This is done through such methods as promoting temperance, having needle exchanges with outreach components, using drug substitution programs (e.g., methadone maintenance), and providing resources to lessen drug toxicity (e.g., designated drivers or free cabs on holidays). Historically, supply reduction and harm reduction (temperance) have been the most widely used methods. In the twentieth century, with the recognition of addiction as a disease process, demand reduction has become a viable method of prevention. In 1996, about 1/3 of the $13.3 billion in federal funds budgeted for drug control was allocated to demand reduction.

HISTORY OF PREVENTION

Temperance Versus Prohibition

Attempts to regulate drugs, and particularly alcohol, have wavered between moderation of use and prohibition. In the United States, eighteenth- and early nineteenth-century attempts to regulate alcohol consumption initially focused on the ideal of temperance. The guiding attitude was that heavy drinking, and especially drunkenness, was destructive, sinful, and immoral but moderate use could improve health and mood. Initial efforts consisted of convincing drinkers to switch from distilled spirits (hard liquor) to beer, wine, and fermented cider.

By the 1850s, the ideal of total abstinence had replaced that of temperance. These efforts eventually led to passage of the Eighteenth Amendment to the Constitution in 1919 forbidding the manufacture, sale, and transportation of alcohol. People's desire to drink again and the growth of crime from illegal trafficking led to the repeal of Prohibition 13 years later.

This conflict between moderate use of psychoactive drugs and moral/legal abhorrence of any use of any amount persists to the present day. Historically, with alcohol, the concept of complete prohibition seems to run on a 70 year cycle: 1780, 1850, 1920, 1990. (Over the last 15 years, all states raised their drinking age to 21 while some states decreased the allowable blood alcohol concentration (BAC) from 0.10 to .08. In 1995, Louisiana became the first state to lower the drinking age back to 18 years. Currently, several states have enacted zero tolerance laws that suspend licenses of youths under 21 convicted of driving with a BAC of just .01, the equivalent of about half a drink.

In the twentieth century, most money consigned to address alcohol and other drug problems in the United States has been spent on interdiction and legal penalties (prison and probation). This effort has stretched from The Untouchables busting stills in the Roaring Twenties and early thirties to the multibillion dollar War on Drugs in the 1980s and '90s.

Scare Tactics and Drug Information Programs

After World War II, concerted attempts to lessen substance abuse didn't begin in earnest until the 1960s when drugs came out of the ghettos and barrios and began to affect middle class kids. In the '60s and '70s, prevention programs assumed that young people lacked knowledge about the dangerous effects of psychoactive drugs. Knowledge-based programs were established to teach students about pharmacological effects, causes of addiction, health effects of drug use, and legal penalties. Pro-

viding factual information with a good dose of scare tactics was considered enough to reduce drug use. Often, the scare tactics overwhelmed the information or made even correct information suspect in the eyes of the students. Unfortunately, early scare tactics also presented nonfactual or distorted information about drugs which destroyed the credibility of their message.

Although factual information produced documentable increases in knowledge and changes in attitude and is still thought to persuade some young people into rational abstention, there is little documented evidence that drug information alone causes changes in behavior.

"I received only one drug education lesson in my ninth grade health class. They talked a lot about all the different types of drugs and drug use. The class actually made me quite aware that I was missing out on a whole lot of drugs. By the time I ended up in therapeutic boarding school, I knew a lot about drug use and abuse but only because of the extensive drug history I had."
Recovering 21-year-old college student

The role of knowledge in comprehensive prevention programs is still unknown. Some studies indicate that among certain adolescent audiences, factual information actually stimulates experimentation. It has been suggested that adolescents' feelings of immortality and invulnerability, a limited view of the future, and an indifference to long-term health consequences all frustrate information-only approaches. School-centered knowledge-based programs may also miss those who skip school frequently and are most at risk. These programs often suffer from underskilled or indifferent teachers and trainers or they are not appropriate to the developmental level of targeted students.

Skill-Building and Resiliency Programs

Prevention efforts then expanded to address the psychological factors that might predispose individuals to turn to drugs and the social skills that might protect them from experimentation and abuse.

- **General competency building:** The aim is to teach people how to adjust to life through training in self-esteem, social mores, decision making, self-assertion, problem solving, and vocational skills. These programs continue to report positive results but once training ceases, the gains are soon lost. Periodic booster shots throughout a student's educational career improve the effectiveness of this kind of prevention education.

- **Special coping skills:** Coping skills, like parenting classes, stress management, and even breathing classes, are taught to people facing stressful situations. Coping skills are seen as ways of developing the self-reliance, confidence, and inner resources needed to resist drug use.

- **Reinforcing protective factors and resiliency:** These are ways to build on natural strengths that people already have available. Factors such as supportive friends and family or opportunities to belong to meaningful groups in their own communities all emphasize the coping resources available to people close at hand.

- **Support system development:** The purpose of this method is to provide sympathetic resources, such as telephone reassurance for elderly living alone or homework hot lines for students struggling with the stress of school.

Changing the Environment

Gradually, prevention programs began to look beyond individuals to the social and environmental influences on drug use, such as family and peer group values and practices as well as media influences. Community organization was stressed as a way to ensure cultural sensitivity and to provide local control over prevention efforts, like billboard and advertising distribution controls. Some community programs focused on societal and organizational changes, such as altering practices in schools, work situations, organizations, cultures, and society at large. These community-based systems-oriented programs have been effective in getting entire neighborhoods to take responsibility for preventing substance abuse.

Public Health Model

As the complexity of prevention efforts increased, a model was needed to better understand the relationships between all elements in society. The result was the public health approach to prevention.

The public health model holds that addiction is a disease in a host (the actual user) who lives in a contributory environment (the social climate) in which an agent (the drugs) introduces the disease. Prevention is designed to affect the relationship of these three factors to control addiction. For example, programs to regulate cigarette advertising are designed to limit the pervasiveness of the agent in the environment. Programs to raise the drinking age or to have drug-free zones around schools are designed to limit the host's access to the agent. National antismoking, drunk driver, and HIV risk reduction campaigns, which

The typical alcoholic American

Doctor, age 54

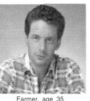

Farmer, age 35

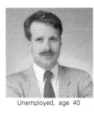

Unemployed, age 40

College student, age 19

Counselor, age 38

Retired editor, age 86

Dancer, age 22

Police officer, age 46

Military officer, age 31

Student, age 14

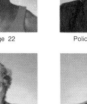

Executive, age 50

Taxi driver, age 61

Homemaker, age 43   Bricklayer, age 29   Computer programmer, age 25   Lawyer, age 52

There's no such thing as typical. We have all kinds.
10 million Americans are alcoholic.
It's our number one drug problem.

For information or help, contact:
CSAP's National Clearinghouse for Alcohol and Drug Information, P.O. Box 2345, Rockville, MD 20847-2345
1-800-729-6686

U.S. DEPARTMENT OF HEALTH AND HUMAN SERVICES • Public Health Service • Substance Abuse and Mental Health Services Administration
Prepared and published by the Center for Substance Abuse Prevention   DHHS Publication No. (ADM) 92-1801

This poster by the Center for Substance Abuse Prevention *emphasizes the fact that alcohol and other drug addictions have no ethnic, economic, age, or sex barriers.*

constitute the bulk of the highly visible programs, seek to limit the influence of the environment on the host. Other prevention activities aimed at the environment-host relationship are designed to reinforce the emotional strengths and protective elements already existing in all people's lives or to improve the economic and emotional environment of those most at risk.

PREVENTION METHODS

Whatever model is used, an excellent method of understanding the effectiveness of various approaches to prevent drug abuse and addiction is to examine supply, demand, and harm reduction in more detail.

SUPPLY REDUCTION

Supply reduction seeks to decrease drug abuse by reducing the availability of drugs through regulation, restriction, and law enforcement. Supply reduction is the special responsibility of state and local police departments as well as the Federal Bureau of Investigation (FBI), the Drug Enforcement Administration (DEA), the Bureau of Alcohol, Tobacco, and Firearms (ATF), the Internal Revenue Services (IRS), and the Customs Service. Precursor chemicals, used in the manufacture of illicit drugs like methamphetamines, are also being regulated. Even branches of the armed services, particularly the Coast Guard, have been enlisted to suppress illegal drug activities, shield U.S. borders from drug trafficking, and break up domestic and foreign sources of supply. Foreign aid to certain countries is tied to their drug eradication or reduction efforts. This complex network of agencies is coordinated by the President's Office of National Drug Control Policy, headed by the federal "Drug Czar."

Legislation and Legal Penalties

To curtail drug availability, drug legislation has been passed which mandates stronger criminal penalties for either suppliers or for users of illicit drugs. The stiffer penalties, which include long prison terms and asset forfeiture, are for the suppliers (those who manufacture, smuggle, and distribute). On the other hand, in the past 15 years, increased jail time just for use has dramatically increased. Legal penalties multiply with each conviction for possession including "three strikes and you're out" laws which require a life sentence for three convictions (usually for violent crimes). As a result, the prison population has more than tripled between 1980 and 1996 to more than 1.6 million. By 1990, the number of drug offenders in federal and state prisons overtook the number of non-drug offenders. Today, between 60–80% of those in all prisons are there for drug-related crimes, such as use and possession, for crimes committed under the influence of alcohol or other drugs, and for crimes committed to raise money for a drug habit.

Sales to minors or near schools may earn a perpetrator up to twice the usual sentence. Supply reduction legislation sometimes extends to laws against products made from hemp and to advertising or sales of drug paraphernalia, i.e., the devices used to prepare or consume drugs, such as roach clips and bongs sold in so-called "head shops."

Governments also promulgate laws that regulate the sale of legal prescription drugs and the availability of alcohol and nicotine. Recent proposals target precursor chemicals, like ephedrine, aimed at preventing illicit manufacture of methamphetamines.

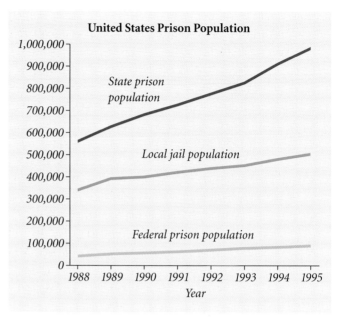

United States Prison Population

State prison population

Local jail population

Federal prison population

Year

Outcomes of Supply Reduction

The effects of law enforcement approaches to the drug problem are debatable. Clearly, the estimated 10–15% of drugs that are kept off the market means that a significant amount of illegal drugs never reaches the streets. The number of people imprisoned for drug crimes cuts down on the use and distribution of drugs and an unknown number of people are dissuaded from becoming involved with drugs by the threat of imprisonment. Strict policies and strong penalties delay the impulse to use, get people to treatment, and keep people in treatment say the advocates of supply reduction.

Some, however, have argued that increased policing, court costs, and implementation of international drug-policing agreements make this an extremely costly approach with relatively minor impact on limiting the supply. In fact, despite a five-fold increase in federal expenditures for supply reduction efforts since 1986, cocaine is cheaper today than a decade ago.

DEMAND REDUCTION

The second major branch of current prevention strategy has focused on reducing the demand for drugs. If individuals never develop an interest in using psychoactive drugs, if those using never progress to abuse or addiction, or if those who abuse drugs or are addicted to them abate their continued use of drugs, then the health and crime problems associated with drug abuse could be greatly lessened at a fraction of the cost of supply reduction efforts.

"We've got one priority, it's goal one. It says if you want to work on the drug issue, you've got to go to the 39 million American kids who are aged 10 and below and influ-

ence their attitudes to cause them to reject smoking cigarettes or abusing illegal drugs until they're 20 because if they don't use when they're young, the odds that they will develop abuse and addiction problems or even use after that are greatly reduced."

Barry McCaffrey, Chief, President's Office of National Drug Control Policy

Three levels of demand reduction (prevention) programs have been developed in the United States to decrease drug abuse. They are primary, secondary, and tertiary prevention.

Primary Prevention

Primary prevention tries to anticipate and prevent initial drug use. It is intended mainly for young people who have little or no experience with alcohol, tobacco, or other drugs, especially those who are most at risk. Its goals are generally to

- promote nonuse or abstinence;

- help young people refuse drugs;

- inform young people about the dangers of drug use;

- delay the age of use, especially of the legal drugs, alcohol, and tobacco;

- promote healthy, nondrug alternatives to achieving altered states of consciousness (Friday night nonalcoholic live dance parties).

Primary prevention involves education about harmful consequences of psychoactive substance use and personal skill-building exercises designed to promote no experimentation with abusable drugs. It attempts to instill resistance by teaching skills in coping, decision making, conflict resolution, and other abilities which assist young people to keep from ever using psy-

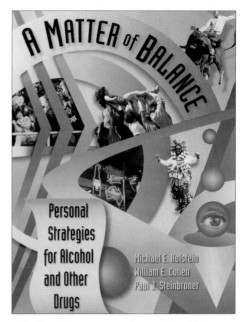

Effective primary prevention, such as this interactive prevention workbook, focuses more on developing personal skills that not only keep students from using drugs but encourage them to develop a satisfying lifestyle.

Courtesy of CNS Publications, Inc.™

choactive substances. It also tries to build self-esteem and teach alternatives to drugs.

In a broad sense, primary prevention also includes nonpersonal strategies such as legislation, policy formulation, and curricular design meant to change opportunities, expectations, and pressures that might encourage initial use.

Though the importance of primary prevention is universally accepted, outcome evaluation of its effectiveness gives mixed reviews of program results and controversy exists over what is the best way to accomplish this important level of prevention. Worse, funding and resources dedicated to primary prevention continue to represent only a small fraction of our national prevention strategy investment.

Secondary Prevention

Secondary prevention seeks to halt use once it has begun. It strives to keep experimental, social/recreational, and habitual use, along with limited abuse, from turning into prolonged abuse and addiction by taking action when symptoms are first recognized. It educates people about specific health effects, legal consequences, and effects on a family. It can also provide counseling.

Secondary prevention adds intervention strategies to education and skill building. Once drug use is recognized, a number of different intervention techniques are employed to engage the user in educational and counseling processes which encourage abstinence and provide skills to avoid further use.

Drug diversion programs for first-time drug offenders have also proven useful and cost-effective. Drug diversion programs route those arrested for possession or use to education and rehabilitation programs instead of putting them in jail.

Secondary prevention is somewhat handicapped by two actions typical of drug abusers and even casual users: concealment, which makes use more difficult to detect, and denial, which prevents the user from acknowledging that there is a problem. On the average, it takes two years for parents to recognize drug use and abuse in their children.

Also complicating secondary prevention is the lag phase, the time between first use of a drug and the development of problematic use. The lag phase is particularly long for tobacco since it may take decades for severe health problems to develop after initial smoking begins. Because most drug users describe their initial use of drugs to be enjoyable and problem free, denial and their sense of invulnerability, along with the lag phase, make them least likely to believe that information about harmful effects applies to them.

Tertiary Prevention

Tertiary prevention seeks to stop further damage from problematic relationships (especially addiction) with drugs and to restore drug abusers to health. It joins drug abuse treatment with strategies employed in primary and secondary prevention, such as intervention and drug diversion programs. Tertiary prevention seeks to end compulsive drug use with such strategies as

- group intervention to engage a person in a treatment program focused on detoxification, abstinence, and recovery;

- cue extinction therapy which desensitizes clients to people, places, or things that trigger use;

- family therapy (especially for younger users), group psychotherapy, or residential treatment by therapeutic communities;

- psychopharmacological strategies like methadone maintenance;

- promotion of a healthy life style;

- development of support and aftercare systems, often 12-step programs.

Advocates of demand reduction, while admitting that interdiction decreases the availability of drugs, point out that young people reported alcohol and other drugs to be more available in 1995 than students did in 1980.

"In our experience over the past 30 years, the best and most cost-effective prevention strategy is treatment on demand."
Darryl Inaba, Director, Haight-Ashbury Detox Clinic

Treatment of alcoholism and drug addiction has been extensively researched and has consistently been documented to be effective. Treatment results in abstinence or decreased drug use in 40–50% of cases, a great reduction in crime (74%), and a savings of $7–$20 for every dollar spent by a community *(1994 California Alcohol and Drug Treatment Assessment, CALDATA).* Despite these results, funding for treatment programs consistently falls short of meeting the needs of those seeking treatment. (The Haight-Ashbury Detox Clinic in San Francisco alone has regularly documented over 400 people on their waiting list every month. Only 20–30% of those on its waiting list ever come into treatment at the Clinic, possibly because they initially came for help at their most vulnerable and treatable moment.)

Drug courts have further increased treatment demand without providing more treatment resources. Drug courts are collaborations of the court, prosecution, public defenders, probation officers, treatment providers, and sheriff's department to coordinate treatment and facilitate criminal proceedings of convicted drug offenders.

HARM REDUCTION

Harm reduction is a growing prevention strategy which recognizes the difficulty of getting and keeping people in recovery. It focuses on techniques to minimize the personal and social problems associated with drug use rather than making abstinence the primary goal.

One example of a harm reduction tactic is providing clean syringes to addicts. In the more effective programs, the needle exchange is used as a point of contact with addicts to try to educate them and get them into treatment. These comprehensive programs seem to be effective in reducing the acceleration of the spread of AIDS and other infections resulting from contaminated needles. A panel jointly convened by the National Research Council and the Institute of Medicine found that bleach distribution and needle exchange efforts operating in 55 U.S. cities in 1996 **can** reduce the spread of the AIDS virus without increasing illegal drug use. It is interesting to note that the study did not say **does** reduce or **has** reduced, only that it **can** reduce. This is because there is much controversy as to whether needle exchange itself actually works.

"The reason why we are so intent on needle use is because it's the route to the heterosexual population and to babies. If you can stop the needle from infecting heterosexual men, then you stop most of the cause of the spread to heterosexual women and to babies." John Newmeyer, Ph.D., drug epidemiologist

Another example of harm reduction involves substituting a legal drug addiction for an illegal one, as in methadone maintenance programs. These programs have been shown to decrease crime and health problems in the user. In 1995, nearly 115,000 patients were enrolled in methadone programs, about one-fifth of all heroin addicts in the United States. A study by the University of Pennsylvania found that comprehensive methadone treatment, combined with intensive counseling, reduced illicit drug use by 79%. Clients were also five times less likely to get AIDS.

In the broad sense of reducing the harm of use without promoting abstinence, some harm reduction tactics for alcohol and tobacco have already been used. Examples include designated driver programs, encouraging eating when drinking, promoting low-tar filtered cigarettes, regulating alcohol and tobacco advertising, and providing users with information on less harmful ways to use drugs.

These legal drug prevention tactics receive some criticism because they may be misapplied: getting even drunker when there is a designated driver, using the idea of moderation as an excuse to break abstinence, or augmenting methadone with alcohol and other drugs to try to get a rush. Harm reduction practices and proposals that are very controversial include

- responsible use education which accepts some level of experimental or social use and seeks to inform people of ways of using drugs that minimize dangers;

- treatment of addicts merely to reduce their habits to manageable levels;

- behavioral management to minimize the amount of drugs used;

- decriminalization or even legalization of all abused drugs.

Some harm reduction tactics also seem to be in conflict with federal drug policy based on zero tolerance and no use of illegal drugs. Changes in laws and policies will probably not be forthcoming soon since many elected officials are afraid of appearing soft on crime and drugs. Drug war advocates fear that any attempt at decriminalization or legalization would introduce the kind of ambiguity about drugs that prevailed in the 1970s, creating confusion about whether drug use is undesirable and leading inevitably to more drug problems. Prevention hawks caution that harm reduction advocates may be contributing to the recent upward trends in drug use in the mid-'90s.

"I had a parole officer who told me to leave those other drugs alone. Drinking is O.K., or smoking a little 'pot' now and then but I have come to believe that I can't take any mood-altering chemical into my body today

and still remain in recovery. That is still what I stick to and believe in."
Recovering heroin addict

Harm reduction and treatment are considered incompatible with recovery by most treatment programs, especially 12-step programs, such as Alcoholics Anonymous or Narcotics Anonymous. The basic tenant of these 12-step programs is that addiction is a chronic, progressive, and fatal disease which is only treatable by total abstinence. Other treatment programs, however, choose limited use as an interim treatment strategy and as a bridge to treatment. They see it as a way to bring abusers and addicts in contact with treatment professionals and drug abuse prevention information.

"For years and years, we've been treated negatively by the medical profession because they say things like, 'Well, this is your fault.' So I avoided doctors and treatment. When I entered this methadone program, I had access to health care and I got some counseling. True, it was originally just to keep the counselors happy but I've been clean of other drugs and I've done no crime for four months." Heroin addict on methadone maintenance

CHALLENGES TO PREVENTION

LEGAL DRUGS IN SOCIETY

We are an alcohol-drinking, tobacco-smoking, prescription- and over-the-counter drug-using society. Looking for quick solutions, we often medicate symptoms rather than solve problems. Legal drugs, such as tobacco and alcohol, are widely available and actively marketed by sophisticated advertising campaigns that attempt to show the fun to be found in psychoactive drugs and that try to establish brand recognition and brand loyalty at an early age. Joe Camel® and the Budweiser® frogs are examples of cartoonlike characters that are familiar to children and that seem to be targeting young potential smokers and drinkers. Alcohol companies spent over $2 billion and tobacco companies over $6 billion on advertising and promoting their products in 1995. This is not surprising since alcohol sales are about $100 billion per year and tobacco sales over $40 billion per year. Billions more are spent advertising over-the-counter drugs, thus promoting the concept that there is a chemical solution for any ailment or discomfort.

This two-tiered approach to acceptable and unacceptable drugs breeds cynicism and disbelief of prevention messages in adolescents and young adults. If prevention messages aren't consistent, they are usually ineffective.

One of the realities of prevention is that there is no quick fix. If the modern reduction of smoking can be said to have begun with the first health warnings issued in the mid-1940s, then the success of the antismoking efforts have taken at least a half a century and are still developing so as to be more effective. First, knowledge must change, then attitudes, and finally practices. These changes can take a generation or more.

A second reality of prevention is that the job is never complete. Each year there is a new group entering grammar school, middle school, high school, and college who need to learn or at least be reminded of the potential dangers of smoking, drinking, or using illicit drugs. The rise in ado-

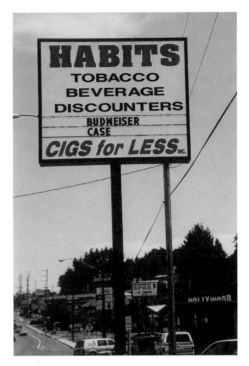

Courtesy Sandra Holstein

lescent smoking in the mid-1990s is due in part to a diminished antismoking campaign, compared with relatively strenuous efforts conducted in the late '60s through the '70s, such things as public service ads on TV, limitations on tobacco broadcast advertising, and increased cigarette taxes.

Third, any prevention campaign becomes progressively more difficult. Prevention techniques succeed with the easiest cases first, those already predisposed to listen and heed warnings. After initial successes, it becomes harder to penetrate deeper into any particular generation to change attitudes and behaviors.

Another challenge to prevention is that no single approach has been shown to work consistently, probably because there are so many variables that contribute to substance abuse and addiction.

FUNDING

Prevention (demand reduction) gets a small share of the total federal expenditure in the War on Drugs, receiving an estimated $4.6 billion in 1996 out of a total budget of $13.8 billion. Prevention is vastly underfunded especially when compared to the cost of alcohol and drug abuse to the United States and the monies committed to the advertising of tobacco and alcohol. It has been estimated that the total national expenditure for primary prevention in 1995 was over $8 billion but drug abuse resulted in a total bill to the nation of $168–$180 billion for health, crime, and other costs in that same period.

FROM CRADLE TO GRAVE

Since drug use affects us from cradle to grave directly or indirectly by examining the patterns of use of different age groups in our society, it is possible to design prevention programs that have a better chance of success.

PATTERNS OF USE

AGE OF FIRST USE

The biggest and most alarming change in drug abuse over the past 30 years is the gradual lowering of the age of first drug use. A 1995 survey by the University of Michigan found that the use of marijuana by 8th, 10th, and 12th graders has been on the rise after more than a decade of decline. From 1991–1995, 12th grade past year use of marijuana rose from 24% to 35%, 10th grade use from 16% to 29%, and 8th grade use from 6% to 16% These are startling figures. Another measure is that the percentage of juvenile arrestees testing positive for any drug except alcohol went from 22% in 1990 to 42% in 1994.

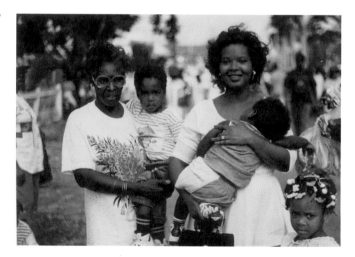

Because the whole family is at risk for problems related to alcohol and other drugs, prevention must be taught from cradle to grave.

Reprinted, by permission, Simone Garlaund.

TABLE 8–1 AVERAGE AGE OF INITIATION OF DIFFERENT SUBSTANCES

These figures show the average age of first use among those who have used various drugs. For example, of the 18 to 25 year olds who have smoked cigarettes, the average age of first use was 18.9 years. For 12 to 17 year olds who have used marijuana, the average age of first use was 13.9 years.

	Age in Years				All Ages	All Ages
Drug	**12–17**	**18–25**	**26–34**	**35+**	**1993–94**	**1994–95**
Cigarettes	11.7	13.9	14.3	15.7	15.0	15.9
Inhalants	12.4	15.6	16.1	18.9	16.4	16.4
Alcohol	12.9	15.3	16.0	18.0	17.0	15.9
Hallucinogens	14.5	17.0	18.0	19.8	18.5	17.0
Marijuana/hashish	13.9	15.8	16.2	20.9	18.2	16.3
Stimulants (illicit use)	14.1	16.2	17.7	20.4	18.8	NA
Sedatives (illicit use)	12.9	16.2	17.6	19.0	19.6	NA
Heroin	14.7	17.6	20.0	20.6	20.1	20.3
Analgesics (illicit use)	12.9	17.3	20.1	26.2	21.7	NA
Cocaine	14.6	17.6	19.9	24.3	21.4	19.0
Tranquilizers (illicit use)	14.4	17.6	19.0	28.5	23.8	NA

Notice that early use of tobacco, even for the 35 and older group, is fairly consistent. All age groups began their use in their early high school years.

(NIDA Household Survey, 1994 and 1995)

USE BY RACE AND CLASS

Often, addicts are portrayed in the media as the weak, bad, stupid, crazy, immoral, poor, or the disenfranchised who have nothing else to turn to except drugs. When drug use is studied on a regional basis, the facts show that the majority of drugs are distributed in rural, not urban, parts of the country. Even in large cities, less than 5% of alcoholics live on Skid Row in the poor sections of cities. When ethnicity was used as a measure, a Gallop Organization study found that in California, the groups most likely to abuse alcohol or other drugs during their lifetime were Anglo-Californians, followed by Hispanics, followed by Asian Californians.

The group least likely to have a substance problem was African Americans. Contrary to common beliefs, urban African Americans who are under 16 years of age and are in school have relatively low rates of use of alcohol and other drugs. The relatively high rate of African Americans in prisons suggests that this ethnic group tends to fall prey more readily to the negative aspects of addiction, including the lure of the drug trade. They may also be the target of greater enforcement efforts. African Americans with drug problems tend to receive treatment through the criminal justice system, whereas others receive treatment from medical and social service programs.

"There's no color barrier. People come from Mill Valley, from Russian Hill, from Pacific Heights. If you go in there and you look at nighttime, you see these people. They come in and supply the money. You know that the Black man only supplies the money the first and the fifteenth and that's that."
Drug counselor

Alcoholics and addicts include not only residents in the inner city but also the most skilled, talented, intelligent, and sensitive individuals in our society. For example, doctors in Canada were found to be 30–100 times more likely to be addicted than members of the general population. Professional groups in health care in general have a much higher addiction rate than society at large. Intelligence is not a guaranteed protection against addiction. Members of MENSA, a high-IQ society, have one of the highest addiction rates, as do gifted high school students. Members of the American clergy also have a relatively high rate of alcoholism. Even nuns had a higher than average incidence of prescription drug abuse. A study in New York showed that the greatest predictor of cocaine addiction was a high annual income. If people use psychoactive substances, they are liable to addictive disease no matter what race, class, or region of the country they live in. Addiction is a nonbiased, equal opportunity disease.

USE BY AGE

Although the absolute numbers of Americans who used illicit drugs in the past month (12.8 million in a population of 211 million 12 and older) may seem small, they have an exaggerated effect on all levels of society, especially in regard to economic loss, accidents, assaults, suicides, crime, and domestic or other violence.

In the rest of this chapter, we examine the consequences of drug use during pregnancy, in school, on the job (includes a section on drug testing), by the elderly and some of the most dangerous consequences of drug use, sexually transmitted diseases and AIDS. We also examine some of the prevention and early intervention programs designed for those groups.

PREGNANCY AND BIRTH

OVERVIEW

Drug and alcohol use during pregnancy continues to be a national problem that results in many infants born with alcohol-related birth defects. Drug abuse during pregnancy occurs in women of all ethnic and socioeconomic backgrounds. From 11–18% of all pregnant women in the United States are using drugs like alcohol, cocaine, "crack," marijuana, sedatives, heroin, amphetamines, and PCP. Fetal alcohol syndrome (FAS) is the third most common birth defect and the leading cause of mental retardation in the United States. Most psychoactive substances may be harmful to the developing fetus. Problems associated with substance abuse during pregnancy are now beginning to be understood.

Maternal Risks

Drug and alcohol abuse during pregnancy puts women at high risk for medical and obstetrical complications, including anemia, sexually transmitted diseases, hepatitis, and poor nutrition. Intravenous use of heroin, cocaine, amphetamines, and other drugs increases risk of additional

TABLE 8–2   DRUG USE BY AGE GROUP–1995

Age Group	Ever Used	Used Past Year	Used Past Month
12–17 (22 MILLION)			
Any Illicit Drug	22.2%	18.0%	10.9%
Cigarettes	38.1%	26.6%	20.2%
Alcohol	41.7%	36.2%	21.1%
18–25 (28 MILLION)			
Any Illicit Drug	45.8%	25.5%	14.2%
Cigarettes	67.7%	42.5%	35.3%
Alcohol	86.3%	78.5%	61.3%
26–34 (36 MILLION)			
Any Illicit Drug	54.8%	14.6%	8.3%
Cigarettes	75.8%	38.4%	34.7%
Alcohol	91.8%	78.8%	63.0%
35 AND UP (125 MILLION)			
Any Illicit Drug	27.9%	5.0%	2.8%
Cigarettes	77.5%	28.7%	27.2%
Alcohol	89.0%	66.2%	52.6%
TOTAL (211 MILLION)			
Any Illicit Drug	34.2%	10.7%	6.1%
Cigarettes	71.8%	32.0%	28.8%
Alcohol	82.3%	65.4%	52.2%

(National Institute of Drug Abuse Household Survey, 1995–released in August, 1996)

complications, such as endocarditis (a heart infection) or even fetal death. Contaminated needles further increase the risk of a woman's becoming infected with the HIV virus and passing the disease to her fetus. Eighty percent of children with the HIV virus in the United States were born to mothers who were or are IV drug abusers or the sexual partners of IV drug abusers. The life expectancy of an infant born with HIV is less than two years. Surprisingly, in the United States, if AZT (AIDS drug) therapy is used, only 8% of the newborns will be infected with the virus. If AZT is not used, there is a 25% infection rate. In underdeveloped countries, that rate jumps to 35–40%.

Multiple drug use is now commonplace and can further complicate a pregnancy. A typical pregnant drug addict is often in poor health and presents herself for treatment late in pregnancy. She often has had no prenatal care or medical intervention and often lives a chaotic life style.

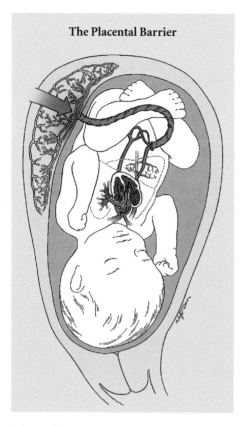

The Placental Barrier

Figure 8-2 •

The developing baby and its circulation are protected by the placental barrier which screens out substances that would affect the fetus. All psychoactive drugs breach this protective barrier and affect the baby, usually more than the mother.

Fetal and Neonatal Complications

Since psychoactive drugs cross the blood-brain barrier, one of the most impervious barriers of the body, they can easily cross the placental barrier, the membrane separating the baby's and the mother's blood (Fig. 8-2). So a fetus is exposed to the same chemicals that a mother uses. After birth, many drugs can pass into a nursing mother's breast milk and expose a nursing infant to dangerous chemicals.

Because of the infant's or fetus' metabolic immaturity, each surge of effects from the psychoactive drug that the mother receives may be prolonged in the fetus, causing greater problems for the fetus than for the mother.

The period of maximum fetal vulnerability is the first 12 weeks. During this first trimester, development and differentiation of cells into fetal limbs and organs take place. This is when drugs pose the greatest risk to organ development. Because the brain and nervous system develop throughout the entire pregnancy and beyond, the fetus is vulnerable to damage no matter when a woman uses drugs. The second trimester involves further maturation of the already developed body parts. Drug exposure at this stage creates a risk of abnormal bleeding or spontaneous abortion. The third trimester includes maturation of the fetus and preparation for birth. Dangerous drugs such as heroin or cocaine can cause severe withdrawal in the newborn and perhaps premature birth.

There is much debate over what level of drug use harms the fetus. For that reason, many professionals recommend that pregnant women abstain from all psychoactive drugs.

Because fetal metabolism is very immature compared to that of the mother, drugs can persist in the fetus for a longer period of time and in higher concentrations than in the adult. Valium® or cocaine and their metabolites may remain in the fetus' or newborn's system for days or even weeks longer than in the mother. Withdrawal or intoxication in a baby born exposed to PCP may last for days, weeks, or even months after birth. The problems of fetal drug exposure extend beyond the period of pregnancy. Definite syndromes of neonatal

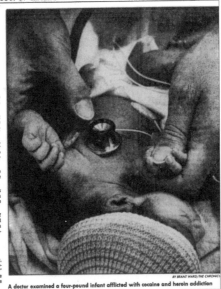

Living Hell Of Infant's Drug Battle

By Elaine Herscher
Chronicle Staff Writer

The tiny baby girl is shrieking nonstop like a trapped bird, her face red and contorted, her body in constant motion.

In her second day of life, she is not snuggling in her mother's arms like other newborns. The four-pound infant is in a plastic chamber, withdrawing from heroin and crack cocaine.

The two drugs cause different symptoms, but it is the crack withdrawal that is making her inconsolable. She is too jittery to eat. She is so irritable and hyperactive that it will take four doses of sedative to calm her down.

She is expected to spend two weeks in the intensive-care nursery withdrawing from the drugs and putting on enough weight to leave.

But that is not the worst. It will be years before it is known how deeply she has been affected by constant exposure to crack in the womb.

"It's very disturbing to see the effects of drug use on both the family and the infant," said Colin Partridge, attending neonatologist at San Francisco General Hospital, where the black-haired newborn lies in an incubator.

Sicker Babies

"These babies are in the hospital longer, they are sicker babies, they may have birth defects or brain damage related to the drug," Partridge said. "It's difficult to be an infant these days as it is, let alone when you have strikes against you."

BY BRANT WARD/THE CHRONICLE

A doctor examined a four-pound infant afflicted with cocaine and heroin addiction

When babies are born prematurely, whether due to drugs or natural forces, the cost of intensive neonatal care is thousands of dollars a day (often paid for by the government).

withdrawal, intoxication, and developmental or learning delays have been attributed to a variety of drugs, including alcohol. Many babies are born with compromised immune systems due to drug use.

Long-Term Effects

Research is still being done on the long-term effects in drug-exposed children when they enter school. Symptoms range from convulsive disorders in the most extreme cases, to poor muscular control and cognitive skills, hyperactivity, difficulty concentrating or remembering, violence, apathy, and lack of emotion. Many of the effects are reversible but the cost of the intensive care that is needed is high. In Los Angeles, which has special educational programs for drug-affected babies, costs to educate one impaired student are about four times higher than the costs to educate an average child. The good news is that recent research indicates that the majority of drug-exposed babies who receive prenatal, perinatal, and postnatal care, along with continued pediatric services, manage to catch up in their development to other nondrug-exposed children after a slow start.

SPECIFIC DRUG EFFECTS

Despite difficulties with scientific research on fetal effects of drug use during pregnancy, medical scientists have identified prenatal and postnatal symptoms and conditions due to specific psychoactive drugs.

Alcohol

Alcohol's effect on the developing fetus is the most widely researched drug in relation to pregnancy. The incidence of fetal alcohol syndrome (FAS), fetal alcohol effects (FAE), and other abnormalities is well documented. Statistics show that anywhere from 0.33 to 1.9 cases per 1,000 live births have FAS. In the United States, African

Americans have an incidence of 6 FAS births per 1,000; Asians, Hispanics, and Whites about 1–2; and Native Americans about 10–30. (See Chapter 5 for complete coverage of alcohol's neonatal effects.)

Cocaine and Amphetamines

Currently in the United States, about 200,000 regular heavy cocaine and "crack" abusers are women (the number is growing yearly) with an average age in the early 20s, the most fertile childbearing years. One can only assume that many of these women use cocaine during pregnancy. From 20–25% of babies born in some inner-city hospitals are born cocaine affected. The recent increase of amphetamine abuse will certainly result in increased numbers of pregnancies affected by this stimulant.

"My one year old was born toxic. She had 'crack' in her system and the hospital called CPS (Child Protective Services) and they kept her. And then I figured it was time for me to stop this. I went into recovery a month after that."
24-year-old recovering "crack" user

The stimulants cocaine and amphetamines increase heart rates and constrict blood vessels, causing dramatic elevations in blood pressure in both mother and fetus. Constriction of blood vessels reduces blood and oxygen in the placenta and fetus, resulting in retarded fetal development. Increased maternal and placental blood pressure can cause the placenta to separate prematurely from the wall of the uterus (abruptio placenta), usually resulting in spontaneous abortion or premature delivery, lifethreatening for both mother and fetus.

Acutely elevated blood pressure in the fetus can cause a stroke in the brain of the fetus. Fetal blood vessels in the brain are very fragile and may be easily damaged by exposure to cocaine. In fact, cases of in-utero stroke and postnatal seizures occur with cocaine use during pregnancy. Third trimester use of cocaine can induce sudden fetal activity, uterine contractions, and premature labor within minutes after a mother ingests cocaine.

Infants exposed to cocaine during pregnancy often go through a withdrawal syndrome characterized by extreme agitation, increased respiratory rates, hyperactivity, and occasional seizures. Because these babies are in withdrawal, intoxicated, or both, they are highly irritable, difficult to console, tremulous, and deficient in their ability to interact with their environment.

Babies exposed to cocaine and amphetamines can be growth retarded with smaller heads, genito-urinary tract abnormalities, severe intestinal disease, and abnormal sleep and breathing patterns. Many of these infants show patterns of neurobehavioral disorganization, irritability, and poor language development. These infants also have a higher incidence of sudden infant death syndrome (SIDS).

There is hope for parents, educators, and others involved with the education and care of these children. Many abnormal neurobehavioral effects improve over the first three years of life. Studies suggest that 60–70% of children prenatally exposed to cocaine will have normal behavior by the age of three. Almost 100% of the children test in the normal cognitive range, meaning they can be taught and learn. Although 30–40% of children exposed to cocaine continue to show hyperactivity and attention deficits, fewer than 5% have attention deficit/hyperactivity disorder (AD/HD).

Opioids

Heroin, morphine, codeine, Demerol®, Dilaudid®, Percodan®, and other opioid addicts have greater risk for miscarriages, abruptio placenta, stillbirths, and severe infections from intravenous use, such as endocarditis, septicemia, hepatitis, and, of course, AIDS.

For pregnant heroin users, the periods of daily withdrawal that alternate with the "rushes" following each drug injection cause dramatic fluctuations believed to harm the fetus and contribute to maternal/fetal complications. Babies born to heroin-addicted mothers are often premature, smaller, and weaker than normal. Prenatal exposure to heroin has also been associated with abnormal neurobehavioral development. These infants have abnormal sleep patterns and are at greater risk for crib death, sudden infant death syndrome (SIDS).

If a mother becomes truly addicted to opioids, so does the fetus. Depending on the mother's daily dose, opioid-exposed infants may exhibit withdrawal sickness, the neonatal withdrawal syndrome, which may appear shortly after birth or take 7–10 days to develop. Symptoms include hyperactivity, irritability, incessant high-pitched crying, increased muscle tone, hyperactive reflexes, sweating, tremors, irregular sleep patterns, increased respiration, uncoordinated and ineffectual sucking and swallowing, sneezing, vomiting, and diarrhea. In severe cases, failure to thrive, seizures, or even death may occur. These withdrawal effects may be mild or severe and may last from days to months.

Most cases of neonatal narcotic withdrawal can be treated with good nursing care, swaddling, and normal maternal/infant-bonding behaviors. Only in severe cases is medication for the infant required. Opioids have been found in breast milk in sufficient concentration to expose newborns.

Marijuana

Most marijuana-exposed newborns go undetected. Studies have reported reduced fetal weight gain, shorter gestations, and some congenital anomalies. In fact, women who use marijuana were found to be five times more likely than nonusers to deliver babies with features and conditions similar to those identified as part of the fetal alcohol syndrome.

Marijuana use can cause difficult labor and delivery, increased incidence of premature labor, prolonged or arrested deliveries, abnormal bleeding, increased cesarean deliveries, abnormal fetal tests, meconium staining (fecal release by the fetus in the womb), and the need for manual removal of the placenta. A Boston city hospital study found babies of marijuana-smoking mothers averaged three ounces lighter and two-tenths of an inch shorter than nonsmoking mothers.

"Smoking marijuana, that was the big one. It has caused behavioral problems for my children. I think that it has affected their ability to learn and remember, based on what I deal with today with them."
35-year-old mother of three

Researchers have also found neurological abnormalities, indicating nervous system immaturity in the newborns of regular marijuana users. These babies had abnormal responses to light and visual stimuli, increased tremulousness, "startles," and a high-pitched cry associated with drug withdrawal. Unlike infants undergoing narcotic withdrawal, marijuana babies were not excessively irritable. New research is needed to reevaluate the risk of current higher-potency marijuana on pregnancy and the fetus.

Over-the-Counter and Prescription Drugs

Over-the-counter and prescribed medications are the most common drugs used by pregnant women. About two-thirds of all pregnant women take at least one drug during pregnancy, usually vitamins or simple analgesics, such as aspirin. Medications to treat maternal discomfort, anxiety, pain, or infection must be prescribed carefully, for a variety of prescription drugs are harmful to the human fetus. Sedative-hypnotics are among the most studied of these drugs.

Drugs such as Valium® or Xanax® (benzodiazepines) accumulate in the fetal blood at more dangerous levels than in maternal blood at dosages normally safe for the mother alone. Besides high fetal drug concentrations, excretion is also slower. The drugs and their metabolites remain in fetal and newborn systems days or even weeks longer than in the mother, resulting in dangerously high concentrations of the drug, leading to fetal depression, abnormal heart patterns, or even death.

A newborn addicted to benzodiazepines may exhibit a variety of neonatal complications. Infants may be floppy, have poor muscle tone, be lethargic, and have sucking difficulties. A withdrawal syndrome, similar to narcotic withdrawal, may also result and may persist for weeks.

Studies have indicated an increased risk of cleft lip and/or cleft palate when Valium® was used in the first six months of pregnancy. Becaue Valium® and its active metabolites are excreted into breast milk, it has been thought to cause lethargy, mental sedation/depression, and weight loss in nursing infants. Because Valium® can accumulate in breast-fed babies, its use in lactating women is ill-advised. Anticonvulsants, such as Dilantin®, markedly increase a pregnant woman's chance of delivering a child with congenital defects. Antibiotics, such as tetracycline, can cause a variety of adverse effects on fetal teeth and bones and can result in other congenital anomalies.

Tobacco

In the overall population, the percentage of females who smoked in the past month has steadily increased from 5% in the 1920s to about 26.8% in 1995 (*NIDA Household Survey, 1995*). By comparison, smoking by males has decreased from 50% to about 31.0% during the same period.

Smoking during pregnancy is particularly dangerous because tobacco smoke contains more than 2,000 different compounds including nicotine and carbon monoxide. Both have been shown to cross the placental barrier and reduce the fetal supply of oxygen.

Recent studies now indicate that women smokers with a heavy habit are about twice as likely to miscarry and have spontaneous abortions as nonsmokers. Nicotine damages the placenta and has adverse effects on the developing fetus. Stillbirth rates are also higher among smoking mothers. It is estimated that if cigarette smoking during pregnancy were eliminated, the infant mortality rate in the United States would decrease by 30%.

As with many other psychoactive substances, smoking decreases newborn birthweights. Babies born to mothers who smoke heavily weigh on the average 200 grams (7 ounces) less, are 1.4 centimeters shorter, and have a smaller head circumference compared to babies from nonsmoking or nondrug-abusing mothers. Although the incidence of physical birth defects is very low in babies born to smoking mothers, there is still a significant increase in cleft palate and congenital heart defects. Smoking leads to potential minor brain and nerve defects which may be hard to detect. Because nicotine is toxic and creates lesions in that part of animal brains which controls breathing, it is given as one possible reason for the increase in SIDS seen in babies born to mothers who smoke heavily.

Babies born to heavy smokers have been shown to have increased nervous nursing (weaker sucking reflex) and possibly a depressed immune system at birth, resulting in more pneumonia and bronchitis, sleep problems, and less alertness than other infants.

Long-lasting effects of smoking exposure before birth can include retarded development and slowed maturation.

Prevention

Since drugs can have such a magnified effect on the fetus throughout pregnancy, it is crucial that pregnant women abstain from all unnecessary drug exposure.

It is estimated that only 55% of women of childbearing age know about fetal alcohol syndrome and as many as 375,000 children every year may be impacted by their mothers' drug use. More than 200,000 pregnant women use illegal drugs and more than 800,000 drink alcohol or smoke during pregnancy according to a survey by the National Institute on Drug Abuse. Reaching pregnant women with appropriate prevention messages, through OB/GYN health professionals, prenatal and well-baby clinics, and public service messages, is essential to reducing the effects of alcohol and drug use on babies.

One doctor feels that if a drug-abusing pregnant woman can be gotten off drugs in the third trimester, there's a chance that the baby will not be born addicted and not have to go through detoxification. Prevention professionals are in general agreement that because the effects of alcohol on a developing fetus are not yet fully known, a clear warning to women not to drink if they are pregnant or planning pregnancy should be given. Complete abstinence is the safest choice.

A challenge to prevention exists in some states where mothers have been convicted of drugging babies or have lost custody of their children. Some fear that such measures encourage pregnant addicts to avoid prenatal clinics and doctors and to give birth outside

In 1988, federal legislation mandated the posting of alcohol warning labels in restaurants and stores that sell liquor, cautioning pregnant women of the dangers of drinking during pregnancy.

hospitals to avoid imprisonment or loss of their children. Other jurisdictions use a treatment alternative to jail. Men use treatment disproportionately more than women. It has been suggested that if women do not have to give up their babies when they enter treatment, the treatment option will be more acceptable. Women in live-in programs have a higher successful completion rate than those in outpatient programs (from 50–70% in one study).

YOUTH AND SCHOOL

In spite of all the headlines about "crack," LSD, and methamphetamine use among adolescents and college students, the most serious drug problem by far is still alcohol. Tobacco is a close second, and marijuana third.

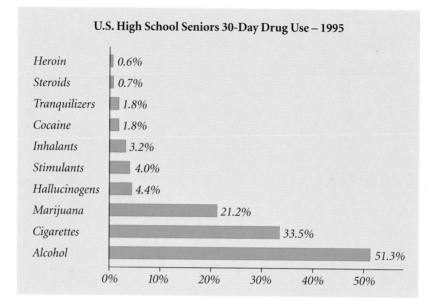

U.S. High School Seniors 30-Day Drug Use – 1995

Drug	Percentage
Heroin	0.6%
Steroids	0.7%
Tranquilizers	1.8%
Cocaine	1.8%
Inhalants	3.2%
Stimulants	4.0%
Hallucinogens	4.4%
Marijuana	21.2%
Cigarettes	33.5%
Alcohol	51.3%

Figure 8-3 •

Since 1992, decreased funding, greater availability of drugs, and a tolerance to drug use have led to high levels of drug use among high school seniors as well as 8th and 10th graders.

"In high school we'd have 'keggers.' We found out whose parents wouldn't be home, have a keg delivered, and have the party there. In college, the drug scene was a little different; besides the alcohol, you could get a better selection of drugs: opium, hashish, mescaline, peyote, LSD, but mostly just marijuana. We were too poor in high school for those." 19-year-old college sophomore

A problem with high school, college, and other drug surveys is that many users lie about or minimize their use of drugs even when assured that the survey is confidential. This is part of the denial process. What has been found is that most figures on current or frequent use of illicit drugs in high schools and colleges are underreported.

"We were supposed to put on a skit about drugs and the minute we sat down we said, 'Now what do the parents want to hear about that?' That's the general attitude all my friends have in dealing with these programs, 'What do the parents want to hear from us?' And a lot of the people teaching these drug programs are also telling us what they think the parents want us to hear. It's all very stereotypical." 15-year-old high school student

The other problem with doing surveys is that problematical use means different things for different people and for different drugs. For example, if a college freshman only gets drunk on Friday and Saturday

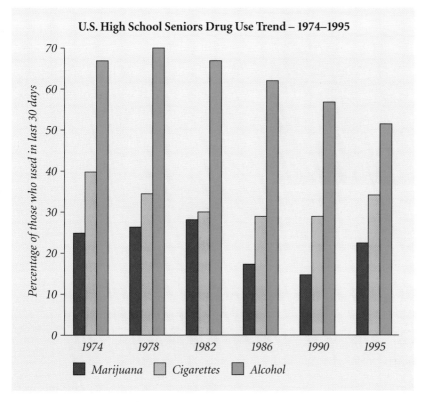

Figure 8-4 •

This graph compares the change in the 30-day use of alcohol, marijuana, and tobacco over the last 20 years by high school seniors.

Monitoring the Future Survey, 1995

nights, usually leading to a fight or unprotected sex, the student would probably swear that he or she doesn't have a drinking problem. But by the definition of abuse, that kind of drinking is a problem. With cocaine, if a student goes on a three-day binge just once a month and spends all his money on the drug and has no money for food or textbooks, that could also be defined as abuse. The true value of youth surveys is that they show trends in drug use, so it is possible to see changes from year to year in order to have a sense of where our society is headed. Surveys also give us a rough benchmark for measuring the effec-

tiveness of the prevention efforts we as a society are expending.

ADOLESCENTS AND HIGH SCHOOL

How Serious Is the Problem?

Several ideas present themselves when we look at the figures about drug use in adolescents (Fig. 8-4). First, there is a high prevalence of the legal drugs, alcohol and tobacco, with all their attendant health consequences. Second, the recent increases in legal and illegal drug use by young people

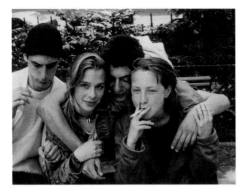

The teenage years are a period of invulnerability, romanticism, and adventure.
Reprinted, by permission, Simone Garlaund.

● ●

show that effective prevention efforts are needed more than ever.

Much of the alcohol and other drug use in high schools is experimental or social and most students haven't had enough time for habituation, abuse, or addiction to occur. They also don't have much experience using, so inappropriate use and use to intoxication are more frequent than with more mature individuals. Another factor that can lead to inappropriate use is that even if people use to control emotional turmoil, they still don't look on drug use as dangerous. Part of the reason is society's benign attitude towards legal psychoactive drugs.

"There is no way that you are going to get a majority of teenagers to say alcohol is an evil substance. That's because it's legal to buy. And how can you say that cigarettes are evil or awful things when everyone over 18 can buy them?"
17-year-old high school student

Finally, adolescents think of themselves as invulnerable to the consequences of use, so their level of concern is lower than with older users. Whereas the majority of teenagers who experiment with drugs will not become addicted, some will and for them, the legal, psychological, and physical effects of psychoactive drugs will cause problems (they also cause problems for nonabusers). Some of the problems are

- 70% of teen suicides involve alcohol or drugs;
- 50% of date rapes involve alcohol (victim and/or rapist);
- 40% of drownings involve alcohol.

Crime

The biggest effect of alcohol and drug use is on crime. In some cities, the youth guidance centers or juvenile halls are overflowing because of crimes related to drugs. For example, as many as 85% of the juveniles in the San Francisco Youth Guidance Center are there because of drugs, either using, under the influence of, dealing, or committing another crime while drunk or high. Nationally, according to the National Institute of Justice, 42% of all juveniles arrested in 1995 while committing a felony tested positive for illicit drugs and over 50% self-reported they had used alcohol in the 72 hours before their arrest.

"We're not immortal. We know that we can die but life for us is not as meaningful as for adults who have kids and responsibilities. If I die, only my friends and my family would be sad but it's not like I'm skipping out on anyone as if I were a parent or had a big position in a company."
16-year-old high school student

The Effects of Drugs on Maturation

In the United States, levels of legal and illegal substance abuse among teenagers are estimated to be the highest found in any developed country in the world. This is particularly alarming from two perspectives: first, drug use among our youth gives us a preview of future levels of drug abuse in our society and second, since teenagers are still maturing and developing physically, drugs are generally more toxic in youth and cause disruption of psychological and emotional growth.

"When you begin to use drugs around 12, 13, or 14, you never have rites of passage. You never get indoctrinated into the adulthood of society. Many people that we talk to who come into treatment actually began using substances at that age, so their rites of passage haven't yet occurred when we see them at 30 or 35. And essentially, we're talking to a 14 to 15 year old in a 30- to 35-year-old body, and that's where we have to begin." Counselor, Haight-Ashbury Detox Clinic

What delayed emotional maturation means is that if students use drugs as a way to avoid feelings, to drown out problems, or as a shortcut to feeling good, then they will not learn how to deal with their emotions and life's problems without drugs. They will not learn patience, they will not learn that emotional pain can be accepted and used to grow on, and they will not learn that being able to do things you don't want to do is part of the maturation process.

Nowhere does prevention play a more important role than in addressing drug abuse problems in young people.

Risk-Focused and Resiliency-Focused Prevention for Adolescents

Recent studies indicate that a number of conditions put adolescents more at risk

for problems and that some who are exposed to multiple risks become substance users. These risks include

- getting pregnant;
- dropping out of school;
- living in poverty;
- having emotional and mental disturbances;
- getting caught in the juvenile justice system;
- lacking self-esteem;
- being exposed to peer group tolerance or encouragement of drug use;
- lacking alternative activities;
- being in a school that has no policies, detection procedures, or referral services for users;
- being in a family that tolerates use, has no rules, has no consistent rules, lacks consistent discipline, and has absent and uninvolved parents or parents who use.

"I believe both my parents were alcoholics. My brother's an addict and alcoholic. It runs in the family. So I basically followed in my father's footsteps—the drinking, the running around." Recovering alcoholic

The challenge to prevention specialists is to develop programs that clearly identify the above risks and eliminate them while enhancing the protective elements that promote healthy life styles and personal accomplishments. Researchers Steven Glenn, Ph.D. and Richard Jessor, Ph.D. present four antecedents or predictors of future drug use in children by age 12 which differentiate future drug abusers from future nondrug abusers.

1. Strong sense of family participation and involvement: By age 12, those chil-

dren who feel that they are significant participants in and valued by their families seem to be less prone towards substance abuse in the future.

2. Established personal position about drugs, alcohol, and sex by age 12: Children who have a position on these issues and who could articulate how they arrived at their position, how they would act on it, and what effect their position would have on their lives seem less likely to develop drug or alcohol problems.

3. Strong spiritual sense and community involvement by age 12: Young people who feel that they matter and contribute to their community and that they are individuals with a role and purpose in society also seem less likely to develop significant drug or alcohol problems.

4. Attachment to a clean and sober adult role model other than one's parents by age 12: Children who can list one or more nondrug-using adults for whom they have esteem and to whom they can turn for information or advice seem less prone to develop drug abuse problems. These positive role models, often persons like a coach, a teacher, activities leader, minister, relative, neighbor, or family friend, play a critical role in the formative years of a child's development.

"There is stuff around you in your life, even if you are just bored, that makes you want to experience the effect of a drug. You can change that if you can make yourself happy. When I'm with friends doing something that's fun or even important, then I don't even think about drugs."
16-year-old student

Primary, Secondary, and Tertiary Prevention for Grades K to 12

When prevention programs are planned, they need to keep the risk and resiliency factors in mind and tailor programs not only for the age groups but also for ethnicity, sex, culture, and any other factors that will get the message across.

Primary Prevention. Primary prevention needs to start as early as kindergarten with parent-educator sessions and the incorporation of established drug prevention lesson plans within the school's overall curriculum. It needs to continue through high school. The most effective prevention programs seem to be where the students are taught self-esteem and confidence and where they are taught not be afraid of their feelings. At the high school level, peer education, class curricula, and risk-focused and resiliency-focused prevention programs are necessary.

Secondary Prevention. School-based prevention programs should include clear formulation and strict policies on substance use, teacher and staff training, parent awareness training, high-risk student counseling, and peer counseling. Additional services include crisis intervention and referral. Other essential (but sometimes neglected) services include follow-up, aftercare, and support to make sure use does not reoccur and that problems that led to substance use are being corrected.

At this level, programs found to be effective in minimizing experimentation with drugs include peer educator programs, prevention curricula, Students Against Drunk Driving (SADD), positive role models, health fairs, and Friday Night Live alternative activities. Mothers Against Drunk Driving (MADD) is one of several groups that has lobbied state and national government for zero tolerance policies. Currently, adults who have a stipulated blood alcohol content (usually .08%) trigger drunk driving laws. Under zero tolerance laws, states would impose DUI penalties, including license revocation, for drivers under 21 with a blood alcohol content of just .02% or the equivalent of one beer, wine cooler, or shot of alcohol. The State of Nevada established mandatory jail sentencing upon the third DUI conviction.

"When I was going through my wild stage, I think what changed my mind about drugs was seeing someone who went through their wild days and never stopped. So I think that there is a point when you cross over from experimentation and go on to abusing."

22-year-old former college student

Tertiary. This program (for students who have had a problem with drugs) uses student assistance programs, teenage Narcotics/Cocaine/Alcohol/Addictions Anonymous meetings, peer intervention teams, and other activities geared at getting drug abusers into early treatment to limit abuse. The honesty of peers seems most effective in reaching students who are in trouble.

COLLEGES

Although illegal drugs appear on college campuses, alcohol is the drug that predominates. In a Carnegie Foundation survey, college presidents ranked alcohol abuse as the "quality of campus life" issue that was their greatest concern. Drinking is embedded in college traditions and norms. College students are particular targets for advertising by the alcoholic beverage industry since a freshman who prefers a particular brand is expected to generate

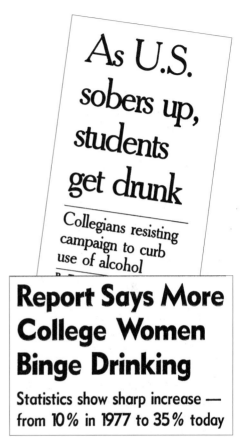

As U.S. sobers up, students get drunk

Collegians resisting campaign to curb use of alcohol

Report Says More College Women Binge Drinking

Statistics show sharp increase — from 10% in 1977 to 35% today

Alcohol is still the number one problem in colleges despite the continued use of marijuana, MDMA, and methamphetamines.

$20,000–$50,000 in sales over his or her lifetime.

Prevalence

Various reports confirm that from 80–90% of students on most college campuses drink at least some alcohol. Research by Harvard University Professor Henry Weschler indicates that 44% of the students surveyed on college campuses binge drink (five or more drinks in a session for men, four or more for women at least once every two weeks). Men bingers outnumber women 50% to 39% but the number of women binge drinkers has been increasing in recent years. The rate of binge drinking is even higher for members of fraternities and sororities: 86% for fraternity members and 80% for sorority members. Fraternity men lag behind nonfraternity men in cognitive development, especially critical thinking skills, after the freshman year.

Secondhand Drinking

Many of the problems that occur on campuses have to do with secondhand drinking, that is, the effect binge drinkers and heavy drinkers have on other students. On campuses where more than 50% of students binge, 87% of nonbinge drinking students reported being victims of assault and unwanted sexual advances, of having sleep and study time interrupted, and suffering property damage. Other secondary binge effects include having to care for or clean up after a drunken student or suffering from the general impairment of the quality of life on campus. Recent efforts include protecting the rights of these students against the damage that other people's drinking does to them.

Prevention in Colleges

College drinking games and songs date back to the Middle Ages, as do attempts to control the damage students did to themselves and to one another. A sheriff still leads the commencement parade at Harvard, a centuries-old tradition to prevent drunken rowdy behavior at graduation. Contemporary college prevention efforts date from the Federal Anti-Drug Abuse Act of 1986 which set aside funds for higher education and designated The Fund for the Improvement of Post-Secondary Educa-

tion (FIPSE) as the granting agency that reviewed prevention grant proposals and dispersed funds. Many current drug courses and campus prevention programs derive from that legislation. Generally, FIPSE programs are believed to work when there is a comprehensive and institution-wide program that establishes consistent messages. These messages can achieve a critical mass which changes environmental norms.

Normative Assessment. One prevention approach that has had success is a program that aims to change common misperceptions that drug and alcohol use among peers is higher than it really is. This process, called normative assessment, recognizes that if students think that heavy drinking or drug use is the normal thing to do, they will be more likely to do it themselves. If they recognize that heavy drinking or illicit drug use is not normal, then they are more likely not to use.

At Hobart and William Smith Colleges in Geneva, New York, researchers found that 68% of the students believed that their peers found frequent intoxication acceptable when in fact only 14% found it acceptable.

Instead of talking about drug and alcohol use, normative assessment emphasizes that prevention efforts should talk about not using. The key is to let students know what constitutes normal use on a particular campus rather than letting their perceptions be formed by sensational stories in the media or exaggerations of their friends and classmates.

Other Programs. Other specific campus programs directed at controlling alcohol use and abuse include the following:

- campus regulation of drinking (25% of campuses ban beer, 32% prohibit liquor on campus, and many campuses ban kegs);

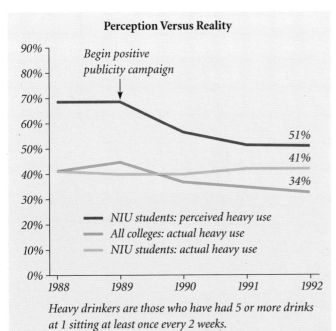

Perception Versus Reality

Begin positive publicity campaign

51%
41%
34%

—— NIU students: perceived heavy use
—— All colleges: actual heavy use
—— NIU students: actual heavy use

1988   1989   1990   1991   1992

Heavy drinkers are those who have had 5 or more drinks at 1 sitting at least once every 2 weeks.

Figure 8-5 •

This study from Northern Illinois University advertised the results of a campus survey that assessed students' perception of the amount of heavy drinking on campus. Students believed that 70% of their fellow students were heavy drinkers when in fact the real figure (and the national average) was about 43%. When the school advertised this fact and showed that heavy drinking wasn't as prevalent as the students thought, heavy drinking dropped even lower, down to 34%.

- no alcohol campus events;
- alcohol-, tobacco-, and drug-free residence halls (wellness dorms);
- requirement that food and some non-alcoholic beverages be served when alcohol is available;
- server training for bartenders at college-sponsored functions;
- banning or regulating alcoholic beverage advertising in campus newspapers;
- curricular infusion (substance abuse education incorporated into many courses);
- announcement and enforcement of campus alcohol and other drug policies;
- higher education prevention consortia where several campuses pool their knowledge and effort; about 90 such consortia exist;
- early detection, intervention, enforcement, and referral by residence hall assistants, peer counselors, the health and counseling centers.

In addition, at the college level, primary prevention includes alcohol-free, tobacco-free, and other drug-free residence halls, well-publicized alcohol-free parties, week-long "red ribbon" alcohol- and drug-free celebrations, and active outreach activities, especially those promoting safe sex.

In an effective college prevention program the three levels of drug abuse prevention (primary, secondary, and tertiary) need to be tailored mostly for 17, 18, 19, and 20 year olds. Experience has shown that as most students mature, their alcohol and drug use becomes more sensible.

"This summer I was talking to some youth counselors at work and one of the things they asked me was where they could get some 'pot.' Not that this bothered me. But

Many colleges have peer education courses for credit.
Those students can then work
as dormitory advisors, peer
educators, or as counselors to
fellow students who are having problems.

Courtesy of The Wellness Center,
University of Illinois at Chicago

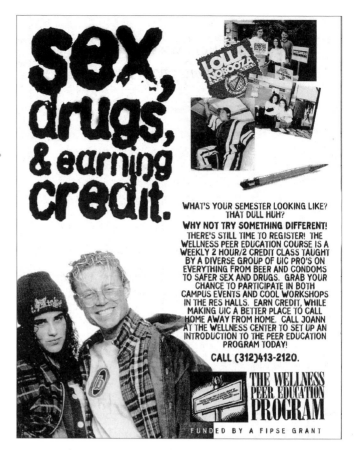

*then again, I was surprised that two guys
who preached not to do drugs were doing
what they had preached against."*
College freshman

It is crucial to recruit peer counselors
who are themselves clean and sober and
will model the kind of attitudes and behavior desirable in a prevention program.

LOVE, SEX, AND DRUGS

*"The deepest human need is the need to
overcome the prison of our aloneness."*
Erich Fromm

Our desire for friendship, affection,
love, intimacy, and sex is a primary driving
force in men and women. That primary
force is affected by drugs in many different
and complicated ways. For example, some
drugs, such as alcohol, marijuana, and "ec-
tasy," lower inhibitions. Some, including
cocaine, amphetamines, marijuana, and
some inhalants, are used to intensify and
otherwise alter the physical sensations of
sexuality and to counter low self-esteem or
shyness.

Drugs generally substitute a simple
physical sensation or the illusion of one for
more complex (yet more rewarding) true
emotions, such as desire for intimacy, comfort, love of children, satisfaction, or release

from anxiety. What psychoactive drugs do is artificially manipulate natural biochemicals, thereby stimulating, counterfeiting, blocking, or confusing true emotions and sensations about romance, love, and sex.

Drugs not only have an impact on all phases of sexual behavior from puberty, to dating, to marital relations but also on sexual aggression, sexual harassment, rape (including date rape), and child molestation. The violence occurs because drugs decrease inhibitions, increase aggressiveness, and disrupt judgment, particularly in those already prone to such behavior. Drugs also encourage high-risk sexual behavior like prostitution, group sex, and anonymous sex which can spread sexually transmitted diseases, like syphilis, gonorrhea, hepatitis B, and HIV disease.

"I'm monogamous. I'm with just one boyfriend at a time. I've been with him for two months now. The one before, I was with for four months."
Teenage "crack" user

The 1960s and '70s signaled an increase in the use and availability of marijuana, along with increased sexual activity. In addition, the onset of the "crack" epidemic in the '80s that continued into the '90s made a low-cost, ultra-compulsive, "fast-food drug" available to a younger population, causing an increase in regular and especially high-risk sexual activity.

"These were women that otherwise I would never even have the nerve to approach. Once I've got 'crack,' then I'm someone who's desirable and I can do with these women anything that I want to. And that's what got me involved with 'crack' cocaine."
"Crack" user

GENERAL EFFECTS

The three main effects of psychoactive drugs on sexual behavior are on desire, excitation, and orgasm. Physically, psychoactive drugs affect hormonal release (testosterone, estrogen, adrenaline, etc.), blood flow, blood pressure, nerve sensitivity, and muscle tension which in turn affect excitation (erectile ability) and orgasm. For example:

- heroin desensitizes penal and vaginal nerve endings;

- alcohol dilates blood vessels, making it harder for excess blood to stay in the genital area, thereby making it difficult to maintain an erection;

- steroids increase testosterone which stimulates the fight center of the brain, making a user more sexually aggressive;

- cocaine and amphetamines release dopamine which stimulates our pleasure center in the limbic system, the same system stimulated during excitation and orgasm;

- many psychoactive drugs affect the hypothalamus which can trigger hormonal changes.

"It's a very euphoric satisfying kind of effect and it's similar to sex—but different. If I have heroin, I don't want or need real sex."
Heroin user

The actual effect of drugs versus what the user hopes they will do can vary radically. In a survey at the Haight-Ashbury Detox Clinic, regular drug users said they combined sex and drugs in order to

- lower their inhibitions;
- try to make themselves perform better;
- increase their fantasies.

"As a teenager, I was sort of shy and the 'coke' made me feel I was super smart, super pretty, a super person. At that age, I felt very awkward and uncomfortable without the drug."
Recovering "crack" user

SIDE EFFECTS

People combine sex and drugs, searching for a shortcut to complex emotions but the reaction to psychoactive drugs is so variable, often escalating into compulsive and addictive behavior, that many of the initial, desired effects on desire and performance change with time. Diminished sexual performance, even to the point of impotence, is experienced by males who are heavy users of a number of drugs, including heroin and alcohol, as is diminished interest in physical and emotional contact.

Sex and love are such complicated processes and so tied in with our mental state that people use drugs not only to enhance their sexuality but also to shield themselves from their sexuality and even from any emotional involvement.

THE DRUGS

Drug-using behavior takes on a life of its own as tolerance, withdrawal, and side effects overwhelm the original intentions of the user.

Uppers

Amphetamines and cocaine are popular with heterosexuals and particularly some male homosexuals because sometimes they can prolong an erection, increase endurance, and intensify an orgasm during initial low-dose use. High-dose and prolonged use however have quite the opposite effect on sexuality.

"The kind of feeling you get when you inject it—it's sort of like the feeling when you're making love with your wife. After a while, when you keep doing it, you're impotent and it doesn't have any effect. The opposite sex can do anything they want to you and you won't react." Recovering cocaine addict

Opioids

Downers are often used to lower inhibitions, though the physiological depressive effects often decrease desire and performance. Some "nod out" when using, some feel "up." These differences can be explained by selective tolerance of different functions of the body to the effects of opioids. For example, with prolonged use, the user's pupils will still be pinned but the depression of emotions will not be as severe.

"You start to look more masculine. You feel out of your skin. You can't really feel yourself anymore. The same sort of people you really loved aren't attracted to you anymore."
Female heroin user

As the habit increases and many users go on the "nod," interest in sex continues to decline. In one study, 60% of heroin addicts reported an overall decrease in desire (impaired sexual desire or libido). While they were high on heroin, that figure jumped to 90%. In another study, 70% reported delayed ejaculation when using, which is why some premature ejaculators self-medicate. Further, the overall rate of impotence (inability to become aroused) in one study of male addicts was 39%, jumping to 53% when they were actually high.

Sedative-Hypnotics

Many sedative-hypnotics, such as benzodiazepines, barbiturates, and street Quaaludes®, have been called alcohol in pill form and touted as sexual enhancers. As with alcohol, it is a case of lowered inhibitions and relaxation versus physical depression that makes one unable to perform or respond sexually.

"Sexually and mentally, everything is so down. If I were a man, I couldn't have an erection. As a woman, I don't have an orgasm. Your mind is just mush but you don't care. The last thing you worry about is sex."
Valium® addict

Along with the disinhibition, sedative-hypnotics also impair judgment, making the user more susceptible to sexual advances. As the dose increases, the sedative effects take over, making the user unable to ward off unwanted sexual advances. The user becomes lethargic and sleepy and experiences extensive muscle relaxation. With abuse comes sexual dysfunction and total apathy towards sexual stimulation. In 1996, the sedative-hypnotic Royhypnol® was labeled the date rape drug and banned in the United States. This benzodiazepine, which is only legally available in other countries, along with prescription Halcion®, which is available in the United States, causes profound amnesia along with lowered inhibitions and decreased physical ability to resist or remember a sexual assault.

Alcohol

"One drink of wine and you act like a monkey, two drinks and you strut like a peacock, three drinks and you roar like a lion, and four drinks, you behave like a pig."
Henry Vollam Morton, 1936

More than any other psychoactive drug, alcohol has insinuated itself in the lore, culture, and mythology of sexual and romantic behavior: champagne to celebrate, the cocktail before sex, or beer swilled before a date. Alcohol's physical effects on sexual functioning are closely related to blood alcohol levels. Its mental effects, however, are less strictly dose related and have more to do with the psychological makeup of the user and the setting in which used. Effects vary from user to user.

Low-dose use:
Males: Usually increases desire (lowered inhibitions, relaxation); slightly decreases erectile ability; delays ejaculation.
Females: Usually increases desire and intensity of orgasm.

High-dose use:
Males: Increases/decreases desire; greatly decreases erectile and ejaculatory ability; causes some impotence.
Females: Greatly lowers desire and intensity of orgasm (lowered inhibitions make a woman more susceptible to coercion and rape).

Prolonged use:
Males: Decreases desire, erectile ability, and ejaculatory ability; causes some impotence.
Females: Decreases desire; decreases intensity of orgasm or blocks orgasm completely.

"Sure I can have sex without alcohol. I've just never had occasion to do it."
Problem drinker

Women and Alcohol

In most societies, more taboos and restrictions are placed on a woman's sexuality than on a man's. In one study, 65% of the women polled said alcohol improved their sexual functioning mostly in regard to the quality of their orgasm.

Many alcoholic females seem to associate their identity as a woman with their sexual activity. Inevitably, because alcohol diminishes sexual arousal, women suffer lowered self-esteem and feelings of inadequacy. Typically, the alcoholic denies that what is happening to her sexuality is related to what is happening with her progressive alcohol use. In one study of chronic female alcoholics, 36% said they had orgasms less than 5% of the time. In both men and women, as the drinking progresses, alcoholic behavior is reinforced and it becomes difficult for the alcoholic to do anything but drink. Sex is merely something to do while drinking.

Men and Alcohol

The familiar release of inhibitions both in words and deeds is the key to alcohol's dual effect on a man's sexual activity, i.e., more desire/less performance. In men, a blood alcohol level of .05 (about three beers in one hour) has a very measurable physical effect on erectile ability and yet legal intoxication in most states is twice that amount. On the other hand, mentally, even one drink can loosen the tongue. Physically, alcohol diminishes spinal reflexes (thus decreasing sensitivity and erectile ability) and dilates blood vessels (interfering with the ability to have an erection or to ejaculate). Even a few drinks lower testosterone levels.

Initially, however, alcohol gives men more confidence because it acts on the area of the brain that regulates fear and anxiety, thereby promoting, not decreasing, aggressiveness. As alcoholism progresses, many men feel less sexual and tend to shy away from the bedroom and even become asexual.

ALL AROUNDERS

Marijuana

Marijuana has been called "the mirror that magnifies" because many of its effects—sensory enhancement, prolongation of time sense, increased affectionate bonding, disinhibition, diffusion of ego, and sex-ualized fantasy—suggest a preexisting desire for these sensations.

Most of the reported effects from marijuana are general comments such as feelings of sexual pleasure rather than specifics like prolonged excitation or delayed orgasm. Marijuana more than any psychoactive drug shows the difficulty in separating the actual effects from the influence of the mindset and setting where the drug is used. If the drug is shared in a social setting, at a party, or on a date, the expectation is that it will make both parties more relaxed, less inhibited, and more likely to do things they wouldn't normally do.

A problem with excessive marijuana smoking is that the user often forgets how to have sexual relations without being high, and so the cycle of excess use is perpetuated. (The loss of sexual interest in other cultures from hashish use is well known.)

MDMA and MDA ("ecstasy," "rave")

Users say MDMA and MDA (at moderate doses), unlike methamphetamines, calm them and give them warm feelings toward others and a heightened sensual awareness. The warm feelings supposedly make closer relations with those around them possible. However, only 25–50% of the users report any of these reactions. Most novice users, 90% in one study, said they would not try the drug again. Also, most of the reports about the sexual effects of MDMA and MDA are anecdotal and since polydrug use is quite widespread (especially involving amphetamine, marijuana, and alcohol), accurate data is lacking.

INHALANTS

"Poppers" (amyl and butyl nitrite)

Volatile nitrites are vasodilators and muscles relaxants. If inhaled just prior to orgasm, they seemingly prolong and enhance the sensation. Abused as orgasm intensifiers by both the gay and straight communities in the 1960s, they too gained the reputation of being yet another "love drug." The side effects however of dizziness, weakness, sedation, fainting, and loss of erection often counteract the desired effects.

Nitrous Oxide (laughing gas)

Nitrous oxide has become popular at "rave" parties and "desert raves" for the giddiness it produces. However, it is not generally looked upon as a sexually enhancing substance. One study of 15 dental personnel who abused the substance over a period of time found impotence in seven cases. The problem eventually was reversed when use of the gas was stopped.

PSYCHIATRIC DRUGS

Most patients who use psychiatric medications have preexisting emotional problems which can impair sexual functioning. By treating the mental condition, the drugs can also affect the sexual problems of the user. For example, an antidepressant can make a patient more able to engage in intimate relations and sexual appreciation, capabilities which were impaired by the depression.

Various studies involving tricyclic antidepressants, such as desipramine (Norpramine®) and amitriptyline (Elavil®), have linked them to decreased desire, problems with erection, and delayed orgasm. Initially, however, in many cases, the relief from depression makes the user more able to participate in sexual activities. Many of the newer antidepressants, such as Zoloft®, Prozac®, and Paxil®, cause delay or inhibition of orgasm. Delayed orgasm often goes away with time. Prozac® has also been associated with a significant incidence of sexual disinterest where sex is possible but interest diminishes.

Antipsychotics, such as thioridazine (Mellaril®), inhibits erectile function and ejaculation. Chlorpromazine (Thorazine®) and haloperidol (Haldol®) can inhibit desire, erectile function, and ejaculation. Impaired ejaculation appears to be the most common side effect of the major tranquilizers (antipsychotics).

With lithium, there are some reports of decreased desire and difficulty maintaining an erection as the dosage increases.

APHRODISIACS

The search for true aphrodisiacs is complicated by the complexity of the sexual response. Are we talking about affection, love, or lust when we discuss drugs that enhance sexuality? Are we talking about drugs that change the mental or the physical aspects of sexuality? Is the drug expected to increase desire, prolong excitation, increase lubrication, delay orgasm or improve its quality? Is a drug that lowers inhibitions an aphrodisiac?

Heroin sometimes delays orgasm, cocaine sometimes increases desire or prolongs an erection, and alcohol lowers inhibitions, thereby increasing desire.

Some purported aphrodisiacs, such as Spanish fly (cantharidin derived from a

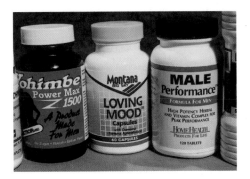

The number of over-the-counter and prescription drugs that contain yohimbe and promise improved sexual performance has grown.

beetle) or ground rhinoceros horn, work by irritating the urethra and bladder, promoting a pseudosexual excitement. But Spanish fly is actually toxic. Pheromones are human hormones discovered in perspiration. The scent or odor of these substances has been shown to increase desire and sexual stimulation. Yohimbine is an alkaloid obtained from several plant sources including the yohimbe tree in west Africa. This psychedelic produces some hallucinations and a mild euphoria. It has been used in high doses as a treatment for impotence in men by increasing blood pressure and heart rate, thereby increasing penile blood flow. It can produce acute anxiety at low dosages.

One problem with purported sexual enhancers is that the body adapts to any drug, so that its effectiveness decreases with time. Next, with illegal substances, controlled use is difficult and side effects start to overwhelm any benefits. Third, and perhaps most important, the psychological roots of most feelings are quite complex and generally more important to sexual functioning than mere enhancement of sensations. Drugs can distort, magnify, or eliminate feelings involved with erotic activities.

SUBSTANCE ABUSE AND SEXUAL ASSAULT

"Richard Allen Davis told police he killed 12-year-old Polly Klaas because he feared he had already slaughtered two other little girls in her Petaluma home while high on alcohol and drugs. Davis said he had entered Polly's home the night of October 1, 1993 after drinking two quarts of beer and smoking a marijuana joint laced with PCP. He said he had little memory of taking Polly."

Excerpt from the San Francisco Examiner, May, 1996 (Davis was found guilty and sentenced to death.)

Some generalizations about the effects of psychoactive drugs on sexual behavior can be made.

• Alcohol lowers inhibitions and muddles rational thought, making the user more likely to act out irrational or inappropriate desires.

• Cocaine and amphetamines increase confidence and aggression, making the male user more likely to impose his will on his date.

• Marijuana and sedatives lower inhibitions, making users more likely to carry out their desires, wanted or not, or making the woman less able to resist.

• PCP and heroin make the user less sensitive or indifferent to pain, making users more liable to damage their partners or themselves.

• Steroids increase aggression and irrational behavior.

In most cases, the male user already has tendencies towards improper or aggressive behavior and the alcohol or other drug is the final trigger. The trigger can also be an emotion such as anger, hate, or in some cases, lust. For example, with date rape, the man may just intend to have sex but when he is refused or doesn't get his way, he becomes angry and takes what he feels is his. In the final analysis, rape is motivated by a need to overpower, humiliate, and dominate a victim not a desire to have sex.

SEXUALLY TRANSMITTED DISEASES (STDs), NEEDLE-TRANSMITTED DISEASES, AND AIDS

Estimates are that worldwide, 330 million cases of sexually transmitted diseases (STDs) occurred last year. Another 24 million people are infected with the HIV

(AIDS) virus. One of the main reasons for this increase is the use of alcohol and other drugs.

Epidemiology

In spite of the fear of sexually transmitted diseases, such as gonorrhea, syphilis, genital herpes, genital warts, chlamydia, hepatitis B, and especially HIV disease, and in spite of a dramatic growth in unwanted pregnancies, the practice of unsafe and unprotected sex by high school students, college students, and young adults continues. About 85% of all STDs occurs in persons between the ages of 15 and 30. Very often, alcohol and other drugs are involved.

The *Youth Risk Behavior Study* in 1994 found that students who drank heavily were much more likely to have had high-risk sexual intercourse than light drinkers or abstainers. Heavy drinkers were also more likely to have had two or more partners. The use of "crack" cocaine, methamphetamine, and marijuana also increases high-risk sexual activity due to stimulation of sensations, lowering of inhibitions, and impaired judgment.

In addition, the very nature of sexual activity clouds judgment as do most drugs. Drugs also affect memory, so even if users do something dangerous while under the influence, they might not remember it or if they do, they will see it in a more benign light and not appreciate the risks they took, thus laying the groundwork for repetition of the behavior.

With this mix, it is no wonder that almost half of all U.S. teenagers who are very active sexually have had chlamydia, the fastest-spreading sexually transmitted disease. In fact, experts think that as many as 4 million Americans have caught the disease (often without knowing it). Perhaps 20% of all very sexually active men and women have genital herpes. Even syphilis, which

had diminished dramatically in the last 50 years, has started to climb again. Most ominously, there were 76,814 new cases of AIDS in 1995.

"This woman was pregnant, she was living on the street, she was prostituting, was HIV positive, and had a $250-a-day habit. I mean she's not a bad looking woman but she was definitely into her 'smack' and her cocaine. She told me she had to sleep with at least five guys a day, minimum, to support her habit. I wonder how many people she's given her diseases to." AIDS patient

The increased risk of STDs, including HIV disease, in the drug-abusing population is also much higher because drug abuse requires money and people will often do anything to raise money to avoid the cocaine crash or heroin withdrawal symptoms. Trading sex for drugs is an all too common practice.

"I was selling dope and made $3 or $4 thousand a week. I had women coming to me. I never 'tossed' a woman in my life. Those women were coming after me. I mean, you've got to look at both sides of it." 22-year-old recovering "crack" dealer/user

One thing to remember about sexually transmitted diseases is that there is a delayed incubation period before symptoms show up and the disease can be transmitted to others. There are also some diseases where symptoms aren't evident but the illness is still transmittable.

Needle-Transmitted Diseases

Many of the same illnesses that are transmitted sexually can be transmitted through contaminated hypodermic needles when drugs are taken intravenously.

TABLE 8–3   SEXUALLY TRANSMITTED DISEASES

Disease	First Symptoms	Typical Symptoms
Chlamydia or NGU (nonspecific urethritis)	7–21 days	Discharge from genitals or rectum
Pelvic inflammatory disease (PID)	Highly variable	Infection of uterus, fallopian tubes, and ovaries, a potential cause of infertility
Gonorrhea ("clap," "dose")	2–30 days	Discharge from genitals or rectum, pain when urinating, sometimes no symptoms
Herpes simplex I or II (cold sores, fever blisters)	2–20 days	Painful blisters/sores on genitals or mouth, fever, malaise, swollen lymph glands
Veneral warts (genital warts)	30–90 days (even years)	Itch, irritation, and bumpy skin growths on genitals, anus, mouth, throat
Syphilis ("syph," "bad blood," "lues")	10–90 days	Primary stage: chancre on genitals, mouth, anus; secondary stage: diffuse rash, hair loss, malaise
Hepatitis B and C (serum hepatitis)	60–90 days	Yellow skin and eyes, dark urine, severe malaise, weight loss, abdominal pain
Trichomonas vaginalis (vaginitis)	7–30 days	Women: vaginal discharge, itching, burning; men: usually no symptoms
Pubic lice ("crabs," "cooties")	21–30 days	Itching, tiny eggs (nits) on pubic hair
Scabies ("7-year itch")	14–45 days	Itching at night, bumps and burrows on skin
Monila (candidiasis, yeast)	Highly variable	White thick vaginal discharge and itching in women, men most often have no symptoms
Bacterial vaginosis (gardnerella, nonspecific vaginitis)	Highly variable	Vaginal discharge, peculiar odor in women, men most often have no symptoms
HIV infection (leads to AIDS)	Many months (up to 5 years)	Weight loss, fever, swollen glands, fatigue, severe malaise, recurrent infections, sore throat, skin blotches

(Courtesy of the Venereal Disease Action Council of Portland, Oregon)

And since high-risk sex is often associated with drug use, the risk of transmitting diseases is even greater.

Needle kits are called "outfits," "fits," "rigs," "works," "points," and many other names. Intravenous drug use is also called "mainlining," "geezing," "slamming," or "hitting up." Problems with needle use come from several sources. Besides putting a large amount of the drug in the bloodstream in a short period of time, needles also inject other substances, like powered milk, procaine, or even Ajax®, which are often used to cut or dilute drugs. They can also inject dangerous bacteria and viruses. One of the most common diseases transmitted is viral hepatitis, an infection of the liver. Besides HIV infection, this is the most common disease in needle users. Another common problem is endocarditis, a sometimes fatal condition caused by certain bacteria that lodge and grow in the valves of the heart. In 1996, several cases of necrotizing fasciitis (a flesh-eating bacteria and wound botulism, or gangrene) were reported in tar heroin injectors in California.

Needle use can also cause abscesses at a contaminated injection site or they can inject bits of foreign matter in the bloodstream which can lodge in the spine, brain, lungs, or eyes and cause an embolism or other problems. Needle users can also contract cotton fever, a very common disease. The symptoms are similar to those of a very bad case of the flu. Its cause is unknown though some believe that it results from bits of cotton (used to filter the drug) which lodge in various tissues or from infections (viral or bacterial) carried into the body by cotton fibers injected into the blood.

Typically, veins of the arms, wrists, and hands are used first. As these veins become hardened due to constant sticking, the user will inject into the veins of the neck and the legs. As it becomes difficult to locate usable veins, addicts will also shoot under the skin ("skin popping"). They will also shoot into a muscle in the buttocks, shoulder, or legs ("muscling"). If they become desperate as they run out of places to inject themselves, they will shoot into the foot and males will even inject in the dorsal vein in the penis.

HIV Disease and AIDS

Definitions. HIV means human immunodeficiency virus, the virus which causes AIDS. AIDS stands for acquired immune deficiency syndrome. AIDS is identified by the incidence of one or more of a group of serious illnesses, such as pneumocystis carinii pneumonia, Kaposi's sarcoma cancer, or tuberculosis, which develop when the HIV virus has taken control of the patient's body. However, since 1993, a new definition of AIDS has been added. AIDS is now also defined as having a T-cell count below 200. T-cell counts measure the level of effectiveness of one's immune system.

AIDS is fatal because the HIV virus destroys the immune system, making it impossible for the body to fight off serious illnesses, such as pneumonia. Usually, death occurs from a combination of many diseases and infections. Many needle users test positive for the HIV (AIDS) virus because they shared a needle used by someone already infected.

"At one 'shooting gallery' in New York that I visited, users came in, shoved their money through one hole in the wall, then shoved their arms through another hole in the wall and received an injection. Russian roulette with real bullets seemed safe compared to this practice." Drug education outreach worker

It is impossible to overemphasize the danger of using infected needles because IV use of a drug bypasses all the body's natural defenses such as body hairs, mucous membranes, body acids, and enzymes. And the HIV virus itself destroys the body's last line of defense, the immune system. In fact, recent research shows that, in and of themselves, opioids and other drugs of abuse can weaken the immune system. This, coupled with the malnutrition and unhealthy habits that compulsive drug use promotes, makes the body unable to fight off any illness.

"I told this guy that was sharing some 'speed' with me that I had AIDS and that

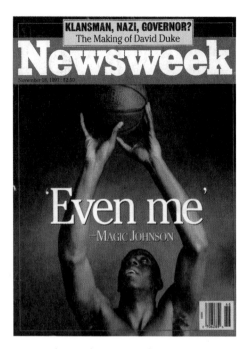

KLANSMAN, NAZI, GOVERNOR?
The Making of David Duke

Newsweek

November 18, 1991 · $2.50

'**Even me**'
—MAGIC JOHNSON

Magic Johnson, former star of the Los Angeles Lakers, contracted HIV disease from unprotected sex, illustrating the spread of the disease into the heterosexual community. In the rest of the world, spread of the disease through heterosexual contact is much more prevalent than through homosexual contact or IV drug use.

he should clean the needle but he was so strung out and anxious to shoot up that he pulled a knife on me and made me give him the needle." Intravenous cocaine user

Epidemiology of HIV and AIDS. One to 2 million people, or one in every 130 to 260 people in the United States are infected with the HIV virus and virtually all of them will develop AIDS.

Through December 1995, about 129,000 intravenous (IV) drug users had full-blown AIDS as a result of injecting themselves with HIV-infected needles. This is about 31% of the 513,486 cases of AIDS in the United States. By the end of 1995,

319,849 had died from AIDS since the epidemic began in 1981. Some have estimated that the infection rate among IV drug users approaches 30%. In addition, approximately 300,000 more needle drug users are infected with the HIV virus. Infected needle drug users spread the disease to non-drug users through unsafe sexual practices.

Prevention of HIV and AIDS. It is important to remember the pattern of the spread of communicable diseases. They start slowly but then rage through the most susceptible groups. In the case of HIV and AIDS in the United States, the gay community that practiced unsafe sex was the most vulnerable compared to other countries where heterosexual high-risk sexual activity spreads the disease. Once the most vulnerable have been infected, there is usually a lull in the increase of the disease. During such lulls, a false sense of security, along with clouded judgment, builds up a new well of infection. Most experts predict that the majority of new cases of HIV in the United States (as in the rest of the world) will be in the heterosexual and drug-using communities. Continuing public education and public health prevention activities are crucial to stem the spread of AIDS and, for that matter, all sexually transmitted diseases.

"The only way the attitudes and practices towards AIDS would change is if everybody got these diseases, you hear what I'm saying? Because it doesn't really sink in unless it strikes close to you. Once the virus is in your own backyard, you become very serious. Kids wanna wear rubbers once they find out their father has it, you know what I mean? People are concerned once they find out their mother has it, or their brother has it, or they have it."
Recovering 43-year-old heroin addict who is HIV positive

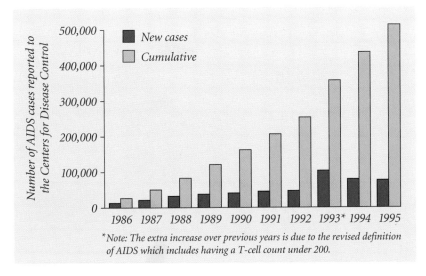

Fig 8-6 •

In 1995, for the first time, the number of new cases of AIDS decreased from the previous year.

Several strategies exist to stop the spread of AIDS, particularly in the drug-using community: education programs teach about the dangers of AIDS, interdiction limits the flow of drugs into the country, needle exchange programs limit the spread of the disease, drug abusers are encouraged to give up IV drug use or taught how to clean needles with bleach. In studies by the Center for Disease Control and other agencies, drug abuse treatment, along with education and needle exchange programs that are tied to outreach components, seems to be the most effective HIV disease or AIDS prevention strategy.

Harm Reduction. In San Francisco, several groups, including the HIV Prevention and Research Center of the Haight-Ashbury Free Medical Clinics, have outreach programs meant to reach IV drug users who are not in treatment. Outreach workers from the Center, armed with AIDS educational material, free bottles of bleach, and free con-

doms, go out to the "shooting galleries," "'crack'/'rock' houses," "dope pads," and other areas to distribute these materials and provide treatment referrals if requested. Other groups distribute free needles. It's an intervention into drug-related behavior without intervening into drug use. The drug use intervention part of the total policy is handled by the other sections of the clinic.

The problem with tying education about the risks of sharing needles too close to treatment is that it may miss the larger segment of IV drug users who are not ready for treatment and therefore at highest risk for AIDS. Users alienated by the treatment community or in denial are hard to educate. At clinics with a more tolerant policy toward relapses and toward users who can't clean up during their first few tries, the user is at least in contact on occasion with a treatment facility that can intervene, present important information, and eventually get the client into treatment, which is the best way to slow the spread of AIDS.

Publicity about the dangers of using dirty needles or having unprotected sex is one of the ways to limit the spread of AIDS.

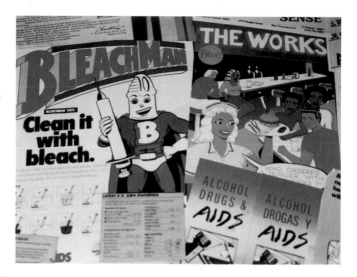

Education however does work. In San Francisco, in just a short period of time, drug users' awareness about the dangers of AIDS and the need to clean needles jumped from a few percent to 85%. The HIV-positive segment of the IV drug-using population in San Francisco is 15–17% compared to 60–80% in New York. Part of this HIV infection rate difference between the two coasts is certainly due to the educational efforts of the Clinic, the San Francisco Health Department, and the gay community. Other differences seem to be the greater presence of "shooting galleries" in New York, the limited number of treatment facilities, the difficulty in obtaining clean needles, and language barriers.

Recently, many new drugs besides AZT, one of the original AIDS drugs, have been developed and are showing promise in slowing or even halting the spread of the HIV virus in the body. New developments with a group of drugs known as protease inhibitors seem especially promising in the treatment of HIV infection. In addition, studies have shown that people who test positive for HIV, who remain clean and

sober, and maintain a healthy life style with plenty of rest, good food, and exercise will avoid full-blown AIDS for years longer. And those who have an AIDS diagnosis will live months to years longer.

"As I've started going into recovery and learning that I'm worth something and learning that I can have a life even though I'm HIV positive, yeah, it scares me to go back out there 'cause I know that when I use, I have unsafe sex, bottom line. And when I'm high, I'm not going to put on a condom. When I'm high, I will let people do things to me that I normally wouldn't let them do."

Recovering amphetamine user who is HIV positive

DRUGS AT WORK

More than 7.4 million of the 12.8 million adults who used illegal psychoactive drugs in the last 30 days were employed and 75% of those full time (*1995 NIDA Household Survey*).

COSTS

Studies on the impact of alcohol and other drug abuse in the American workplace have resulted in estimates that substance abuse cost our industries about $43 billion in 1979, $60 billion in 1983, and $140 billion in 1995 ($60 billion for drug-related costs, $80 billion for alcohol-related costs). Detailed analysis of these substance abuse-related costs reveals not only an impact on industry but also an impact on the substance abusers themselves, their families, and their coworkers.

Loss of Productivity

A substance abuser compared to a non-drug-abusing employee is

- late 3–14 times more often;
- absent 5–7 times more often and 3–4 times more likely to be absent for longer than 8 consecutive days;
- involved in many more job mistakes;
- likely to have lower output, make a less-effective salesperson, experience work shrinkage, that is less productivity despite more hours put forth;
- likely to appear in a greater number of grievance hearings.

Medical Cost Increases

Substance abusers as compared to non-drug-abusing employees

- experience 3–4 times more on-the-job accidents;
- use 3 times more sick leave;
- overutilize health insurance for themselves and for their families;

- file 5 times more workers' compensation claims;
- increase premiums for the entire company for medical and psychological insurance;
- endanger the health and well-being of coworkers.

Legal Cost Increases

As tolerance and addiction develop, a drug-abusing employee often enters into some form of criminal activity. Crime at the workplace brought about by drug abuse results in

- direct and massive losses from embezzlement, pilferage, sales of corporate secrets, and property damaged during commission of a crime;
- increased cost of improved company security, more personnel, urine-testing costs, product monitoring, quality assurance, intensified employee testing and screening;
- more lawsuits, both internal and external, expanded legal fees, court costs, and attorney expenses;
- loss of customer good will and negative publicity from drug use and trafficking at the workplace, employee arrests, the perception that there are more substance abusers than just those arrested, and manipulation of client contracts or goods.

PREVENTION AND EMPLOYEE ASSISTANCE PROGRAMS (EAPs)

Businesses attempt to control drug abuse in two ways. One method is through preemployment drug testing and on-the-job testing and the other is through employee assistance programs (EAPs).

Purpose of EAPs

In response to the increased problem of drugs in the workplace and the resultant drain on profits and productivity, many employers have instituted an employee assistance program, or EAP. Successful EAP programs balance the needs of management to minimize the negative impact drug abuse has on their business with a sincere concern for the better health of employees.

Designed as an employee benefit, an EAP can assist with a wide range of life and health issues and not just substance abuse problems. These programs often encourage self-referral for the employee as well as a supervisor's referral as an alternative to more stringent discipline for poor work performance. The successful EAP brings to the workplace a broad-based strategy to address the full spectrum of substance abuse prevention needs. The most successful EAPs share two overall design features.

1. They frame the EAP drug abuse services as part of a full spectrum prevention program which minimizes employee attraction to drugs and helps those with problems get into treatment.

2. They provide a diverse range of services for a wide spectrum of employee problems (emotional, relationship, financial, wage garnishment, and burnout).

These two design features lessen employees' apprehension about being labeled a drug abuser. They prevent drug problems before they start and they identify drug problems for employees in denial who don't accept the fact that they have a problem and often first approach the EAP about another problem area. The EAP is comprised of six basic components:

1. prevention/education/training;
2. identification and confidential outreach;
3. diagnosis and referral;
4. treatment, counseling, and a good monitoring system (including drug testing);
5. follow-up and focus towards aftercare (relapse prevention);
6. confidential record system and effectiveness evaluation.

In a full-spectrum prevention program, the EAP provides primary, secondary, and tertiary prevention.

Primary Prevention. In the most effective EAP programs, both corporate and individual denial are addressed with a systems-oriented approach to prevention. Education and training about the impact of substance abuse are provided at all levels in the corporation: to the administration, unions, and line staff. These segments agree on a single corporate policy on drugs and alcohol abuse.

Secondary Prevention. Both education and training focus on drug identification, major effects, and early intervention, which are incorporated into the prevention curriculum. The corporation's legal, grievance, and escalating discipline policies are redesigned in light of EAP goals. Security measures (e. g. testing, staff review, monitoring) are established in a manner which is legal, appropriate, and humane. These measures operate both as deterrents to use as well as methods of identifying the abusers and getting them help.

Tertiary Prevention. The EAP formalizes its intervention approach, allowing for confidential self-referral, peer referral, and supervisor-initiated referral to the EAP. A diagnostic process is established along with a number of appropriate treatment referrals. Treatment is confidential but the EAP monitors treatment to insure proper follow-up aftercare and continued recovery efforts. The employment status of workers is evaluated on work performance and not on their participatory effort in the EAP.

Effectiveness of EAPs

Well-conceived, successful programs that strike a balance between the corporation's security needs and a genuine concern for the health and welfare of each individual employee have demonstrated great effectiveness and cost savings to businesses. Several studies in major corporations, such as Southern Pacific, General Motors, Alcoa Aluminum, Eastman-Kodak, and others, have documented a 60–85% decrease in absenteeism, a 40–65% decrease in sick time utilization and personal/family health insurance usage, and a 45–75% decrease in on the job accidents, as well as other cost savings once the EAP system was put into operation.

DRUGS IN THE MILITARY

One example of reducing the use of psychoactive drugs in the workplace is the experience of the military. Since 1980, the use of illicit drugs has dropped nearly 90%. In the same period, cigarette smoking dropped by one-third. The rate of heavy drinking showed a smaller drop. In a survey of American military personnel, psychologist Robert Bray of the Research Triangle Institute in North Carolina found that from 1980–1995, 30-day illicit drug use dropped from 27.6% to just 3% of military personnel.

The reasons for the drop are varied. Probably the strongest reason was an intensified program of urine testing, starting in the early 1980s, with a positive result as grounds for discharge. The message was zero tolerance. In the past, drug users had been treated and kept in the military but with zero tolerance, they decided that there was no margin for having impaired people. A second reason for the drop in

drug use was that drugs, in general, became less popular in society over that period of time. The drop in smoking from 51% to 32% over the same period of time was attributed to military smoking bans and stop-smoking programs, as well as a general smoking decline in society as a whole. Heavy drinking still occurs at a higher rate than the general public: 17.1% versus just 12% in the general public. Part of the difficulty in reaching heavy drinkers who are mostly among young enlistees is because there is such a high turnover rate in the ranks.

The military has the advantage of being able to fire almost anyone they define as being dangerous to other military personnel. In addition, because it is the military, they can conduct testing whenever and almost wherever they choose.

DRUG TESTING

Increasingly, drug testing has appeared in all walks of life, not just in business. Drug testing has long been used to determine the blood or breath alcohol level of drivers suspected of drunk driving, of ex-convicts or felons on probation, of others suspected of a crime, or to test for compliance in addicts who are in treatment. The federal government has even issued a mandate for a drug-free workplace. Recently though, some laws have been enacted to regulate or control random testing of special groups, testing of job applicants, testing of all federal employees, and even random testing of teachers and students.

At present, the most widespread use of drug testing is in the military, in preemployment drug testing, and in drug treatment facilities. The military tests potential enlistees but it also uses extensive random testing to identify and treat or discharge users. Most medium and large businesses

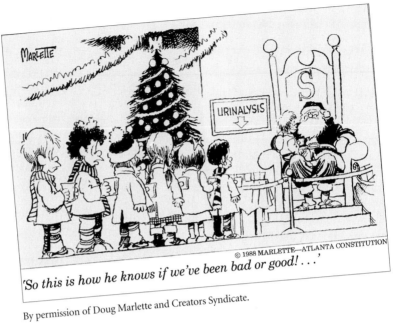

'So this is how he knows if we've been bad or good!...'

By permission of Doug Marlette and Creators Syndicate.

routinely use preemployment testing to keep drug users out because the problems they engender once in the company can be very expensive. There have also been so many challenges to random testing that many businesses are leery of using it. However, random testing is still used in jobs which involve public safety, such as bus drivers, policemen, and pilots.

THE TESTS

Many different laboratory procedures are used to test for drugs in the urine, blood, hair, saliva, sweat, and even different tissues of the body. Each test possesses inherent differences in sensitivity, specificity, and accuracy as well as other potential problems. Currently, some two dozen methods are used to analyze body samples for the presence of drugs. None is totally foolproof. The following are the most common methods.

Chromatography, Especially Thin Layer Chromatography (TLC)

TLC, a urine test, searches for a wide variety of drugs at the same time and is fairly sensitive to the presence of even minute amounts of chemicals. The major drawback is its inability to accurately differentiate drugs that may have similar chemical properties. For example, ephedrine, a drug used legally in over-the-counter cold medicines, may be misidentified as an illegal amphetamine.

Enzyme Multiplied Immunoassay Techniques (EMIT)

EMIT urine tests are extremely sensitive, very rapidly performed, and fairly easy to operate. However, they cannot usually distinguish the concentration of the drug present. Also, a separate test must usually be run for each specific suspected drug. EMIT tests can also mistake nonabused chemicals for abused drugs, mistaking, for example, opioid alkaloids in the poppy seeds of baked goods for heroin or another opioid. The chemical in Advil® or Motrin® may be mistaken for marijuana and the form of methamphetamine in Vick's Inhaler® is sometimes mistaken as "crank." This method is so sensitive that a rock concert goer can show a positive trace of marijuana even though he or she didn't smoke. This oversensitivity is corrected by raising the sensitivity level of the test so only current users will test positive.

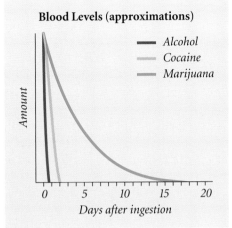

Gas Chromatography/Mass Spectrometry Combined (GC/MS)

The GC/MS test is currently the most accurate, sensitive, and reliable method of testing for drugs in the body. However, it is very expensive, requires highly trained operators, and is a very lengthy and tedious process in comparison to other methods. Being very sensitive, it can detect even trace amounts of drugs in the urine and therefore requires skilled interpretations to differentiate environmental exposure from actual use.

Hair Analysis

Hair analysis employs hair samples to detect drugs of abuse. Chemical traces of most psychoactive drugs are stored in human hair cells, so the drugs can be detected almost as long as the hair stays intact, even decades after the drug has been taken. This gives a picture of the degree of drug use (to differentiate occasional use from addictive use) and decreases the frequency of testing.

DETECTION PERIOD

Many factors influence the length of time that a drug can be detected in some-

Figure 8-7 •

This graph compares the length of time cocaine, marijuana, and alcohol remain in the blood. For purposes of testing, there is a cutoff level when testing for certain drugs, so that even when there is still some of the drug in someone's blood or urine, it will not be detected by the standard test.

one's blood, urine, saliva, or other body tissues. These include an individual's drug absorption rate, metabolism rate, distribution in the body, excretion rate, and the specific testing method employed. With a wide variation of these and other factors, a predictable drug detection period would be, at best, an educated guess. Despite this, the public interest requires that some specific estimates be adopted. For urine testing, these estimates can be divided into three broad periods: latency, detection period range, and redistribution.

Latency

Drugs must be absorbed, circulated by the blood, and finally concentrated in the urine in sufficient quantity before they can be detected. This process generally takes about 2 to 3 hours for most drugs except

TABLE 8–4 DETECTION PERIOD RANGE CHART

Drug	Period Range
Alcohol	1/2–1 day
Amphetamines ("crank," "speed")	2–4 days
Barbiturates	
amobarbital, pentobarbital,	2–4 days
phenobarbital	up to 30 days
Benzodiazepines	
e.g., Xanax®, Royhypnol®	up to 30 days
Cocaine ("coke," "crack")	12–72 hours
Marijuana	
casual use to 4 joints per week	5–7 days
daily use	10–15 days
chronic, heavy use	1–2 months
Opioids	
Dilaudid®	2–4 days
Darvon®	6–48 hours
heroin (morphine is measured)	2–4 days
methadone	2–3 days
PCP	
casual use	2–7 days
chronic, heavy use	several months
Quaalude®	2-4 days

alcohol, which takes about 30 minutes. Thus, someone tested just 30 minutes after using a drug would probably (but not always) test negative for that drug. A chronic user or addict, however, should have enough chemicals already present to test positive even if tested within 30 minutes.

Detection Period Range

Once sufficient amounts of a drug enter the urine, the drug can be detected for a certain length of time by urinalysis. The rough estimates for the more common drugs of abuse are shown in Table 8–4. Again, these are merely rough estimates

with wide individual variations. Thus, an individual delaying a urine test five days because of cocaine abuse will probably, but not definitely, test negative for cocaine.

Redistribution, Recirculation, Sequestration and Other Variables

Long-acting drugs like PCP, ethchlo-vynol (Doriden®), and possibly marijuana can be distributed to certain body tissues or fluids, concentrated and stored there, then be recirculated back into the urine. While not common, this can result in a positive test following negative tests and several months of abstinence.

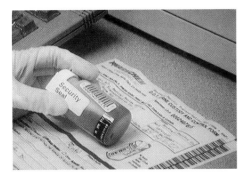

There is a rigid chain of custody for urine samples in good drug-testing laboratories. Detailed paperwork follows each sample.

ACCURACY OF DRUG TESTING

Despite many claims of confidence in the reliability of drug testing, independent blind testing of laboratory results continues to document high error rates for many testing programs.

False positive tests could result from the limitations of testing technology. For example, phenylpropanolamine and dextromethorphan, found in many cold products, have been misidentified as amphetamines and opioids respectively. Herbal teas have been implicated in producing a false cocaine-positive result.

Errors also can result from the mishandling of urine and other specimen samples taken. Tagging the specimen with the wrong label, mixing and preparing the testing solutions incorrectly, calculation errors, coding the samples and solutions, logging and reporting of results, and exposure of samples to destructive conditions or to drugs in the laboratory have all resulted in inaccurate tests.

False negative results, not false positives, constitute the bulk of urine-testing errors. These result from laboratories being overly cautious in reporting positive results and from specimen manipulation by the

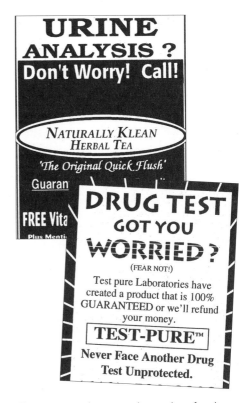

For every security precaution against cheating on urine tests, someone is bound to come up with a method to try to bypass it.

testee. Many manipulations, some effective and some just folklore, have been used by drug abusers to prevent the detection of drugs in their urine.

Attempts to manipulate urine testing have grown to such proportions that "clean pee" (drug-free urine) has become a profitable black market item. Further, recent designer drugs create a major problem in drug testing. Many have no standard to test against and some are so potent (the effective dose so small) that they will be impossible to identify in the body. Inaccurate tests also result from disease states, pregnancy, medical conditions, interference of prescribed drugs, and individual metabolic conditions.

With the technology available at this time, the best chance for a reliable drug-testing program would include direct observation of the body specimen, rigid chain of custody over the sample, use of the most accurate testing methods available (e.g., GC/MS) with a mandatory second confirmatory test via a different method, testing for a wide range of abused drugs, and use of a detailed medical and social history in the interpretation of lab results to determine any prescription or over-the-counter drugs which interfere with testing.

Consequences of False Positives and Negatives

Concerns about false positive test results are well-publicized, debated, and feared. People could lose their jobs, be denied unemployment, lose their freedom, or even be thrown out of the Olympics over an erroneous positive result. Less publicized or feared but just as critical are the false negative results. These prevent the discovery of drug abuse and feed the already strong denial process in the user. They permit the addict to become progressively more impaired and dysfunctional until a major life crisis occurs.

Nevertheless, drug testing is still an effective intervention, treatment, and monitoring tool, especially to intervene with heavy users and to discourage casual use. Addicts often state that they wished they had been tested and identified before their lives had been destroyed. Drug abusers in treatment often request increased urine testing to help them focus on abstinence and resist peer pressure. They can say, "Hey, I can't use. I have to be tested." Treatment programs use testing to overcome denial and dishonesty in addicts during early treatment. Recovering addicts in jobs that expose the public to high risk would not be acceptable without a reliable drug-testing program.

DRUGS AND THE ELDERLY

SCOPE OF THE PROBLEM

Overall Drug Use

The number of elderly has doubled since 1950. At present, 13% of our population is 65 years or older and that figure will increase to 20% by the year 2030. As the population grows, the problems with drug overuse, abuse, and addiction will increase as well. As the body ages, the use of all kinds of drugs increases, from over-the-counter medications, to prescription drugs, alcohol, and even street drugs. But since initiation to drug use usually occurs in adolescence and the main drug available in the 1920s, '30s, and '40s was alcohol, the use of drugs like cocaine, marijuana, and heroin is quite small among the elderly.

- In 1995, 30-day marijuana use for Americans over 35 was only 1.8% versus 6.7% for 26–34 year olds.

- Cocaine use for those over 35 is just 0.4% compared to 1.2% for 26–34 year olds.

- Alcohol use in those over 35 is 52.6% versus 63% in the younger group.

From 363 million prescriptions in 1950 to over 2 billion in 1995 (*National Prescription Audit*), the increase in the use of prescription drugs has been fueled by a greater life span and the discovery of hundreds of new compounds. This surfeit of available remedies for the illnesses and problems of the aging process have also increased the chances of adverse reactions from mixing drugs along with the chances of abuse of those drugs with psychoactive properties. In addition, peak use of over-the-counter medications occurs at age 65 and these too can have adverse reactions.

Nursing Home Drug Abuse

BY STEVEN FINDLAY
Special to The Chronicle

utting a relative into a nurs.

Innocent Victims of Drugs

Over-medication kills thousands of old people

BY LEE SIEGEL
ASSOCIATED PRESS
Los Angeles

They take too many drugs, and sometimes plead for more. They get confused, shaky and sick, and feel like they're going crazy. At least 200,000 end up in hospitals each year. Untold thousands die.

Dope-shooting junkies? Hard-core crack cocaine smokers? No. Just folks taking their medicine.

"Most older people are taking too many drugs, and are taking doses that are dangerously high," said Dr. Sidney Wolfe, director of the Washington, D.C.-based Public Citizen Health Research Group, founded by consumer advocate Ralph Nader.

"The greatest epidemic of drug abuse in American society is among our older people," who suffer 9 million adverse reactions to medicine a year, says "Worst Pills, Best Pills," Wolfe's 1988 book on over-medication of older people.

Side effects include depression, hallucinations.

BY LOS ANGELES TIMES

BY STEVE RINGMAN/THE CHRONICLE

overused to keep nursing home patients docile

at most homes   bly before they are," says Avorn.
se given antip-
In fact, mental-   In too many homes, however,
the system invites lack of consent.

Isolation, ill health, and financial worries are some of the problems that can lead the elderly to drug abuse.

Chemical Dependency

From 2% to 10% of the elderly population have a chemical dependency problem. Often the elderly abuse psychoactive drugs to deal with physical or psychological problems, their feelings of loneliness, being unwanted, not respected, and rejected by their families and the workplace. Events such as the death of a spouse, retirement, illness, loss of physical appearance, financial worries, and ageism can also increase drug use and abuse.

Overuse (as opposed to occasional use) of psychoactive drugs by the elderly is often overlooked, ignored, or passed off as a minimal health concern of old age.

In addition, abuse and addiction of drugs by the elderly often go unrecognized by the medical community. Many manifestations of drug abuse can be attributed to other chronic illnesses often present in those over 55. In addition, since so many

drugs are being used legally, adverse reactions due to the misuse of psychoactive drugs can be masked. Even family members of someone over 55 misattribute the symptoms of drug abuse to the normal effects of aging or the effects of legal prescription drugs.

All too often, the attitude of society is one of, "They've lived a full life and made their contribution to society, so why disturb their lives now? If they want to abuse drugs at this age, who will it harm? They deserve to be able to abuse drugs now." This attitude assumes that the unhindered abuse of psychoactive drugs is desirable. But since addiction is a progressive illness for the elderly as well as the young, continued use leads to progressive physiological, emotional, social, relationship, family, and spiritual consequences that users find intolerable. Addiction means unhappiness and lack of choice, no matter what the age of the addicted person.

Costs mount up for untreated elderly chemical abusers. From 20% to 50% of hospitalized elderly adults suffer from alcoholism. Failure to prevent and then treat chemical abuse among this population leads to huge costs in treating the high blood pressure, cardiac and liver disease, gastrointestinal problems, and all the other diseases resulting from the abuse of drugs.

PHYSIOLOGICAL CHANGES

The human body's physiological functioning and chemistry are not as efficient in the elderly as they are in young people and midlife adults. This results in an abnormal response to drugs in the aged as compared to younger adults. Generally, elderly people's enzymes and other bodily functions become less active, conditions which impair their ability to inactivate or excrete drugs. This makes drugs more toxic in older people. For example, Valium® is deactivated by liver enzymes but after the age of 30, the liver slowly loses its ability to make these deactivation enzymes. Thus, a 10 milligram dose of Valium® taken by someone age 70 will result in an effect equal to a dose of up to 30 milligrams taken by someone age 21.

Older people are also more likely to have concurrent illnesses which may greatly alter the effects of drugs in their bodies or make them more sensitive to the toxic and adverse side effects. Conditions like diabetes, liver, heart, and kidney disease all affect or are affected by drug abuse. Further, drugs used to treat these concurrent illnesses, along with a greater use of over-the-counter drugs by the aged, give rise to a greater potential for drug interactions. Such interactions frequently have synergistic effects on psychoactive drugs (actions which exaggerate their effects).

The most commonly abused drugs in the elderly are alcohol, prescription sedatives like Valium®, codeine, Darvon®, and other opioid analgesics, narcotic cough syrups, and over-the-counter sedatives or sleep aids.

Age does not endow a person with an immunity to the negative effects of drugs or chemical dependence. Thus prevention, education, and treatment services targeted for the aged are as important as those for adolescents.

PREVENTION ISSUES

Primary Prevention

Because social drinkers and even abstainers develop late onset alcoholism, often in response to problems of aging, older people need to be reeducated about the dangers of excessive alcohol or other psychoactive drugs. Since events, such as loss of a loved one, retirement, the effects of aging, and enforced idleness can lead to drug abuse, elderly people need to receive information and counseling about ways to manage the problems associated with growing older without using psychoactive drugs at all or at least, in the case of alcohol, in moderation. Drawing on their talents as volunteers in the community, providing social occasions for them, continuing their education are also ways that primary prevention can work for this group. Information about primary prevention, customized for the elderly, needs to be given to those who provide services to this population, such as nurses, physicians, and social workers.

Secondary Prevention

Secondary prevention for this age group focuses on recognition of early stages of alcoholism or drug abuse and appropriate intervention tactics. Frequently, there is strong denial by this age group, particularly because many of this generation see alcohol and other drug abuse as a sin or moral failure. Drug abuse tends to be secretive or hidden, particularly because of the seclusion and solitude many live in, so that a mobile professional staff and vigorous outreach program are necessary. Home visits are particularly effective. It is especially important to recognize alcoholism as a primary disease which must be treated, along with addressing other needs.

Tertiary Prevention

Treatment frequently involves different procedures from those used with younger clients. This age group is not used to abrupt coercive confrontational therapies. The pace of therapy has to be slower, more reassuring, and more patient. Bringing in the entire family to create an understanding sympathetic support group helps. Detoxification needs more time and the time period for recovery extended, often to two years or more. Thereafter, out-patient counseling, peer group work, and a protective environment (safe from alcohol and other drugs) provide continuing care and reinforce recovery.

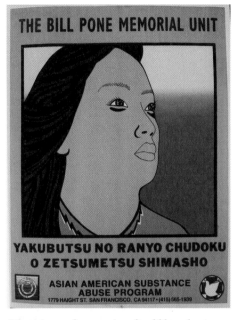

Education and prevention should be culture specific.
Courtesy of the Haight-Ashbury Free Clinic

CONCLUSION

NO SIMPLE SOLUTION

There is no simple solution to substance abuse prevention, no optimum prevention program or formula for prevention. Alcohol, tobacco, and other psychoactive drugs are all around us. The roots of the problems they cause are often multiple and complex, dealing with personal, interpersonal, and environmental elements. They begin early in life, sometimes at conception, and continue throughout life.

There is profound disagreement about drugs and drug policy in our society. Some see all drugs as inherently evil substances that must be regulated by laws. Some see drug use as a matter of choice, of free choice in the case of legal drugs or eventual decriminalization or legalization in the case of illicit drugs. Some see drug abuse as a pathological disease requiring treatment. Drug use is seen as a behavior that some say should be criminalized and that others say should be permitted. The various attitudes about what drugs are have profound and differing implications for what prevention should be. For instance, should the target of a prevention program address drug abuse itself, specific drugs (alcohol, tobacco), personal problems, or underlying social or environmental problems for which drug abuse is a symptom?

CURRENT PROMISING DIRECTIONS

It is impossible to prevent abuse unless family, school, and environment are involved. As we finish the twentieth century, prevention is seen as a shared responsibility. The most promising approaches are the comprehensive ones in which various segments of a community work in unison—youth, merchants, police, professionals, schools, parents, and the media. An entire community arrives at a consensus about what it must do to prevent drug abuse, then agrees on the specific model(s) that would best serve individuals and the whole community. Not allowing alcohol sales near schools or at street fairs is an example of a starting point. Ideally, any program will be designed to reach all members of the community.

People are at risk throughout their lives. If they are going to be exposed from cradle to grave, then prevention has to extend over a lifetime.

- Early primary prevention can help a baby who has an addicted mother by giving the mother parenting skills, teaching her to show unconditional love, teaching the importance of holding her baby, and making her aware of all the resources available to her. Toddlers can be given activities that increase bonding with their parent or caregiver.

- Parents may decide not to drink or use during their child-rearing years and model good alcohol and other drug behavior. The family is a crucial prevention delivery system at this stage.

- Grammar schools can integrate prevention into the curriculum. Since children up to 10 years old generally listen to parents, teachers, and authority figures, information and skill-building lessons are of great value. In addition, developmental skills can be taught, including resistance skills, decision-making skills, processing moral dilemmas, and talking about feelings.

- By middle school, many children stop listening as much to adults and start listening to other children. Peer educator programs can identify natural leaders who will serve as models, leaders, teachers, and guides for in-school prevention with peers.

- In high school and college, since there is greater exposure to drugs, prevention must assume a higher level to counter experimentation and social use. Prevention at this level must make a continual effort, involving curriculum infusion, support services, environmental change, policy formulation, promulgation, and enforcement, as well as alternatives to alcohol and other drug use in social occasions.

- For the work force, prevention needs to be continued through EAPs. They must be proactive and provide ongoing prevention, referral, and treatment opportunities. Prevention education should be provided in the normal course of job training and parallel such educational programs as safe-lifting techniques and sexual harassment training.

- For older people, preretirement training sessions and grief counseling can help prevent alcohol and other drug use. Outreach programs need to take the prevention message to the people who are housebound or are not part of the school-workplace-community avenues of access.

- Finally, prevention must be adapted to the needs of specific audiences. A program for a rural midwestern town may not be consistent for a school in inner-city Los Angeles. Secondary prevention designed for experimenters who need to know effects of drugs might actually stimulate experimentation in a primary audience. Since no single prevention program can demonstrate universal reproducible results, modifications of existing programs must be made to fit a particular situation.

CHAPTER SUMMARY

Introduction

1. Psychoactive drugs affect people at all ages from the "crack"-affected baby to the elderly woman who borrows a friend's prescription painkiller.

PREVENTION

Concepts of Prevention

2. The goals of prevention are to prevent abuse before it begins, stop it where it has begun, and treat people where abuse and addiction have taken hold.

3. The three methods of prevention are supply reduction, demand reduction, and harm reduction.

4. Historically, prevention has wavered between temperance and prohibition.

5. Scare tactics, drug information programs, skill-building and resiliency programs, environmental change programs, and the public health model are some of the prevention tactics that have been tried.

6. The public health model uses the concepts of the host (the actual user), the environment (the social climate), and the agent (the psychoactive drug) to explain all the combinations of prevention programs.

Prevention Methods

7. Supply reduction by law enforcement and other government agencies, augmented by the passage of laws, tries to dry up the supply of drugs on the streets. The effectiveness of supply reduction is open to debate.

8. Demand reduction tries to reduce people's desire for drugs either through treatment or through prevention.

9. Primary prevention for drug-naive young people aims to prevent use from beginning.

10. Secondary prevention seeks to halt drug use once it has begun.

11. Tertiary prevention, usually some form of treatment, seeks to stop further damage from drug abuse and addiction. Though intervention, individual and group therapy, medical intervention, cue extinction, and promotion of a healthy life style, recovery is encouraged.

12. Harm reduction's primary goal is not abstinence but rather reduction of the harm that addicts do to themselves and to society.

13. Drug substitution programs, designated driver programs, and outreach needle exchange programs are some examples of harm reduction. These programs conflict with zero tolerance government programs.

14. The concept of controlled use conflicts with most treatment programs, especially 12-step groups.

Challenges to Prevention

15. The legality of alcohol and tobacco along with large amounts of advertising limit the believability of many prevention programs.

16. Prevention that works takes time, must be carried on throughout people's lifetimes, and must be adequately funded.

FROM CRADLE TO GRAVE

Patterns of Use

17. The age of first use of drugs has gotten lower and lower, particularly since 1992. Caffeine, cigarettes, inhalants, and alcohol are generally the first drugs used.

18. Neither intelligence, income, nor social class protect one from abuse and addiction.

Pregnancy and Birth

19. About 11% of all pregnant women in America are using psychoactive drugs, such as alcohol, cocaine, cigarettes, and marijuana.

20. Drugs are particularly dangerous to the fetus because its defense mechanisms, e.g., drug-neutralizing metabolic system, immune system, and mature organs, are not yet developed. For example, each surge of effects from a drug the mother takes gives multiple surges to the defenseless fetus.

21. Major problems from drug use during pregnancy include a higher rate of miscarriage, blood vessel damage, severe withdrawal symptoms, and a much higher risk of sudden infant death syndrome (SIDS).

22. The problems of drug abuse during pregnancy last well beyond the birth of the baby. Withdrawal, intoxication, and developmental delays are commonplace.

23. Fetal alcohol syndrome (FAS) is the third most common cause of mental retardation in the United States.

24. Cocaine and amphetamines cause increased blood pressure and heart rate, stroke, and premature placental separation. Opioids cause physical addiction to the fetus. Heavy marijuana use, heavy smoking, and over-the-counter drug use also affect the fetus.

25. Eighty percent of children with AIDS are born to addicted mothers who use drugs intravenously.

26. Prevention includes prenatal education, drug education, and medical care.

Youth and School

27. Alcohol and tobacco are still the major problems in high schools and colleges.

28. The levels of substance abuse among youth in the United States are among the highest of any developed country.

29. A sense of invulnerability, the lag time between initial drug use and severe consequences, and especially delayed emotional maturation are major reasons for increased psychoactive drug use in junior high, high school, and college.

30. Identifying risks and teaching resiliency are two important prevention strategies for students.

31. A strong sense of family, established personal positions on drugs, strong spiritual sense, active community involvement, and attachment to a good role model help prevent drug abuse and addiction.

32. Primary, secondary, and tertiary prevention must be continued throughout school and beyond.

33. Heavy drinking and secondhand drinking (e.g., noisy dorms) are the two biggest drug problems in college.

34. Normative assessment (understanding real levels of abuse), having nonalcohol activities, and having alcohol and drug-free dormitories are good college-level prevention techniques.

Love, Sex, and Drugs

35. Those who use drugs to achieve sexual gratification are usually looking for a quick sensation rather than enduring emotions.

36. Drugs affect desire, excitation, and orgasm, often in diverse and contradictory ways.

37. The social effects of combining drugs and sexual activity, usually caused by lowered inhibitions or the need to support a drug habit, are increased sexual activity, high-risk sexual practices, sexual aggression, and an increase in sexually transmitted diseases.

38. Physical effects of drugs include hormonal changes, blood flow and blood pressure changes, nerve stimulation or desensitization, and muscle tension changes, all of which affect sexual response.

39. Cocaine and amphetamines in low doses can stimulate desire but in high doses, they make orgasm more difficult. In females, they can either increase or decrease desire and orgasm but in high doses, a decrease is much more likely.

40. Opioids generally suppress sexual activity. Sixty percent report a general decrease of desire; 90% report decreased desire while they were high.

41. Sedative-hypnotics enhance desire by lowering inhibitions and inducing relaxation. But with abuse, sexual dysfunction and apathy have been reported.

42. There has been a cultural link between love, sex, and alcohol. Initially, alcohol lowers inhibitions and often increases aggressiveness. Long-term abuse causes a decrease in performance.

43. Because of the distortion of the senses involved with psychedelics, their effect on sexual experience can be very unpredictable.

44. Psychotropic medications, such as antidepressants, may enable patients to engage in sexual activities that their depression or psychosis kept them from doing.

45. The search for a true aphrodisiac may be illusive because sexuality is more a matter of mental attitude than physical sensation.

46. By lowering inhibitions, distorting judgment, and increasing aggressive impulses, sexual assault increases with alcohol and drug use.

47. Worldwide, over 330 million cases of sexually transmitted diseases occurred last year.

48. The use of contaminated needles and the increased incidence of high-risk sexual behavior due to drug abuse have increased the incidence of sexually transmitted diseases, such as chlamydia, pelvic inflammatory disease, gonorrhea, venereal warts, and AIDS.

49. AIDS is a disease which destroys the immune system, so the user is susceptible to any infection. Drugs also lower the body's defenses indirectly.

50. The best AIDS prevention program is substance abuse treatment for those who want it, and education on the dangers of sharing dirty needles and engaging in high-risk sex practices.

51. Other diseases caused by dirty needles include hepatitis, cotton fever, endocarditis, abscesses, malaria, tuberculosis, and syphilis.

Drugs at Work

52. Drug abuse in the workplace costs American business more than $140 billion a year.

53. Drug abuse in the workplace causes loss of productivity, medical cost increases, and legal cost increases.

54. The most effective answer to drug abuse in the workplace seems to be EPAs (Employee Assistance Programs).

55. Good EAP programs have been documented to decrease absenteeism 60–85% and to decrease on-the-job-accidents 45–75%.

56. Testing, zero tolerance, and drug education have drastically reduced drug use in the military.

Drug Testing

57. The major uses of drug testing are preemployment testing, testing to see if a client in treatment is being abstinent, and testing in jobs that are hazardous to the public.

58. The major types of drug tests are thin layer chromatography (TLC), enzyme multiplied immunoassay technique (EMIT), and gas chromatography/mass spectrometry (GC/MS).

59. The important aspects of testing are the length of time it takes for drugs to leave the body, the accuracy of the various methods, and the consequences of false positives and false negatives.

60. It takes 2 or 3 hours for most drugs to enter the urine and be detectable. Alcohol, the exception, takes 30 minutes.

61. False negative tests can be as damaging as false positives. Failure to recognize a serious addiction can be more serious than damage to one's reputation from a false positive.

Drugs and the Elderly

62. As drug users get older, they become less able to neutralize and metabolize drugs.

63. Drug abuse in the elderly is often overlooked. Continuing education, recognition of the signs of abuse, and appropriate treatment need to be directed at the elderly.

Conclusion

64. Prevention has no simple answer, no one program that will work for everyone.

65. Special programs need to be directed at each age group and then further directed to specific ethnic, cultural, sexual, and educational groups where possible.

Treatment

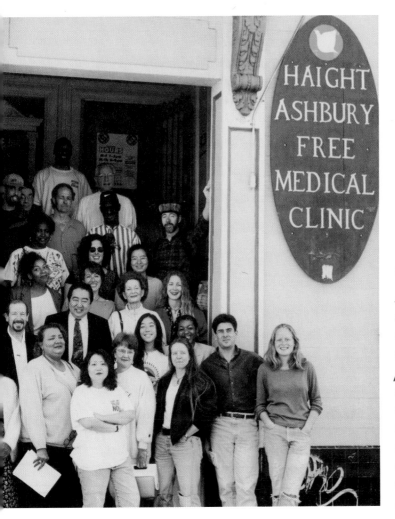

*T*he Haight-Ashbury Free Clinics opened their doors in 1967 to help take care of the influx of young people during the "Summer of Love." Since that time, they have treated more than 85,000 clients with one of the highest success rates in the country. There are 130 people on staff.

- **Introduction:** The most prevalent mind disorder is substance abuse.
- **Treatment Effectiveness:** Treatment has a 50% success rate and saves $7 in costs related to unchecked addiction for every $1 spent on treatment. Prison recidivism drops three- to fourfold with treatment.
- **Broad Range of Techniques:** Providing a wide range of treatment approaches, plus customizing treatment for culture, sex, ethnic, and other target populations, dramatically improves outcomes.
- **Beginning Treatment:** Breaking through denial is the crucial first step. Hitting bottom, especially with health, family, work, financial, or legal problems, often gets the user into treatment. Direct intervention is also used to get the person into treatment.
- **Treatment Goals:** Motivating clients towards abstinence and reconstructing their lives in ways that exclude drug abuse as an option are the two main treatment goals.
- **Selection of a Program:** Correct diagnosis, a delicate process with drug abuse, helps treatment professionals match the client to the best program.
- **Treatment Continuum:** Once addiction has occurred, treatment becomes a lifetime process.

  Detoxification uses medical care, emotional support, and medications to control withdrawal symptoms, reduce craving, and help the client to begin abstinence.

  Initial Abstinence uses counseling, anticraving medications, drug substitution, and desensitization techniques to rebalance body chemistry, continue abstinence, and prevent relapse due to environmental triggers.

  Long-Term Abstinence involves participation in group, family, and 12-step programs to prevent relapse and to recognize that addiction is a lifelong danger.

  Recovery is a lifelong process which involves rebuilding one's life style to live sober and drug free.
- **Individual Versus Group Therapy:** Individual counseling, peer groups, 12-step groups, facilitated group therapy, and educational groups are all used in treatment.
- **Treatment and the Family:** Treatment should involve the whole family. The problems of codependency, enabling, and being a child of an alcoholic or an addict must be addressed.
- **Drug-Specific Treatment:** Certain psychoactive drugs call for specialized medical and counseling treatment techniques, e.g., methadone maintenance, stimulant abuse groups, or dual diagnosis groups.
- **Target Populations:** Treatment should be culturally specific (i.e., address ethnicity, sex, language).
- **Treatment Obstacles:** Developmental arrest, lack of cognition, conflicting goals, poor follow-through, and lack of facilities are the main problems in treatment.

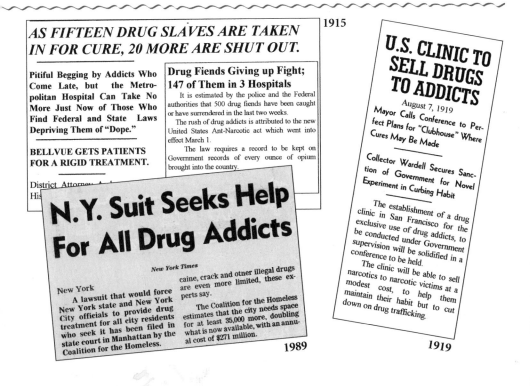

1915

AS FIFTEEN DRUG SLAVES ARE TAKEN IN FOR CURE, 20 MORE ARE SHUT OUT.

Pitiful Begging by Addicts Who Come Late, but the Metropolitan Hospital Can Take No More Just Now of Those Who Find Federal and State Laws Depriving Them of "Dope."

BELLVUE GETS PATIENTS FOR A RIGID TREATMENT.

District Attorney
His

Drug Fiends Giving up Fight; 147 of Them in 3 Hospitals

It is estimated by the police and the Federal authorities that 500 drug fiends have been caught or have surrendered in the last two weeks.

The rush of drug addicts is attributed to the new United States Ant-Narcotic act which went into effect March 1.

The law requires a record to be kept on Government records of every ounce of opium brought into the country.

N.Y. Suit Seeks Help For All Drug Addicts

New York Times

New York
A lawsuit that would force New York state and New York City officials to provide drug treatment for all city residents who seek it has been filed in state court in Manhattan by the Coalition for the Homeless.

caine, crack and other illegal drugs are even more limited, these experts say.

The Coalition for the Homeless estimates that the city needs space for at least 35,000 more, doubling what is now available, with an annual cost of $271 million.

1989

U.S. CLINIC TO SELL DRUGS TO ADDICTS

August 7, 1919

Mayor Calls Conference to Perfect Plans for "Clubhouse" Where Cures May Be Made

Collector Wardell Secures Sanction of Government for Novel Experiment in Curbing Habit

The establishment of a drug clinic in San Francisco for the exclusive use of drug addicts, to be conducted under Government supervision will be solidified in a conference to be held.

The clinic will be able to sell narcotics to narcotic victims at a modest cost, to help them maintain their habit but to cut down on drug trafficking.

1919

INTRODUCTION

Addiction is a disease of loss and only when the losses become unbearable will most people seek treatment on their own.

"My experience was that it got so bad, so fast, and I mean so bad, I lost everything I had. I lost my dignity, I lost my job, I lost my children, I lost my home, I lost the trust and respect of everyone in my family and every one of my friends around drugs and specifically around the methamphetamine use that came at the end of my addiction. I lost everything I had to live for. That was my primary motivation for recovery. And it took that depth of pain and misery for me to get the message. Somehow, in all my years of using drugs, I never heard the word absti-

nence. I never heard the word recovery. I never knew another way."

33-year-old recovering cocaine and methamphetamine abuser

When one examines the range of conditions which impair the human mind, it becomes very evident that chemical dependency is the most prevalent disorder. For example, the national incidence of schizophrenia is about 0.7%; major depression, bipolar disease, and affective disorders, about 4.2%; and unspecified mental illnesses, another 2%. This compares to alcoholism, which affects 10% to 12% of the U.S. population over the age of 12; addiction to heroin or cocaine devoid of alcohol problems, another 6%; other primary drugs of addiction, about 8%; and nicotine addiction, about 25%. Further complicating the picture is the fact that most addicts today are poly-substance abusers.

Chemical dependency may also be America's number one continuing public health problem. More than 400,000 Americans die prematurely every year due to nicotine addiction. Another 130,000 die prematurely from alcohol dependence and overdose; 6,000 to 10,000 die of cocaine, heroin, and recently methamphetamine dependence. Even inhalant abuse kills 1,200 inhalant abusers every year. Further, 35% to 40% of all hospital admissions are related to nicotine-induced health problems and 25% to alcohol-induced health problems. These figures are staggering when compared to other major health problems like AIDS, prostate or breast cancer, and even stroke.

Finally, psychoactive drug abuse has profound effects on social systems, family relationships, crime, violence, mental health, and a dozen other areas. Certainly, if we could reduce the impact of addiction, we would have a major impact on the quality of life in the United States and around the world.

TREATMENT EFFECTIVENESS

The good news is that even though chemical dependency is America's and possibly the world's number one health and social problem, it is also the most treatable. Several studies have confirmed that treatment outcomes for drug and alcohol abuse result in abstinence, along with tremendous health, social, and spiritual benefits to the patient.

Past studies conducted by the Rand Corporation and Research Triangle Institute support the current findings of the California Alcohol and Drug Treatment Assessment (CALDATA) Executive Summary, the most comprehensive and rigorous study on treatment outcome conducted by the State of California and duplicated by several other states. All of these studies monitored the effect of treatment on several hundred thousand addicts and alcoholics treated in a variety of programs.

THE CALDATA STUDY (1994)

The CALDATA study monitored patients for a period of three to five years following treatment. Continual abstinence in these patients approached 50% of all those treated. It further demonstrated that crime was abated in 74% of those treated and that the State enjoyed an actual $7 savings for every $1 spent on treatment. (Other studies have shown the savings to be as much as $20 for every $1 spent on treatment.) The study also looked at a number of variables which, when examined, supported many concepts and practices in the treatment field.

- Treatment was most effective when patients were treated continuously for a period of six to eight months.

- Shorter periods of time resulted in poorer outcomes and longer treatment duration resulted in continuously better outcomes but not at the same rate. There is a point of diminishing returns.

- Group therapy was shown to be much more effective than individual therapy.

- Drug of choice also seemed to affect outcomes. For example, those who listed alcohol as their primary drug of choice had more than two times better treatment outcomes than those who listed heroin as their primary drug of choice. Cocaine users' outcomes fell between these two drugs.

- Better treatment outcomes were linked to program modifications directed at

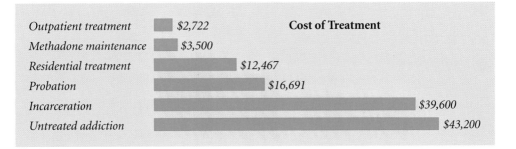

Figure 9-1 •
The cost of treatment for an addict is less than one-tenth the cost of incarceration.
McLellan et al., 1994, Lewin-VHI, unpublished estimates.

being culturally consistent with a specific target population. For example, programs which targeted women and added child care services to their treatment programs had much better outcomes than generic treatment programs for women. Those programs which then added transportation services had better outcomes than those that just had child care. Every additional innovation that was target-group specific improved the outcome of treatment.

TREATMENT AND PRISONS

The percentage of arrestees testing positive for drugs (not including alcohol) is many times the percentage of drug use in the general population. Arrests for drug offenses soared from 470,000 in 1980 to 1,350,000 in 1994. Juvenile arrests for drug crimes doubled from 1990 to 1994. Despite the high percentage of drug problems among the inmate population, treatment is available for fewer than 10% of federal inmates who have serious drug habits.

Recent studies of prisoners and those involved with the criminal justice system have shown that drug abuse treatment reduces recidivism dramatically. Normally,

60% to 80% of criminals are rearrested after being released from prison. Drug abuse addiction treatment lowers that number to only 20% and since the cost of keeping a felon in jail runs between $25,000 to $40,000 a year, not including any assistance for the felon's family, compensation for human and property damage, and a dozen other costs, the savings for keeping people out of prisons is quite large (Fig. 9-1). In contrast, outpatient treatment costs between $2,000 to $4,000 a year, depending on the treatment approach.

"In California during the early '90s, we built nine new prisons but we built no new universities and actually suffered a decrease in drug treatment slots due to reduced funding. Yet 80% to 85% of our prisoners listed a drug problem as a major reason for their offense. I think we have our priorities backwards."
Education consultant

TREATMENT WORKS

Over the past 25 years, many innovations have been developed to improve the effectiveness of treatment for chemical de-

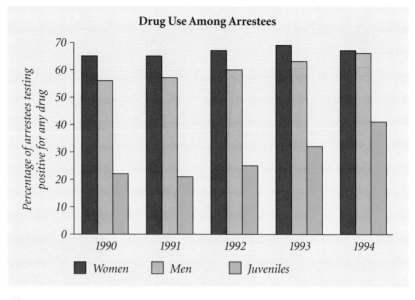

Drug Use Among Arrestees

Figure 9-2 •

Testing at jails is for illicit drugs. Besides alcohol, the most common drugs are cocaine and marijuana. National Institute of Justice.

pendency. Addicts can and do enter recovery life styles which are much more rewarding than their previous lives. The sooner addicts recognize, accept, and surrender to the treatment process, the less suffering and damage will occur during their lives. The recovering community now represents a significant portion of the population of most cities in the United States. This community offers practicing addicts hope that they too can change their lives should they choose to enter treatment.

"I'm not the same person that I was when I entered this fellowship. Through my recovery and the 12 steps, I have found meaning and purpose in my life. It feels especially good with my kids because they know that I'm here for them. There's no catch-up anymore. I keep my promises. The challenge of a sober parent is keeping promises."
Recovering "speed" addict

BROAD RANGE OF TECHNIQUES

Horace B. Day concluded his 1886 book on the problems of opium dependence in the United States with this statement, "There is no agreement among the medical profession as to the proper treatment of opium disease or morphinism." This statement is still applicable today in a much broader sense in relation to treatment of all chemical dependencies. As we have noted throughout this book, addiction is a complex interaction between biologic, social, and toxic factors—heredity, environment, and psychoactive drugs. Given these multiple influences, treatment has evolved along various paths, all of which enjoy some success. However, since each person is unique and the level of addiction different, no treatment has proven to be universally effective for everyone who has an addiction. Often, effective treatment requires a variety of techniques in a variety of settings.

"I'm considering going into inpatient treatment. I've talked it over with my counselor and he said 'Anybody can stay clean in the closet.' I'm good as far as bullshitting and manipulating. I could pass a 30-day and probably a 60-day situation. But you know, when I come outside, there's things which I'm going to have to deal with, so an outpatient program still makes sense."
24-year-old "crack" addict in group therapy meeting

Besides matching the treatment protocol to the level of addiction and the user's personality, it is very important to factor in the physical withdrawal syndrome produced by a drug or a combination of drugs, because withdrawal from drugs, especially alcohol and sedative-hypnotic drugs (e.g., Valium® or Klonopin®), may produce life-threatening seizures which require medical and hospital management. Cocaine or amphetamine withdrawal usually requires less medical intervention but clients need intense psychosocial intervention to prevent relapse.

"My mother swore off the gin and the Valium® for my wedding. She was too good to her word. She started withdrawing and having convulsions at my reception and almost died in the ambulance. It put somewhat of a damper on the honeymoon."
23-year-old bride

TREATMENT OPTIONS

A wide range of options exists for the treatment of alcohol or other chemical addiction. The range is

- from medically assisted detoxification to "cold turkey" or "white knuckle" dry outs;

- from expensive medical or residential approaches to free peer groups, 12-step groups, or social-model group therapy;

- from outpatient treatment to halfway houses to residential programs;

- from long-term residential treatment (two years or more) to seven-day hospital detoxification with aftercare;

- and from methadone maintenance to acupuncture, aversion therapies, or a dozen other methods.

"I believed there were only AA and NA for my 'crank' use and I knew—I just knew these wouldn't work. Then after a particularly nasty run which I thought I kept from my probation officer, he gave me a choice of getting into treatment or going back to prison. I was startled when he handed me a full page list of different places I could go. There was a medical program. There was a NA program made up of 'speed freaks' like myself. There was a mental health program near my apartment. There were places I could go to live while kicking."
35-year-old recovering "crank" addict

Treatment programs which focus their development on a specific target population and provide culturally relevant services have demonstrated the ability to attract, bond, and shepherd addicts into a recovery process much better than a general program with no specific focus. Models for such an approach have been developed based on ethnicity, age, sex, profession, sexual orientation, mental status, drug of choice, and even specifically for those with HIV infection or AIDS.

BEGINNING TREATMENT

It is vital to remember that addiction is a dysfunction of the mind. Brain cells, unlike all other cells, are the only nonrenewable cells in the human body. We are born with all the brain cells we will ever have, unlike tissues such as skin cells which are totally replaced every eight days or so. Thus, the brain cell disease of addiction is a chronic progressive process which can be treated and arrested but not one that can be reversed or cured. Recovery is a lifelong process not a 30-day wonder. Addicts must refrain from ever abusing and, in most cases, even using small amounts of any psychoactive drugs if they want to avoid relapsing into addiction.

"Friday, I was feeling good. I even went to a meeting. I'd been in this program for two years. I thought I could have one drink to relax with some friends I ran into. I had about five scotches and ended up using all night long in a hotel with two prostitutes. I went through about $700 and was broke and then I stole $150 from my roommate. I was ripped off a couple of times buying stuff and at the end of it, I was tweaked and I still wanted more."
Recovering 24-year-old "crack" user

RECOGNITION AND ACCEPTANCE

Treatment starts with a recognition and acceptance of addiction by the addict. This self-diagnosis often requires the addict to hit bottom or be the subject of an intervention with an assessment to support and validate the need for treatment. Only then can an addict be entered into a continuum of lifelong processes to assist her or him in a quest for recovery.

Hitting Bottom

Addiction is a progressive illness which leads to severe life impairment and dysfunction when left to proceed without disruption.

"It had gotten to the point where the depression was so great that I didn't want to go to work anymore. I had just neglected all my responsibilities. It was just a lot of depressing days that I couldn't take anymore." Recovering polydrug abuser

The earlier it is recognized, accepted, and treated, the more likely the recovering user will have a rewarding life and good health. All too often, users come in for treatment after they have hit rock bottom, leaving their hopes for a quality life handicapped.

"I got up and I looked at my pipe. And then I said, 'No,' and I put it down and I put it in the trash—I didn't break it—and I rocked myself and I said, 'No dope, no dope, no dope,' and I rocked myself until I could not rock myself anymore." Recovering "crack" addict

Denial

Overcoming denial, the essential first step in all treatment, is also the most difficult to accomplish. Denial is the universal defense mechanism experienced not only by addicts but also by their families, friends, and associates. Denial prevents or delays the proper recognition and acceptance of a chemical dependency problem. Denial is a refusal to acknowledge the negative impact that the addiction is having on

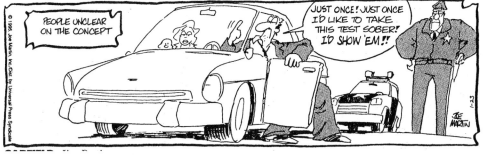

MISTER BOFFO *Joe Martin*

PEOPLE UNCLEAR ON THE CONCEPT

JUST ONCE! JUST ONCE I'D LIKE TO TAKE THIS TEST SOBER! I'D SHOW 'EM!!

one's life. It is also the shifting of responsibility of negative consequences to other causes rather than addiction.

The medical profession also has a tendency to deny or overlook addiction. How deeply does a physician inquire about a patient's alcohol or other drug use history? How often is a caffeine intake assessment done by a physician who is treating anxiety and insomnia in a businessman? Denial, plus the toxic effects that psychoactive drugs have on judgment and memory, makes the addict likely to be the last person to recognize and accept her or his addiction.

"I woke up after passing out in a friend's home and they had taken my money away from me and they had posted somebody at the door and my mother came and said, 'I will not watch your children for you while you go out and party. If you do something about your problem, I'll take care of your kids for a week.' That was the first time anybody had said to me I had a problem and that was the first time anybody said, 'Stop. You can't do this anymore.' Of course, it was also the first time anybody in my close circle of my family had found out that I *was an IV drug user although they knew I used drugs."* 37-year-old recovering "speed" user

Breaking Through Denial

Usually, those closest to the addict, the family or spouse, have the best chance to make the earliest recognition of addiction (not just use) and to help the person break through denial. Besides close relations, others able to recognize addiction include friends, coworkers, employers, ministers, medical professionals, the IRS, and the law. On the other hand, addiction is the only illness which requires a self-diagnosis for treatment to be effective. Normally, when physicians tell patients that they have high blood pressure, they usually accept that diagnosis without question and make changes in their lives to improve their health. But when addicts are first confronted with their addiction, they almost always deny any drug problem and continue to abuse drugs.

There are several ways to break through denial.

- *Legal Intervention:* The threat of loss of property or freedom forces users to accept that they are having a problem with drugs. Legal requirements may mandate treatment while incarceration can limit drug use and promote abstinence in prisons where drug trafficking is kept to a minimum. Unfortunately, some prison personnel estimate that, if tested, from 10% to 30% of inmates would test positive for an illicit psychoactive drug.

- *Workplace Intervention:* Poor performance and the threat of the loss of one's livelihood may break through denial. Strong employee assistance programs can work with the at-risk employee.

- *Physical Health Problems:* Deteriorating health and doctors' warnings can make the user consider drug problems as a possible cause or complicating factor.

- *Mental Health Problems:* Emotional and mental trauma, like depression, anger, and mental confusion, that affect day-to-day functioning can also act as a warning signal.

- *Financial Difficulties:* Problems such as paying bills, buying food, or covering the rent which are affected by escalating drug costs force the user either to deal drugs, turn to other crime, or cut back on use, thus compelling the user to recognize the financial damage of addiction.

- *Health Problems:* The existence of lung cancer, high blood pressure, or heart, liver, kidney, and other diseases caused by drug toxicity can be a powerful tool to confront a patient's denial to addiction.

Intervention

Special strategies have been developed to attack the denial in drug abusers and addicted people and help them recognize their dependence on drugs. Generally re-

ferred to as intervention, these strategies have been documented since the late 1800s to effectively bring those who are addicted into treatment and hold them there. Further, there are now specialists who help to organize and implement intervention.

"When my dog died, I got a prescription for Xanax® to help because I felt so bad. Then I got Dalmane® to help me sleep, Valium® for my muscle tension, Librax® for my upset stomach, Klonopin® for my headaches, and even Ativan® to help me cut down on my drinking, all on Medicare. And because they were prescribed, I never thought I had a problem until they literally dragged me into the living room for an intervention."
Recovering benzodiazepine addict

Most intervention strategies consist of various elements.

Love. An intervention should always start and end with an expression of love and genuine concern for the well-being of the addicted person. Multiple participants should be recruited from various aspects of the addicted person's life—all of whom share a sense of true affection for the user but recognize the progressive impairment of the addiction and are bold enough to commit themselves to participation in the intervention. Generally, this intervention team consists of two or more of the following: family members, close friends and coworkers, other recovering addicts, a representative of the user's spiritual community (clergy or community leader), and a lead facilitator.

Facilitator. A professional intervention specialist or a knowledgeable chemical dependency treatment professional is selected to organize the intervention, educate the participants about addiction and treatment options, train and assist team members in the preparation of their statements, and support or confirm the diagnosis of addiction. The team meets and prepares its intervention without revealing their activities to the user.

Intervention Statements. Each team member prepares a statement that he or she will make to the addicted person at the time of the intervention. Each statement consists of four parts:

* a declaration of how much they love, care for, and respect the user;
* specific incidents they have personally witnessed or experienced related to the addiction and the pain they have personally experienced from the incidents;
* personal knowledge that the incidents occurred not because of the user's intent but because of the effects that the drug has caused on the user's behavior;
* reassurance of their love, concern, and respect for the user with a strong request that he or she recognize and accept the illness and enter treatment immediately.

Anticipated Defenses and Outcomes. The facilitator prepares the team to deal with expected defense mechanisms like denial, rationalization, minimization, anger, and accusations. The team also prepares for all logistics (reserving a program or hospital admission, packing clothing and toiletries, covering work and home duties) so that the user will have no excuse or delay in entering treatment immediately should a successful intervention ensue. The team also prepares for contingencies and alternative treatments other than the ones they selected should the addict refuse to accept their first recommendation. It is important that the user accept one of the treatment programs selected by the team and not delay entry by selecting a different program.

The Intervention. Timing, location and surprise are crucial components of the actual intervention. A neutral, nonthreatening, and private location must be secured for the intervention. It should occur at a time (usually early Sunday morning) when the user is most likely to be sober or not under the influence of a drug. The evidence presented in statements should include current incidents. A reliable plan should be developed to get the addicted person to the location which does not cause her or him to suspect what is about to occur. Finally, the facilitator should prepare the order of the statements which have been rehearsed by the team prior to the intervention.

Contingency. Successful or not, it is important for the intervention team members to continue to meet after the intervention to process their experiences. This also provides the opportunity for team members (especially family members) to explore their own support or treatment needs for issues such as codependency, enabling, or adult children of addicts syndrome.

Despite the inherent risks of anger or rejection which may result from an unsuccessful intervention, the potential benefits from these strategies far outweigh the risks. At a very minimum, the pathological effects of secrecy which pervade an addiction have been brought out to all those who are most affected by it, allowing a chance for successful treatment.

TREATMENT GOALS

Most treatment experts agree that the two most important goals for treatment outcome are first, to motivate clients towards abstinence from their drugs of abuse and second, to reconstruct their lives once their focus is redirected away from substance abuse.

To accomplish these and other goals, several elements need to be addressed through an understanding that addiction treatment is a lifelong process for addicts. Treatment merely motivates, initiates, and provides some tools which help them to have uninterrupted abstinence from their addiction throughout their lives.

"Well basically, I'd like to stay off drugs. I'd like to get my family life together again and have a relationship with my children—a good one— and if nothing else, I'd just like to know that when I do die, I did have a life, you know, aside from being just another dope fiend in the gutter."
24-year-old recovering heroin addict

PRIMARY GOALS

A comprehensive treatment model will include the capacity to accomplish the following goals.

Motivation towards Abstinence. Components of these efforts consist of education, counseling, and involvement with 12-step or self-help groups. This might include harm reduction approaches like methadone maintenance whereby an addict is provided with an alternate medically controlled drug to promote abstinence from the street drug of choice.

Creating a Drug-Free Life Style. This covers all aspects of an addicts' lives, including the ability to address social/environmental issues, like homelessness, relationships, family, and friends, in order to develop drug-free life interactions. They are connected to drug-free activities, like clean and sober dances, and most important, they learn relapse prevention skills, such as stress reduction, cue resistance, coping, decision making, and conflict resolution.

SUPPORTING GOALS

Enriching Job or Career Functioning. Often neglected in treatment, jobs and career comprise a major portion of someone's life. This goal is accomplished through vocational services, management of personal finances, and maintenance of a drug-free workplace.

Optimizing Medical Functioning. Besides treatment of withdrawal and other acute medical problems associated with addiction, many addicts have undiagnosed or existing medical problems which have been neglected through their use of drugs. The comprehensive treatment program includes the ability to assess and treat such conditions.

Optimizing Psychiatric and Emotional Functioning. Many studies suggest that greater than 50% of all substance abusers also have a coexisting psychiatric condition. Identification and appropriate treatment of psychiatric problems are an essential element of the modern treatment program (see Chapter 10).

Addressing Relevant Spiritual Issues. Although the inclusion of either spirituality or religious beliefs in addiction treatment is controversial, the most effective long-term treatments of addiction are the spiritually based 12-step Alcoholics Anonymous and Addictions Anonymous programs. Further, many of the other treatment programs in operation base their interventions on the 12-step traditions. Thus, it has become essential for programs to at least help clarify this issue with their clients and provide appropriate referrals.

"I don't have hopes of living forever. I never have. I mean, to be my age is a complete shock to me, so it's not about that but the issue is about the quality of life."
40-year-old recovering heroin addict

SELECTION OF A PROGRAM

Most program selections occur on the spur of the moment based upon cost, familiarity, location, and convenience of access. The current era of managed health care has made pretreatment assessments essential because they can better match addicts to programs that address their specific needs and thus promote better outcomes.

In making a program selection, one should be knowledgeable about the addicted person's specific needs, his or her resources to afford treatment, the specific components and deficiencies of available programs, and the ultimate client goal of these potential programs.

It is important to note that program selection should be completed before a formal intervention is performed on an addicted person. Successfully getting someone to accept and address a drug problem can be completely undermined by having no immediate resource for the addict to address his or her problems.

DIAGNOSIS

Once addiction is suspected, various diagnostic tools can be used to help verify, support, or clarify the potential diagnosis of chemical addiction. Several diagnostic criteria have been developed to assist clinicians in making a diagnosis of chemical dependence. These are some of the more common ones used.

- The American Psychiatric Association *Diagnostic and Statistical Manual of Mental Disorders (DSM-IV)* relies on the pattern and duration of drug use, the negative impact of drugs on the social or occupational functioning of the user, and the pathological effects (e.g., tolerance or withdrawal symptoms) to confirm a diagnosis of addiction.

- The Selective Severity Assessment (SSA) evaluates 11 physiologic signs (e.g., pulse, temperature, tremors) to confirm the severity of the addiction in an addict.

- The National Council on Alcoholism Criteria for Diagnosis of Alcoholism (NCA CRIT) and its Modified Criteria (MODCRIT) outline two bases on which to make the diagnosis of alcoholism:
  1. physical and clinical parameters;
  2. behavioral, psychological, and attitudinal impact.

- The simplest diagnostic aid, the Michigan Alcoholism Screening Test (MAST), uses just 25 questions which are primarily directed at the negative life effects of alcohol on the user (see Chapter 5). There is also the short Michigan Alcoholism Screening Test with just 13 questions.

- The Addiction Severity Index (ASI) represents the most comprehensive and lengthy criteria for the diagnosis of chemical dependency. One hundred and eighty items cover six areas that are affected by substance use and abuse.

TYPES OF PROGRAMS

Available and funded treatment programs usually concentrate only on the very first phase of treatment called detoxification. Though highly variable, this phase of

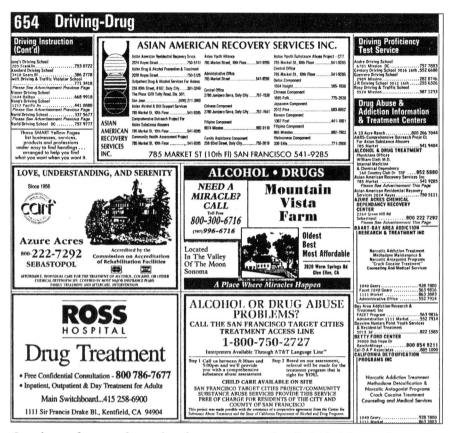

Over the past five years, the number of treatment centers has diminished due mostly to managed care and less insurance coverage for addiction and alcoholism care.

treatment ranges from as little as five days to as long as several years.

There is a wide range of treatment models and settings for accomplishing detoxification or more extensive treatment. These vary from inpatient hospitalization to outpatient programs and from medical models to social-model (nonmedical) approaches. Program selection is based upon the need and financial resources of the client.

"Someone asked me, 'Where would you go to get off drugs? Where would you feel comfortable?' If I had everything I needed, life-time supplies, and I was shipwrecked on an island, that would be fine."

Recovering 22-year-old methamphetamine abuser

Hospital detoxification programs are inpatient medical model programs which are generally the shortest in duration (7 to 28 days). These are usually the most expensive type of program but have the advantage of being able to do a more comprehensive assessment and treatment of the addict's overall physical and mental health.

Social-model detoxification programs are nonmedical programs which are either inpatient or outpatient. These are also very short term (7 days to 3 months) aimed at providing a safe and sober environment for addicts to detoxify from their drug, thus enabling them to enter into a full recovery program.

Therapeutic communities are generally long-term (1 to 3 years) residential (inpatient) programs which provide full rehabilitative and social services within the confines of the facility. Many addicts are often put off by making such a long commitment to being cut off from society. Many programs divide the treatment into 3 to 6 month phases which permit making commitments to each phase of treatment rather than the full 1 to 3 years all at one time.

Halfway houses permit addicts to keep their jobs and outside contacts while being involved in a residential treatment program. Addicts receive educational and therapeutic interactions after work hours and live within the facility. Weekends or nonworking days are reserved for more intensive program work which continues for a long duration (1–3 years).

Sober-living or transitional-living programs are generally for clients who have completed a long-term residential program. They consist of apartments or co-ops for groups of recovering addicts with strong house rules to maintain a clean and sober living environment which is supportive of each person's recovery effort. Minimal to moderate treatment structure is provided for those living arrangements, and programs merely monitor compliance to protocols which allow the addicts themselves to reenter the broader society with a drug-free life style.

Partial hospitalization and day hospitals are medical outpatient programs which involve the client in therapeutic activities for 4 to 6 hours per day while the client still lives at home. These programs provide medical services for detoxification and for medically assisted recovery with medications that either treat withdrawal symptoms, modify craving, or help prevent relapse. Counseling and education are part of these programs.

Harm reduction programs consist of pharmacotherapy maintenance approaches, such as methadone maintenance clinics, behavioral training programs to control drug use, education programs on how to minimize problems from use, partial detox clinics to minimize damage to the user, and even designated driver programs.

PROGRAM UTILIZATION

In 1994, a total of 1,847,000 people were treated in various programs and facilities. It is estimated that another 1,706,000 hard-core users also needed treatment and possibly another 3,537,000 less hard-core but still problematical users needed some kind of treatment. The totals mean that in 1994, about 7 million Americans had serious enough drug and alcohol problems to need treatment.

TREATMENT CONTINUUM

"I know it sounds strange but the best thing that ever happened to me was that I became an addict. That's because my addiction forced me into treatment and the recovery process and through recovery I found what was missing in my life."
Nurse with 20 years of recovery time

The chronic progressive and relapsing nature of addiction is a depressing and degrading process. Addicts invariably lose self-esteem and a large percentage (34–38%) develop suicidal depression by the time they enter treatment. Recovery is a spiritually

TABLE 9–1   ONE DAY CENSUS OF CLIENTS IN TREATMENT BY INSTITUTION

Type of Institution	1980	1987	1993
Free standing/outpatient	197,255	306,406	503,684
Community mental health centers	95,086	89,182	140,685
General hospital (including VA hospitals)	49,529	63,039	95,826
Other specialized hospitals	18,907	26,852	22,714
Halfway houses/recovery houses	17,891	17,049	24,343
Other residential facilities	31,112	45,320	70,398
Correctional facilities	12,143	9,434	38,353
Others and unknown	66,929	56,841	48,205
Totals	**488,852**	**614,123**	**944,208**

- 70% of all clients were male.
- 4.9% of female clients were pregnant.
- Close to half of all clients resided in urban areas.
- 1/4 of all clients were IV drug users at the time of admission.
- About 10% of all clients in units were reported as HIV positive.
- 105,000 were under 20 years old.
- 698,000 were between 21 and 44 years old.
- 131,000 were between the ages of 45 and 64.
- 9,700 were over 65 years old.

(National Drug and Alcoholism Treatment Unit Survey [NDATUS], 1994)

uplifting and motivating process through which individuals gain a sense of purpose, community, and meaning for their lives. As mentioned, there are multiple modalities developed to treat addiction but whatever the method used, treatment should address four major phases that lead one to health: detoxification, initial abstinence, sobriety, and continuous recovery. It is necessary for the addict to commit to abstinence from the abused drug through all phases of treatment.

DETOXIFICATION

The first step is to get the drug out of the body's system. The user's body chem-istry has become so unbalanced that only abstinence will give it time to metabolize the drug and begin to normalize neuro-chemical balance. It takes about a week to completely excrete a drug such as cocaine and perhaps another 4 weeks to 10 months until the body chemistry settles down.

Assessment of the severity of addiction is important to determine whether the addict requires detoxification through hospitalization or residential treatment, or whether the addict can be managed on an outpatient basis. Physical dependence on alcohol or sedatives, major medical or psychiatric complications, pregnancy, or an overdosed addict are all indications for initiating detoxification in a hospital-based program.

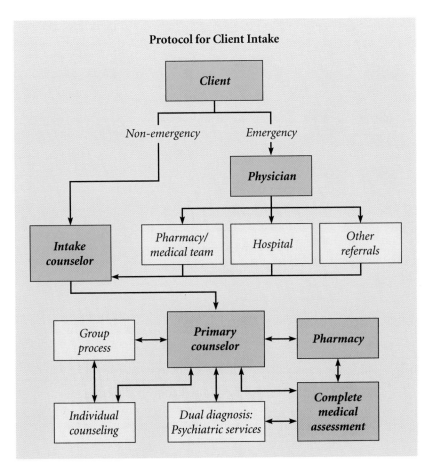

Figure 9-3 •

This is the protocol for the Haight-Ashbury Detox Clinic. It emphasizes the complexity of treating a compulsive drug user who comes in for treatment, particularly if other problems, such as medical complications, mental problems (dual diagnosis), or HIV disease are involved. The limiting factor for many clinics is their budget.

"Something told me I had to stop, so I did. And I stopped by myself for seven days straight. I didn't know what I was going through. I was having flashes, I heard people talking to me, I was sweating. I had the shakes real bad. So I called General Hospital. They gave me poison control and they transferred me to the Haight-Ashbury Clinic." 23-year-old recovering cocaine addict

Medication Therapy

A variety of specific medications is used during the detoxification phase to ease the symptoms of withdrawal and minimize the initial drug cravings which occur.

- Clonidine (Catapres®) dampens the withdrawal symptoms of opioids, alcohol, and even nicotine addiction.

- Phenobarbital is used to prevent withdrawal seizures and other symptoms associated with alcohol and sedative-hypnotic dependence.

- Methadone is the federally approved medication for opioid addiction treatment while l-alpha acetyl methadol (LAAM) and buprenorphine are being developed as alternatives for methadone in the detoxification (or maintenance) of opioid addictions.

- Antipsychotic medications, like halperidol (Haldol®), and antidepressants, like desipramine and imipramine (Tofranil®), have been used in the initial detoxification of cocaine, amphetamine or other stimulant drug addictions.

- Bromocriptine (Parlodel®), amantadine (Symmetrel®), and L-Dopa® have been used to treat the craving associated with cocaine and stimulant drug dependence; naltrexone (Revia®) and ritanserine have been used to dampen alcohol cravings.

- Nicotine patches (Nicoderm® or Prostep®) are approved to treat the withdrawal symptoms of tobacco, whereas nicotine-laced gum (Nicorette®) helps to lessen craving.

- Antabuse® (disulfiram) helps to prevent alcoholism relapse by creating unpleasant side effects if alcohol is used while it is being taken.

- Naltrexone (Revia®) blocks the effects of opioids. The addict will have a minimal response to heroin if she or he happens to slip while in treatment. It is also being used to prevent craving in recovering alcoholics.

- Finally, a number of amino acids are used individually or in combination with each other to alleviate withdrawal and craving symptoms from addiction to various drugs. The theory is that these amino acids are used by the brain to make neurotransmitters that were depleted by the drug addiction. It is believed that the imbalance or depletion of neurotransmitters is the cause of the withdrawal and craving. Common amino acids used for this purpose are tyrosine, taurine, tryptophane, d,1-phenylalanine, lecithin and glutamine.

Psychosocial Therapy

Medical intervention alone is rarely effective during the detoxification phase. Indeed, most programs forego medical treatment when the addict is not in any health or emotional danger from drug withdrawal. Intensive counseling, group work, and 12-step group participation have proven to be the most effective measures of engaging addicts into a recovery process and should be the main focus of all phases of treatment despite the many medical innovations being developed.

Psychosocial client interactions during detoxification are usually intense (daily encounters in an outpatient program) and highly structured for a two to six week duration. The aim of this treatment phase is to break down residual denial and engage the client into the full recovery process. This is accomplished through mandated participation in educational sessions, task-oriented group work, therapy groups, peer recovery groups, 12-step groups, and individual counseling. Treatment focuses on helping the addict to learn about the disease concept of addiction, the harmful effects of the disease, and the intensity of detoxification symptoms being experienced by the addict. The clients also receive information about their treatment and any medications used in detoxification. Clients develop their recovery or treatment plan with their primary counselor and initiate activities to accomplish their goals. Some programs have also begun to use structured treatment manuals which have a developed curriculum for each phase of treatment with individual daily lesson plans, exercises, and homework assignments.

"I knew I could do it myself. I tried those programs in AA. I stopped using drugs a million times and I never needed one of those programs. I figure if you're going to do it, you're going to do it anyway."
Recovering heroin addict/alcoholic

INITIAL ABSTINENCE

Once the addicts have been detoxified, their body chemistry must be given the opportunity to regain balance. Continued abstinence during this phase is best promoted by addressing both the continuous craving for drugs and the problems in their lives which may put them at risk for relapse.

Anticraving medications, such as those used during the detoxification phase, can be continued during the initial abstinence phase when more traditional approaches, like voluntary isolation (staying away from slippery places like bars, slippery people like co-users, and slippery things like drug paraphernalia), counseling, group and 12-step meetings, are ineffective in controlling the episodic drug hunger.

Medication Therapies for Initial Abstinence

Medical approaches like Antabuse® for alcoholism, naltrexone for opioids and alcohol, and various amino acids like tyrosine or d, l-phenylalanine for many of the drug addictions have been used to support the work of the self-help groups by suppressing or reversing the pleasurable effects of drugs or decreasing the drug craving, all of which help encourage the addict to stay clean.

Recently, an injection of a benzodiazepine antagonist, flumazenil (Mazicon®), has been used for the treatment of benzodiazepine overdose. Research into a cocaine and a true alcohol antagonist may lead to treatments for these addictions in the same manner that naltrexone is effective in preventing readdiction to opioids.

Environmental Triggers and Cue Extinction

Environmental triggers or cues often precipitate drug cravings. Addicts must learn to recognize their triggers which can be anything from drug odors to even hearing a song about drugs. They must then develop mechanisms to avoid those cues. Finally, they must learn to cope with cues or be prepared with a strategy to prevent themselves from using. It is important to note that drug craving is a true psychological response which is manifested by actual body changes of increased heart rate and blood pressure, sweating, dilation of the pupils, specific electrical changes in the skin, and even an immediate drop of two degrees or more in body temperature.

Deconditioning techniques, stress reduction exercises, expressing one's feelings, and long walks or cold showers are all strategies used by addicts to dissipate the craving response when it arises.

Techniques such as Dr. Anna Rose Childress's Desensitization Program retrain brain cells to not react when confronted by an environmental cue. The procedure involves exposing an addict to progressively stronger environmental cues over 40 to 50 sessions in a controlled setting. This technique gradually decreases response to the cues until there are no physiologic signs of a craving response even when the addict is exposed to heavy triggers. Every time an addict refrains from using while craving a drug, it lessens the response to the next trigger experience. Desensitization has also been called cue extinction.

"I did it myself. Every day I would take out my Librium® pills and look at them, touch them, and even smell them. Then, I would put them back in the bottle because I knew I couldn't ever use them again. After a while, I lost interest in them altogether."
Recovering Librium® addict

Psychosocial Support

Initial abstinence is also the phase during which addicts start to put their lives back in order, working on all the things they neglected to take care of while practicing their addiction. A comprehensive analysis of an addict's medical health, psychiatric status, social problems, and environmental needs must be conducted and a plan developed to address all issues presented.

Most importantly, addicts need to build a support system that will give continuing advice, help, and information when the user returns to job and home and is subject to all the pressures and temptations that made drug abuse begin. The support groups and 12-step programs like AA (Alcoholics Anonymous), NA (Narcotics Anonymous), CA (Cocaine Anonymous), and others are essential to maintaining a clean sober drug-free life style. Involvement in group therapy and continued recovery counseling have been demonstrated to have the most posi-

Environmental cues that trigger drug craving can include anything from paraphernalia, drug-using partners, old neighborhoods, or money.

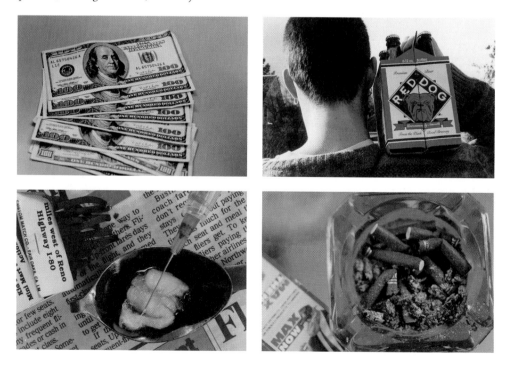

tive treatment outcomes during the initial abstinence phase.

LONG-TERM ABSTINENCE

The pivotal component of this phase occurs when an addict finally admits and accepts her or his addiction as lifelong and surrenders to the long-term, one-day-at-a-time treatment process. Continued participation in group, family, and 12-step programs is the key to maintaining long-term abstinence from drugs. The addict must accept that addiction is chronic, progressive, incurable, and potentially fatal and that relapse is always possible.

"We always say, 'I know that I have another relapse in me. I don't know if I have another abstinence in me.'"
7-year member of Alcoholics Anonymous

It is also vital for recovering addicts to accept that their condition is chemical dependency or drug compulsivity and not just that of alcoholism, or cocainism, or opioidism. Individuals who manifest addiction to a particular drug, such as cocaine, are well advised to abstain from the use of all psychoactive substances, especially alcohol. Even a seemingly benign flirtation with marijuana will probably lead to other drug hunger and relapse. It is a common clinical observation that compulsive drug abusers often switch intoxicants only to find the symptoms of addiction resurfacing through another addictive agent. Drug switching does not work with recovery-oriented treatment.

RECOVERY

Treatment and a continued focus on abstinence are not enough to assure recovery and a quality life style. Recovering addicts also need to restructure their lives and find things they enjoy doing that give them satisfaction, that give them the natural highs instead of the artificial highs they came to seek through drugs. Without this, they may have sobriety but they will not have recovery. This integral phase of treatment has been validated experimentally by Harvard Medical School Professor of Psychiatry Dr. George E. Vaillant in studies in 1983. He indicates four components necessary to change an ingrained habit of alcohol dependence. In the following model, the generic term drug is substituted for Dr. Vaillant's specific reference to alcohol:

1. offering the client or patient a non-chemical substitute dependency for the drug, such as exercise;
2. reminding her or him ritually that even one episode of drug use can lead to pain and relapse;
3. repairing the social, emotional, and medical damage done;
4. restoring self-esteem.

Continued and lifelong participation in the fellowship of 12-step programs along with the concerted effort to seek out natural healthy nondrug rewarding experiences is the formula that most recovering addicts have found to be successful in achieving their treatment goals.

"I have to look deep inside me. I'm hungry and I don't know why I'm hungry but I know I don't want no cocaine today. I used to be hungry for cocaine. I used to get angry because I couldn't do as much cocaine as I wanted. Then I got the cocaine and I'm lonely because I don't have no friends. So I'm tired of being sick and tired and I'm here. My sobriety is number one. That comes before anything in my life today."
Recovering 26-year-old "crack" addict

OUTCOME AND FOLLOW-UP

Primarily promoted by government and other funding sources to justify spending for addiction treatment, client outcomes and follow-up evaluations have become a major element in treatment program activities. What seems to be neglected by this process is an opportunity for treatment programs to utilize the data obtained to modify their treatment protocols and interventions to promote better outcomes for clients. Since addiction by nature is a chronic, multivaried, and relapsing condition, there is a need to develop outcome measures which evaluate different phases of the recovery process including long-term follow up.

Indications most often evaluated for successful addiction treatment include

- prevalence of drug slips and relapses (duration of continuous sobriety);
- retention in treatment;
- completion of treatment plan and its phases;
- family functioning;
- social and environmental adjustments;
- vocational or educational functioning including personal finance management;
- criminal activity or legal involvement.

What is important to note is that in general, all types of addiction treatment have demonstrated positive client outcomes when evaluated by rigorous scientific methods.

INDIVIDUAL VERSUS GROUP THERAPY

There are two main integrated components of addiction treatment: psychosocial therapy and medical (especially medication) therapy. Recent developments in understanding the neurobiological process of addiction have resulted in an explosive growth of medication treatments and the new medical specialty of addictionology. However, it is important to remember those treatments are not effective unless they are integrated with psychosocial therapies.

There are two general types of counseling therapies: individual and group. Most treatment facilities will use a combination of these counseling therapies.

INDIVIDUAL THERAPY

Individual therapy is a process usually conducted by trained chemical dependency counselors often credentialed to work with substance abusers. They deal with clients on a one-to-one basis to explore the reasons for their continued use of psychoactive substances and identify all areas of intervention needs. This may lead to a referral for specialized treatment, such as psychiatry, medical care, family counseling, and others. The therapist is able to work with addicts to help them gain a perspective on their usage and to identify tools and mechanisms that will keep them abstinent from drugs.

A treatment plan is developed with the client to guide in this process and individual treatment may continue from one month to several years. Although the majority of treatment is based on group and peer interaction, individual treatment may be more effective for certain types of drugs, such as heroin and sedatives.

A drug counselor and a heroin addict in a counseling session at the Haight-Ashbury Detox Clinic in San Francisco

Addict: "When I'm going through withdrawal, it's a physical thing and then after

I'm clean, I have the mental problem having to say no every time I get money in my hands: 'Should I or shouldn't I? No, I shouldn't. Go ahead, one more time won't hurt.' After I've passed withdrawal and I pass by areas where I used to hang out and I see other people nodding, in my mind, I start feeling like I'm sick again. I want to stay clean."

Counselor: "You can stay clean for a while. Is that what you want? You want to stay clean for a while or for the rest of your life?"

Addict: "I want to stay clean permanently."

Counselor: "Permanently drug free?"

Addict: "But I can do it without attending those [Narcotic's Anonymous] meetings."

Counselor: "All by yourself?"

Addict: "I mean with the medication that I take."

Counselor: "But the medications are only going to last you 21 days. They'll help you for a little while with the withdrawal of getting off heroin. But what are you going to do when the urges come up?"

Addict: "I guess I'll deal with that when the time comes."

Counselor: "So you're just going to wait for it? You're going to wait for the urges to come on and start using then?"

Addict: "Nah, I can deal with it."

Counselor: "You're being highly uncooperative. As a matter of fact, we're going to stop the medications today because we know you're still using heroin and we can't have you using on the program."

Addict: "I need those medications."

Counselor: "What for? It's just another drug. What you're doing is using it like another drug. I'd like for you to come back to get into that group meeting we have at three o'clock. Also, I want you to go to an NA (Narcotics Anonymous) meeting every day. I want you to go to these meetings and participate. Talk every opportunity you can. And also what I want you to do is bring back the signed participation card that you attended. I want you to do that. That's just part of the requirement of being in the program. See, I'm going to assume that you want to stop using drugs."

Addict: "Why can't I just get the detoxification drugs?"

Counselor: "Because we're not just a medication program. It's a counseling and full recovery program too."

It is also observed that individual treatment is less threatening for many individuals and therefore can be used as a short-term initial treatment in addiction.

GROUP THERAPY

There are several types of group therapies. They are facilitated, peer, 12-step, educational, topic-specific, and targeted. Generally, a major focus of group therapy is having clients help each other to break the isolation that chemical dependency induces, so they know they are not alone. Addicts are able to gain experience and understanding from each other about their addiction and learn different ways to combat craving which helps prevent their abuse or relapse. As peers, they are also better equipped to confront one another on issues which may lead to relapse or continued use.

"The group keeps me honest with myself. I get to look at a lot of things and behaviors that are going on with me and I try and keep in the now, keep thinking about staying clean today and the group keeps me focused on my goal of each day trying to stay clean." Recovering "crack" cocaine user

Facilitated Groups

Group therapy usually consists of six or more clients who meet with one or more therapists on a daily, weekly, or monthly basis. Therapists may facilitate the group by actively leading it, bringing up topics to be discussed, and processing all issues with their clinical insight. The facilitator (counselor) helps to establish a group culture where sharing, trust, and openness become natural to the participants.

Stimulant abuse peer group which uses confrontational techniques and a facilitator

William: "I have two sets of friends. People I use with and people who don't use at all. We've got together and had dinner and so forth."

Facilitator: "That's real safe for you, William. Listen to me, William. They don't know what to look for. They don't know what to expect and you can manipulate them real easy."

Maria: "The same thing happened to me. You still think you can sit around with alcoholics, with people who drink, like you think you can hang around with dope dealers?"

William: "So the only people I can associate with are people in recovery?

Maria: "I had to give up my sister."

William: "Okay, admit it. Everybody out there doesn't have a problem."

Maria: "But, you do."

William: "That's true."

Facilitator: "Let me ask you a question. Can you see your ears?"

William: "No."

Facilitator: "So that means we can see something you can't see, right? Okay. So far, this group, with your issues, we're batting a thousand. Yes or no?"

William: "Yes."

Peer Groups

Peer group therapy consists of therapists playing a less active role in the dynamics. They observe interaction and are available to process any conflicts or areas of need but they do not direct or lead the process.

Drug abuse recovery peer group

John: "I didn't want to come here this morning and then to come here and be faced with, 'Well, you gotta think whether you really want to be here.' It's like I'm ready. And I'm scared."

Counselor: "What's scaring you?"

John: "I feel like I'm failing myself."

Bob: "When did you fail before?"

John: "When have I failed before? Oh, I would say the last time was when I got busted buying 'crack'. Just going out there is failing. Knowing I shouldn't be doing that."

Bob: "You gotta put that out there. You gotta deal with that."

John: *"The thing is I'm scared of when I'm going to snap again."*

Tom: *"Yeah. I believe you. Going out, getting mad, getting in trouble, hurting yourself."*

John: *"I don't know where it could lead. It used to be getting high."*

Tom: *"Well, beating the crap out of somebody might be the first step but then you go use."*

John: *"I haven't beat the crap out of anybody lately."*

12-Step Groups

The most widely used group process is a peer group based on the 12-step model first developed by Alcoholics Anonymous in the 1930s. These groups have no professional therapist present to interact with their members. Each group is independent and relies on the members knowledge and successes to help curb alcohol and other drug use. The parent group provides literature, suggestions for meeting format, and general structure. The core book is called *Alcoholics Anonymous* (usually referred to as *The Big Book*) which was written by Bill Wilson and Dr. Bob Smith, the founders of AA, along with 100 recovering alcoholics who tell their stories.

"When I went to my first meeting, a 30-year-old beautician was running [telling] her story about how her drinking started, the pain she suffered because of it, and what happened to change her. I was a 49-year-old male with my own business and yet her story was my story. Her reaction to alcohol was the same as mine. Her helplessness after the first drink was mine. Her denial was mine. Her divorce was mine. Her reaction to life's problems were mine. The familiarity and the sheer power of her running her story has kept me in the group for five and one-half years. In AA they say, 'We only have our stories and all we can do is tell what worked for us to stay sober.' But that way, I could listen and accept (or reject) ideas rather than being lectured at and told what to do or walking out on my wife whenever she dared to talk about my drinking. I got a sponsor that first night. He was about my age and he showed me the ropes. He also told me the first night that the only way he stays sober is by helping me and his two other sponsorees to stay sober. Since I've been in the program, I've relapsed three times but I've gotten sober four times." Recovering 54-year-old alcoholic

Some of the other 12-step groups that have formed are Cocaine Anonymous (CA), Narcotics Anonymous (NA), Marijuana Anonymous (MA), Gamblers Anonzymous (GA), Overeaters Anonymous (OA), Sexaholics Anonymous, Emotions Anonymous, Relationships Anonymous, and Shoppers Anonymous. In addition, Al-Anon, ACoA, and Alateen use the 12-step process.

All 12-step programs are free. They pay their minimal costs through voluntary donations. The only requirement for membership is a desire to stop the addiction.

The 12-step process engages addicts at their level of addiction, breaks the isolation, guilt, and pain, and shows them they are not alone. The process also fully supports the idea that addiction is a lifelong disease and must be dealt with for the remainder of a person's life. It promotes a program of honesty, open-mindedness, and willingness to change. Those are the key elements in sustaining lifelong abstinence from drugs, alcohol, and other addictive behaviors. It breaks down denial and supplies a structure through which people can continue to work on their addiction. The basis of 12-step programs is spirituality.

"People misunderstand spirituality. They mistake it for religion. Spirituality is people's personal relationship with their higher power as they define him, her, or it. Religion is the way they practice their spirituality. My higher power is God as I learned of him in my youth. For others, their higher power could be an ideal, a philosophy, the goodness within them, a great person they met in their lives, the stars, or the 12-step group itself. It's something outside of themselves that they can turn to, to get help for their smothering addiction and to reconstruct their lives. It's only when they give up the need to try to control everything in their lives and give up control to their higher power that they gain the power to overcome their addiction and say no to the first drink."

51-year-old ex-priest who gives talks on spirituality and his recovery from alcoholism

Although most 12-step groups understand and accept spirituality, some users cannot accept the idea of a higher power. For those people, *The Big Book* of Alcoholics Anonymous says take what you want and leave the rest. These people can get a lot out of meetings and learn from the experiences of others.

The 12 Steps of Alcoholics Anonymous

Step 1: We admitted we were powerless over alcohol [cocaine, cigarettes, food, gambling, etc.] and that our lives had become unmanageable.

Step 2: Came to believe that a power greater than ourselves could restore us to sanity.

Step 3: Made a decision to turn our will and our lives over to the care of God *as we understood Him.*

Step 4: Made a searching and fearless moral inventory of ourselves.

Step 5: Admitted to God, to ourselves, and to another human being the exact nature of our wrongs.

Step 6: Were entirely ready to have God remove all these defects of character.

Step 7: Humbly asked Him to remove our shortcomings.

Step 8: Made a list of all persons we had harmed and became willing to make amends to them all.

Step 9: Made direct amends to such people wherever possible, except when to do so would injure them or others.

Step 10: Continued to take personal inventory and when we were wrong, promptly admitted it.

Step 11: Sought through prayer and meditation to improve our conscious contact with God *as we understood Him*, praying only for knowledge of His will for us and the power to carry that out.

Step 12: Having had a spiritual awakening as the result of these steps, we tried to carry this message to alcoholics and to practice these principles in all our affairs.

What is important to understand is that the 12 steps work for any addictive behavior. This is because the roots of addiction lie first, in the character and life style of the user and second, in the use of psychoactive substances.

There are also secular versions of the peer group process used in 12-step groups. These groups do not believe that a higher power is necessary for recovery.

A group like **Rational Recovery (RR)** believes that if you learn to like yourself for who you are, then you will not need to drink or use other drugs. They believe that all addictions come from the same roots. Their approach is based on rational emotive therapy developed by Albert Ellis.

Another group, **Secular Organization for Sobriety (SOS)**, also makes no distinction among the various chemical addictions. Their goal is sobriety, one-day-at-a-time, like AA's and NA's goal.

Women for Sobriety (WFS) does have a spiritual basis but feels that AA principles work better for men. WFS emphasizes the power of positive emotions. **Men for Sobriety** (MFS) has also been formed.

Educational Groups

These groups focus primarily on providing information about the addictive process in recovery. Trained counselors provide the education and often bring in other experts to promote individual lesson plans to help addicts gain knowledge about their conditions.

Homework assignments are often included to help addicts understand the information. A variety of workbooks and manuals, such as recovery workbooks, have been written to assist this process. They also teach relapse prevention, coping skills, and even support therapy.

Targeted Groups

These groups can either be part of a formal program or a nonfacilitated peer group and are directed at specific populations of users. Such targeted groups include men's groups, women's groups, gay and lesbian groups, skinhead groups, dual diagnosis groups, bad girls groups (targeted at prosti-

tutes), and priest/minister/rabbi groups (targeted at the clergy). The key element to the success of any group is its ability to develop a group culture which provides relevant, meaningful, acceptable, and insightful knowledge for that selective gathering of participants.

Topic-Specific Groups

Whereas target groups are aimed at certain cultures, topic groups are aimed at certain issues, e.g., AIDS recovery, early recovery, relapse prevention, maintenance, relationships, and codependency. The advantage of these groups is that they allow the participants to focus on key specific issues that are a threat to their continued recovery.

From most studies, group therapies seem to promote better outcomes and sustain abstinence than individual therapies. Specifically, alcohol and cocaine addiction are more responsive to the group process than to individual counseling. From an administrative standpoint, group processes are also much more cost-effective since attracting a large number of clients can be served by a minimal amount of staffing.

TREATMENT AND THE FAMILY

Addiction is a family disease. Abuse of drugs and alcohol greatly impacts every member of addicts' families regardless of whether or not they participate in the abuse of psychoactive substances. Analysis of employed addicts and alcoholics demonstrates that their families use the employer's health insurance at a rate of 5 to 10 times more than the families of nonaddicts. This is indicative of the great emotional, physical,

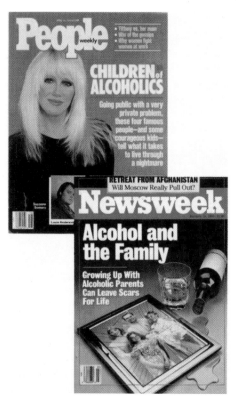

Addiction is not confined to the addicts.

and social strain that addicts place on their families.

"Addicts don't have families, they take hostages." Anonymous

Despite this well-established relationship, the family is often ignored and neglected in the treatment of addictive disease. This has resulted in family members seeking treatment on their own through traditional family and mental health services or through self-help family treatment systems, like Tough Love, Al-Anon, or Nar-Anon.

More importantly, continued stress from family problems or troubled family members makes it difficult for the recovering addict to remain abstinent.

"A family is ruled by its sickest member."
Moss Hart, dramatist

GOALS OF FAMILY TREATMENT

Treatment of addicts and their families has four major goals:

1. acceptance by all family members, including the addicts themselves, that addiction is a treatable disease, not a sign of moral weakness;

2. establishing and maintaining a drug-free family system which often includes treatment of the spouse's drug problems or those of the addict's children;

3. developing a system for family communication and interaction which continues to reinforce the recovery process of the addict. This is accomplished by integrating family therapy into addiction treatment;

4. processing the family's readjustment after cessation of drug and alcohol abuse.

DIFFERENT FAMILY APPROACHES

Family therapists employ a wide variety of techniques and tools to accomplish these goals once all family members have been motivated to participate. The following are some of the more commonly used models.

Family Systems Approach

This model explores and recognizes how a family regulates its internal and external environment making note of how these interactional patterns change over time. Three major areas of focus of this approach are daily routines, family rituals (e.g., holidays), and short-term problem-solving strategies.

Family Behavioral Approach

This approach operates under the concept that interactional behaviors are learned and perpetuated by reinforcements for continuing the behavior. Thus, the therapist works with the family to recognize those family behaviors associated with drug use, to categorize the interactions as either negative or positive in reinforcing drug usage, and then to provide interventions to support and reinforce those behaviors which promote a drug-free family system.

Family-Functioning Approach

This approach first helps the addict or treatment programs classify the family system into one of four different types, then uses the classification as a guide for a therapeutic intervention best suited to the functioning of that system.

- *Functional family systems* are those in which the family of the addict has maintained healthy interactions. Interventions in this system are therefore targeted directly at the addict. Other family members receive limited education and advice to support the recovery of the addict.

- *Neurotic or enmeshed family systems* usually require intensive family treatment aimed at restructuring the way the family interacts.

- *Disintegrated family systems* call for a separate yet integrated treatment of addicts and their families. Al-Anon may be attended by the family while an alcoholic is engaged in an intensive medical detoxification program. Though separated in treatment, this approach needs to be integrated at some point into the common goal of maintaining a drug-free life style by the addict.

- *Absent family systems* are those in which family members are not available for treatment.

Social Network Approach

The social network approach focuses mainly on the treatment of the addict and establishes a concurrent and integrated support network for the family to assist it with the issues caused by the addiction. Through participation in multiple family support or therapy groups, the family breaks its isolation and develops skills which help it support the recovery effort of its addicted member.

Tough Love Approach

Though controversial, this movement has grown on the West Coast. The Tough Love approach addresses the major obstacle of denial in both the addict and his or her family. When the addicted family member refuses to accept or deal with dysfunctional drug-using behavior, the family members seek treatment and support from other families experiencing similar problems. The family learns to establish limits for its interaction with the addict. This has included even kicking that family member out of the home and severing all contact until the addict agrees to treatment.

OTHER BEHAVIORS

"Even though it was my dad that drank till he got sick, doing the intervention was harder for me than for him. I knew he denied his drinking. I didn't realize that I did too, even though I didn't drink myself, and that I had almost as many problems as he did."

31-year-old adult child of an alcoholic (ACoA)

The stress of living with an alcoholic or drug abuser causes dysfunctional behaviors in the nonusing family members. The most prevalent conditions are

- codependency;
- enabling;
- manifesting symptoms caused by being children of addicts or adult children of addicts.

Codependency

Just as addicts are dependent upon a substance, codependents are dependent on the addicts to fulfill some need of their own. For example, a wife may be dependent on her husband maintaining his addiction in order for her to hold power over the relationship. As long as he's addicted, she has an excuse for her own shortcomings and problems. In this way, it creates dysfunction in the addict because it promotes the addiction. Codependency can also be extremely subtle. For example, a person who has been abstinent from alcohol for a week or so has a spouse who offers a drink as a reward for the abstinence. In this kind of household, the chances of recovery are greatly reduced unless the codependents are willing to accept their role in the addictive process and submit to treatment themselves.

Enabling

When a family becomes dependent upon the addiction of a family member, there is a strong tendency to avoid confrontation about the addictive behavior and a subconscious effort to perpetuate the addiction, often led by a person who benefits greatly from that addiction, the chief enabler. Although enablers may be disgusted with the addict and the addictive behavior, they continue paying off drug debts, paying rent, providing money, or even continuing emotional support for a practicing addict. As with codependents, the enablers need to accept the role they are playing in this cycle and seek therapy so they can be more effective in the addict's recovery.

Children of Addicts and Adult Children of Addicts

Children of addicts take on predictable behavioral roles within the family which "co" the addiction and which continue on into their adult personalities. In addict families, children usually take on one or more of the following roles.

- *Model child:* These children are high achievers and are overly responsible. They become chief enablers of addicted parents by taking over their roles and responsibilities.
- *Problem child:* These children experience continual multiple personal problems and often manifest early drug or alcohol addiction. They demand and get most of what attention is left from parents and siblings.
- *Lost child:* These children are withdrawn, "spaced-out," disconnected from the life and emotions around them. Often avoiding any emotionally confronting issues, they are unable to form close friendships or intimate bonds with others.
- *Mascot child or family clown:* These children use another avoidance strategy which is to make everything trivial by minimizing all serious issues. They are well-liked and easy to befriend but are usually superficial in all relationships, even those with their own family members.

What is important to remember about children of alcoholics (addicts) is that although they may not abuse drugs, their behavior and emotional reactions can be as dysfunctional as that of an addict. Often they learn very early on that they cannot control the addiction of a loved one, so they often resort to trying to control all other aspects of their life, leading to strained and inappropriate relationships later in life.

Adult children of alcoholics (ACoA) or addicts also

- are isolated and afraid of people and authority figures;
- are approval seekers who lose their identity in the process;
- are frightened by angry people and personal criticism;
- become or marry alcoholics or find another compulsive person to fulfill abandonment needs;
- feel guilty when standing up for themselves instead of giving in to others;
- become addicted to excitement and stimulation;
- confuse love and pity; tend to love people who can be pitied and rescued;
- repress feelings from traumatic childhoods and lose the ability to feel or express feelings;
- judge themselves harshly and have low self-esteem;
- are reactors rather than actors.

ACoA is a 12-step group to help adult children of alcoholics work through the emotional baggage that followed them into adulthood. ACoA and other similar groups try to help members

- understand the disease of addiction and alcoholism because understanding is the beginning of the gift of forgiveness;
- put themselves on top of their priority list;

- detach with tough love;
- feel, accept, and express feelings and build self-esteem;
- learn to love themselves, enabling them to love others in healthy ways.

Al-Anon or **Nar-Anon** are 12-step-oriented groups targeted for the families of addicts or alcoholics. They involve peer interaction and often the addict is not present. The group meets to support and provide resources to families of addicts to deal with their addicted relatives or lovers. It is common for families to participate in these groups prior to their addicted family member participating in any treatment. **Alateen** is a division of the Al-Anon Family Group. Alateen focuses mostly on 14 to 17 year olds who have an alcoholic in their family and feel more comfortable with just their peers.

DRUG-SPECIFIC TREATMENT

POLYDRUG ABUSE

Experience at the Haight-Ashbury Detox Clinic and treatment centers across the United States shows that although addicts may identify a drug of choice, they are more often than not polysubstance abusers who are using a wide range of substances either concurrently or intermittently. The profile of alcoholics, for example, often includes sedatives, cocaine, and even opioids in addition to their abuse of alcohol. Treatment programs need to be aggressive about identifying the total drug profile of their clients. Heroin addicts will often minimize or lie about their use of alcohol even though their use of that drug may be at a problematic level.

"I have cleaned up off of dope though I've been a drug addict for 23 years. And I have no desire whatsoever to do drugs but alcohol is still there and I do it out of boredom."
42-year-old recovering heroin addict

By addressing addiction as chemical dependency rather than a drug-specific problem, treatment is effective in promoting recovery, preventing relapse, and preventing a switch to alternate drug addictions. When treatment doesn't address all addictions, a heroin addict might come back as an alcoholic a few months later.

It must be observed that tissue dependence to alcohol and other sedatives is a medical emergency. Untreated withdrawal will result in life-threatening symptoms. For example, when sedatives are mentioned in the drug profile in addition to what addicts identify as their drug of choice, a medical assessment must be done to determine the tissue dependence level. If someone is indeed physically addicted, antiseizure medication and medical management are needed in the treatment process.

STIMULANTS (cocaine and amphetamines)

Stimulant abuse is often accompanied by a wide range of psychiatric symptoms. Acute paranoia, schizophrenia, major depression, and bipolar disorder are often the initial presentations by a stimulant addict, particularly at the end of a long run. These symptoms require psychiatric intervention to prevent harm and to assess whether they have been caused by the drug itself or whether the mental illnesses are preexisting and will continue to be a problem after detoxification and initial abstinence.

Besides psychoactive symptoms or dual diagnosis, other key symptoms to watch for in cocaine or amphetamine abusers who are detoxifying are prolonged craving, anergia (exhaustion), anhedonia (lack of an ability to feel pleasure), and euthymia (a feeling of elation which occurs three to five days after stopping use). Euthymia makes users feel that they never were addicted and that they don't need to be in treatment. The anergia and anhedonia start to overtake the euthymia at about two weeks after starting detoxification and these feelings, particularly the total lack of ability to feel pleasure, often lead to relapse.

"I think when you're using the drug, it's real easy to deny everything that's going on and put everything on the shelf and not cope with it. Your whole world becomes the acquiring of whatever drug you happen to be using. But when you stop, it's all there waiting for you. And, eventually, you have to deal with it."
Methamphetamine user

Detoxification and Initial Abstinence

After detoxification and treatment for any psychotic symptoms and any life-threatening symptoms, such as extremely high blood pressure and heart rate, the vast majority of stimulant abusers respond positively to traditional drug counseling approaches.

However, a number of stimulant addicts have not been able to respond to these traditional approaches and initially require a more intensive, medical approach to bridge the detoxification/withdrawal period prior to their engagement into recovery.

Medical treatments include the use of antidepressant agents, such as imipramine, desipramine, amitriptyline, doxepin, trazodone, or fluoxetine (Prozac®). These affect serotonin, the neurotransmitter in the brain that deals with both depression and mood.

Antipsychotic medications, such as haloperidol (Haldol®), chlorpromazine (Thorazine®), and others, are also used to buffer the effects of unbalanced dopamine. Sedatives, such as phenobarbital, chloral hydrate, Dalmane®, Librium®, or even Valium®, are prescribed very carefully, on a short-term basis, to treat anxiety or sleep disturbance problems.

Nutritional approaches aimed at enhancing the production of those neurotransmitters which have been depleted by heavy stimulant use have been used to decrease craving and counteract many of the withdrawal symptoms seen in stimulant addiction.

Long-Term Abstinence

A lot of work is currently being put into the treatment of craving and particularly stimulant craving. Two major types of craving have been addressed: endogenous craving and environmentally triggered craving.

Endogenous craving is believed to be caused by the depletion of dopamine in the nucleus acumbens of the limbic system. To treat this situation, many medications, like amantadine, bromocryptine, and L-Dopa®, have been used to simulate dopamine in the nucleus acumbens, thereby diminishing craving for stimulants. Animal research suggests that the dopamine imbalance may last for up to 10 months after cessation of cocaine or amphetamine use.

Environmentally triggered craving, which is particularly intense in stimulant addiction and is more likely to lead to relapse than endogenous craving, has to be treated by intense counseling, group sessions, or desensitization techniques. This type of craving may last throughout one's life but evidence indicates that continued abstinence weakens the craving response. This weakening can lead to the extinction of craving caused by environmental triggers.

TOBACCO

The only guaranteed successful therapy when it comes to tobacco is to never smoke, chew, or use it in any form. Abstinence is necessary because many of the neurologic and neurochemical alterations which cause nicotine addiction are permanent. This means that even 10 years after cessation of smoking, a single cigarette can trigger the nicotine craving in some users.

The failure rate for most therapies to stop smoking is 70% to 80%, this in spite of the fact that 80% of all smokers want to quit. In the past, the focus on treatment was the psychological components of addiction, particularly the habit of smoking. Unfortunately these approaches didn't fully take into account the lifetime nature of nicotine addiction and therefore recovery. They tried to apply short-term fixes (e.g., 21-day smoking cessation programs) to a long-term problem.

Recently, in recognition of the very real alterations in brain chemistry that trigger nicotine craving during withdrawal, the treatment community has focused on pharmacological treatments.

Nicotine Replacement

Since the main mechanism that causes craving is the drop in blood levels of nicotine which then triggers withdrawal symptoms, such as irritability, anxiety, drowsiness, and lightheadedness, research has been aimed at nicotine replacement systems. The purpose of these systems is to slowly reduce the blood plasma nicotine levels to the point where cessation will not trigger withdrawal symptoms that will cause the smoker to relapse.

The four types of nicotine replacement systems are transdermal nicotine patches, nicotine gum, nicotine sprays, and nicotine nasal inhalers. One of the main advantages of all of these systems is that users are no longer damaging their lungs with some of the 4,000 chemicals found in cigarette smoke. This alone could save almost 200,000 lives per year in the United States. The main problem is that if relapse prevention, counseling, and self-help groups are not used in conjunction with nicotine replacement therapy, then the chances of smokers returning to their old habits are high.

Nicotine Patches. Nicotine patches, such as Nicoderm® and Habitrol®, are nicotine-soaked adhesive patches that are applied to the skin. Patches can be worn intermittently (daytime only) or continuously. Most of them contain enough nicotine to last for 24 to 72 hours. The advantages of patches are the steady rate of release of nicotine, the ease of compliance, and the lack of toxic effects to tissues in the mouth or digestive track. The disadvantages are the cost, the inability to alter the amount being absorbed, and the 4 to 6 hours it takes for a patch to raise the nicotine level enough to dull nicotine craving. Also, if the user starts smoking while wearing the patch, extremely high and dangerous plasma levels of nicotine can occur.

Nicotine Gum. Nicotine gums, such as Nicorette®, have the advantage of slowing the rise in nicotine levels that smoking brings. The 10-second rush of an inhaled cigarette gives way to the 15- to 30-minute slow rise that nicotine gum provides when absorbed through the gums and other mucosal tissues. A slower rise means that craving, which is triggered by the sudden drop in nicotine levels after smoking, doesn't occur. The 15- to 30-minute rise, however, is considerably faster than the 4 to 6 hours it takes for a transdermal patch to work, so the user has more control over the dose. The disadvantages are the user can cram a lot of gum into the mouth or not use it at all, the gum can irritate mucosal tissues, and an oral habit is maintained (users are still putting something in their mouths when the craving hits or when they are agitated rather than learning other behaviors).

Nasal Spray. Nasal sprays (still undergoing clinical trials) are self-administered and reach the brain in 3 to 5 minutes, thereby giving faster relief to the nicotine craving and giving more control to the user. Disadvantages include irritation to the nasal passages and reinforcement of nicotine addiction.

Nicotine Inhalers. Nicotine inhalers (still undergoing clinical trials) give the fastest relief of nicotine craving without involving the inhalation of all the chemicals present in smoke. The problem seems to be that misuse can produce plasma levels similar to those produced by smoking, thereby perpetuating the addictive process.

Treating the Symptoms. The purpose of symptomatic treatment is to reduce the anxiety, depression, and craving that accompany nicotine withdrawal and therefore trigger relapse. Benzodiazepines, buspirone, Prozac®, and other antidepressants, such as mecamylamine, propranolol, naltrexone, and naloxone, have been used to try to alleviate the symptoms of nicotine withdrawal. Even clonidine, often used to control symptoms of heroin withdrawal, has been used effectively to control nicotine withdrawal.

Most behavioral therapies, which include one-on-one counseling, group therapy, educational approaches, aversion therapy, hypnotism, and acupuncture, have a one-year success rate of 15% to 30%. Many of the techniques used in stimulant abuse recovery are directly applicable to quitting smoking. These include

- desensitizing the smoker to environmental cues that trigger craving;
- practicing alternate methods of calming oneself when under stress or going through withdrawal;
- avoiding environments and situations, such as bars, where smoking is rampant;
- finding other ways of getting the small rush or mild euphoria that nicotine provides;
- teaching the smoker the physiology of nicotine use and addiction along with the medical consequences of smoking or chewing tobacco;
- and teaching the smoker the extraordinary benefits of quitting.

OPIOIDS

Along with treatment for nicotine addiction, treatment for opioid addiction has the highest rate of relapse. This is partially because physical withdrawal from opioids is more severe than withdrawal from stimulants. For this reason, most opioid abusers who want to recover need to be involved in a detoxification and treatment program.

Detoxification

Programs may use mild opioids like Darvon® to detoxify and taper the habit. This allows addicts to have less fear of the pain of withdrawal, less pain during withdrawal, and it encourages them to stay in treatment. An alternative is clonidine which quiets the part of the brain that gets hyperactive when one goes through withdrawal. Methadone and LAAM are used for detoxification (or for long-term substitution treatment known as maintenance pharmacotherapy).

"The physical part of the treatment for opioid addiction is only a tiny portion of the process. It's what happens after you get off, after you detox, that's important. Everyone around you is using, and in a lot of cases you may have financial problems. You may not even have a place to stay. There are other kinds of things that build up and cause you to use again." Drug counselor

Initial Abstinence and Long-Term Abstinence

Long-lasting opioid antagonists, such as naltrexone (Revia®), which decrease craving for the drug and block opioids from activating brain cells, are used after detoxification to insure abstinence.

As with all other treatments, initial abstinence and long-term abstinence are supported by participating in individual counseling sessions, group sessions, or self-help groups, such as Narcotics Anonymous. During the first four to eight weeks of abstinence, daily attendance in these programs is crucial in maintaining a drug-free state when the craving is strongest. As successful treatment continues, fewer sessions are necessary.

Recovery

Since opioid addiction is so time-consuming and involving, the key to recovery from heroin or other opioid addiction is learning a new life style. Instead of waking up every morning with the need to raise $100 to $200 to support a heavy habit, instead of nodding off or feeling drugged, and instead of trying to get clean needles to avoid hepatitis, cotton fever, or HIV infection, addicts have to learn how to enjoy nondrug activities, how to have a relationship, and even how to get a driver's license.

"I'm not used to having a room. For the last two years I was on the streets. I spent $200 a day on heroin and couldn't even manage to find enough money to get a room at the end of the night. That's pretty sick. I've never actually had a checking account and such because I started using and dealing heroin when I was 12 and I always had to hide my finances."
Recovering 42-year-old heroin addict

Other Opioid Treatment Modalities

Methadone Maintenance. Much controversy has swirled around the concept of opiate or opioid substitution ever since morphine addiction became a problem in the nineteenth century. Because of the large number of morphine addicts following the Civil War, opiate maintenance clinics multiplied. At this time, morphine was used in China to treat opium addiction. In the early 1900s, heroin was used to treat morphine addiction in Europe. This practice of using opiates to treat opiate addiction was ended in the United States (though it continued in England and other countries) at the end of World War I and was not revived until methadone maintenance was developed in the late 1960s in New York City. This treatment modality eventually spread to hundreds of methadone maintenance clinics nationwide in the '70s and '80s. Today, there are more than 115,000 heroin addicts in methadone maintenance programs.

The theory is that methadone, a synthetic opiate, while not as intense as heroin, is longer lasting, and thus, will keep the user from having heroin-like withdrawal symptoms for 36 to 48 hours. Heroin, on the other hand, causes withdrawal symptoms in a few hours, so the user goes through the roller coaster of highs and lows and the pain of withdrawal on a daily basis.

With methadone maintenance, the highs and lows that promote addiction are avoided. The user doesn't have to hustle for money to pay for a habit, get drugs and needles on the street, or be exposed to a high-risk life style. With HIV infection rates in intravenous heroin users as high as 80%, this method of harm reduction has certain benefits, including forcing the addict to come to a certain location every day where counseling, medical care, and other services are available which might reduce the harm addicts do to themselves and others.

The controversy arises because many chemical dependency treatment personnel don't believe drug abuse should be treated with another addicting drug on a long-term basis. Since many users seek treatment after only a short period of addiction while their dose is still relatively low, the immediate use of methadone will further ingrain their opioid addiction. The pro-methadone advocates believe that keeping addicts from their harmful life style is more important than focusing on total recovery from opioid addiction which, in any case, is extremely difficult. It also reduces crime and other social problems by providing access to stabilized doses of a legal drug. Methadone maintenance has often been referred to as a political solution for a medical problem.

LAAM. Recently, the use of LAAM (levo acetyl alpha methadol), a long-acting methadone-like drug, has been used in much the same manner. LAAM will stay in the body for up to three days, so users further avoid withdrawal and the ups and downs of opioid addiction. In addition, they do not have to go to a clinic every day. The negative side of LAAM is that it is still an addictive drug and though fewer clinic visits mean lower treatment costs, they also mean fewer opportunities to encourage recovery.

Buprenorphine. Another drug that is being tried for treating opioid addiction is buprenorphine. It is an opioid agonist-antagonist. What this means is that, at low doses, it is a powerful opioid, almost 50 times as powerful as heroin but strangely enough, at high doses, it blocks the opioid receptors. It enables an addict to be started on methadone, then switched to buprenorphine as a transition to a true antagonist, like naltrexone.

SEDATIVE-HYPNOTICS (barbiturates, benzodiazepines)

Withdrawal from sedative-hypnotic addiction results in life-threatening seizures if not medically managed. Thus, intensive medical assessment and specific medical treatment are necessary when treating people who have become addicted to "reds" (secobarbital), Xanax® (alprazolam), other benzodiazepines, "loads" (glutethimide plus codeine), and any one sedative or even muscle relaxants, like Soma® (carisoprodal).

Detoxification

Substitution therapy (using a drug which is cross tolerant with another drug) is needed to detoxify a sedative-hypnotic addict. Although many drugs in this class of substances can be used, outpatient programs often utilize phenobarbital because of its long duration of action and its more specific antiseizure activity. A dose of phenobarbital sufficient to prevent any withdrawal symptoms without causing major drowsiness or sedation is established as a baseline to begin detoxification. Butabarbital is also used as an alternate to phenobarbital in the detoxification process. Phenytoin may be added to either medication therapy to further prevent any seizures from developing.

The initial detoxification from sedative-hypnotics requires intensive and daily medical management which also provides the opportunity to get the addict into intensive counseling and social services which are vital to their recovery once detoxification is completed.

Initial Abstinence

Continued abstinence from sedatives requires intensive participation in group, individual, and educational counseling as well as specific self-help groups or Narcotics Anonymous. Many sedative addicts, and especially those addicted to benzodiazepines, complain of bizarre and prolonged symptoms, such as taste or visual distortions, for several months after detoxification. Also, many experience inappropriate rage or anger during the early months of abstinence which requires skilled mental health intervention.

After detoxification, some sedative addicts experience the reemergence of withdrawal-like symptoms even though they have remained totally abstinent. This reaction can occur anywhere from one to several months after detoxification and may occasionally require medical intervention in treatment.

Two controversial explanations have been offered to explain this phenomena. One asserts that long-acting benzodiazepines, like diazepam (Valium®) or alprazolam (Xanax®), produce active metabolites which persist in the body, resulting in additional withdrawal symptoms once their levels decrease, even after several months of abstinence from the parent drug. Another explanation asserts that these are not true withdrawal symptoms but merely the reemergence of an original anxiety disorder which was controlled by the use of sedatives. Under this second explanation, psychiatrists need to initiate maintenance pharmacotherapy treatment to address the underlying psychiatric problems. Since many antianxiety medications are abusable sedative-hypnotics, this requires skillful medical management to prevent excessive, inappropriate use or relapse to sedative-hypnotic addiction.

Although flumazenil (Mazicon®) has been developed as an effective benzodiazepine antagonist, it is currently available only in injectible form to treat overdoses of these drugs. Future developments may lead to effective oral and long-acting benzodiazepine or barbiturate antagonists to help those addicted to sedative-hypnotics to accomplish initial abstinence.

Recovery

Continued participation in self-help or Narcotics Anonymous groups has been the most effective means of promoting continuous abstinence and recovery in sedative-hypnotic addiction.

As with cocaine and other addictions, the sedative-hypnotic addicts are vulnerable to environmental cues which trigger drug hunger and relapse throughout their lifetimes. Treatment, which includes cue or trigger recognition, avoidance tools, and coping mechanisms, is vital to addressing sedative-hypnotic addiction.

ALCOHOL

Denial

Denial on the part of the alcoholic or compulsive drinker is the biggest hindrance to beginning treatment. One reason that denial is so common with the use of alcohol is the long time it can take for social or habitual drinking to advance to abuse and addiction (10 years on the average). Denial also occurs because alcoholics have no memory of the negative effects they experienced while in an alcoholic "blackout." Thus, they don't believe that alcohol has harmed them. Further, alcohol impairs judgment and reason in all users, making them less likely to associate any problem with their drinking.

Detoxification

For a heavy drinker, physical withdrawal is very uncomfortable but usually not dangerous. Symptoms can often be handled by aspirin, rest, liquids and any

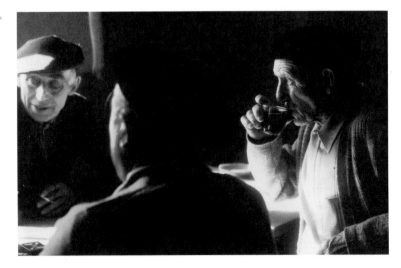

Since alcohol is so much a part of cultures around the world, the transition from social drinking to habituation, abuse, and addiction can be hard to recognize.

Reprinted, by permission, Alain Labrousse, Observatoire Geopolitique Des Drogues.

one of hundreds of hangover cures that have been handed down from generation to generation.

For the alcoholic, the potentially life-threatening symptoms of withdrawal can be medically managed with a variety of sedating drugs, e.g., barbiturates; benzodiazepines, such as Librium®; paraldehyde; chloral hydrate; and the phenothiazines. Since several of these drugs are addictive, they should be used sparingly and on a very short-term basis. Normally, tapering is done on a 5- to 7-day basis but can be extended to 11 to 14 days.

Along with emergency medical care, withdrawal and detoxification can be handled through emotional support and basic physical care, such as rest and nutrition (thiamin, folic acid, multi-vitamins, amino acids, electrolytes, and fructose). Many of the problems will start to abate with detoxification but for the long-term drinker, some damage is irreversible: liver disease, enlarged heart, cancer, and nerve damage among others.

Initial Abstinence

A common treatment for initial abstinence is the use of Antabuse®. Antabuse® is a drug that will make people ill if they drink alcohol. This is used for about 6 months or longer to help get alcoholics through initial abstinence when they're most likely to relapse. A more important part of this process is encouraging them to go to Alcoholics Anonymous meetings or other support group meetings in addition to individual therapy. One procedure is to have the user go to 90 Alcoholics Anonymous meetings in 90 days (called a 90/90 contract).

In 1996, naltrexone (Revia®) was approved by the FDA for the treatment of alcohol addiction. When used during the first three months of the recovery process,

it decreased alcohol relapse by 50% to 70% when combined with a comprehensive treatment program.

Long-Term Abstinence and Recovery

In treatment, one often encounters someone known as a "dry drunk." This means that the person is not actually drinking alcohol but still has the behavior and mindset of an alcoholic. Thus, the purpose of this stage of treatment, besides avoiding relapse, is to begin healing the emotional scars, confusion, and immaturity that had kept the person drinking for so many years.

Many treatment centers advertise 30-day drying out programs, implying that detoxification is the key to recovery rather than being a small initial step in a long process. As with all addictions, working on recovery throughout one's lifetime is necessary to prevent relapse. Brain cells have been permanently changed by years of drinking, so the recovering alcoholic is always susceptible to relapse.

PSYCHEDELICS

Many psychedelics will mimic mental conditions, such as schizophrenia, and so the clinician or intake counselor has to make a tentative diagnosis when first seeing the patient and give the drug time to clear before making a more definite diagnosis. Antipsychotic medications, sedatives, and other medications are used to stabilize the client.

Bad Trips (acute anxiety reactions)

The amount of "acid" or other psychedelic, the surroundings, the user's mental state and physical condition all determine the reaction to all arounders. Because of

TABLE 9–2   TREATMENT FOR BAD TRIPS

The Haight-Ashbury Detox Clinic uses the following ARRRT guidelines in dealing with a person experiencing a bad trip:

A   acceptance: first, gain users' trust and confidence;

R   reduction of stimuli: get users to quiet, nonthreatening environments;

R   reassurance: educate users that they are experiencing a bad trip and assure them that they are in a safe place, among safe people, and that they will be all right;

R   rest: assist users to relax using stress reduction techniques which promote a calm state of mind;

T   talk-down: discuss peaceful, nonthreatening subjects with users, avoiding any topic which seems to create more anxiety or a strong reaction.

their effect on the emotional center in the brain, a user is open to the extremes of euphoria and panic. Inexperienced or even experienced users who take too high a dose of LSD or other psychedelics can feel acute anxiety, paranoia, fear over loss of control, delusions of persecution, or feelings of grandeur, leading to dangerous behaviors like bungee jumping without a cord.

"You would all of a sudden look at a clock and say, 'All right, I'll come down now.' And then, the writing would still be on the wall and you'd still be hearing the sounds and you'd go, 'No, I'm not going to come down. I'm never, never going to come down. I'm never going to be sane again. They're going to lock me up.'" Ex-"acid" user

Over the years, the Haight-Ashbury Detox Clinic has developed a set of steps to help detoxify a psychedelic user having a bad trip.

There are two things to remember when using the ARRRT talk-down technique.

• First, if the user seems to be experiencing severe medical, physical, or even emotional reactions which are not responding to the talk-down, medical intervention is needed. Get the person to a hospital or bring in emergency medical personnel experienced in treating that kind of reaction.

• Second, although most psychedelic bad trip reactions are responsive to ARRRT, PCP may cause unexpected and sudden violent or belligerent behavior. Caution must be exercised in approaching a "bum tripper" suspected of being under the influence of PCP.

The best treatment for someone on a bad trip is to talk him or her down in a calm manner without raising one's voice or appearing threatening. Avoid quick movements and let the person move around so there is no feeling of being trapped.

Some of the "rave" club drugs, like MDMA, "ecstasy", GHB, and ketamine, have created addictive behaviors in users which are treated with traditional counseling, education, and self-help groups.

TARGET POPULATIONS

MEN VERSUS WOMEN

Research at the Haight-Ashbury Detox Clinic has discovered that the process of addiction and especially recovery varies dramatically for men and women. Men are often external attributers, blaming negative life events like addiction on things outside their control, whereas women are more often internal attributers, blaming problems on themselves. For example, if a man slips on a banana peel, he might say, "Who's the idiot who left that peel on the ground?" A woman who slips on a banana peel might say, "I should have looked where I was going. Boy, am I clumsy." When this is extended to their views of addiction, men often blame a wide variety of external forces for their dependence on drugs, whereas women often blame themselves for being bad or crazy.

The counseling and intervention used in treatment have focused on early confrontation to break down addicts' denial and make them accept their condition. While appropriate for men, this treatment approach merely reinforces women's guilt and shame and often prevents them from engaging in treatment or has them leave treatment early. Treatment approaches which are more supportive and less confrontive result in better outcomes for women.

Women have been also found to be the primary child care provider in a family, so for a woman to be able to participate in treatment, child care must be provided. Further, it has been found that women lack transportation more often than their male counterparts. Therefore, bus tokens, vans, car pooling, or other means of transportation provided to women clients also result in higher success rates among clients.

YOUTH

Young people often have the perception of invulnerability to drugs and therefore are often in much greater denial about their addiction than adults. Further, studies confirm that young people are much less willing to accept guidance or intervention from adults but are more willing to listen to their peers. Both of these factors call for programs to develop around peer interaction and guidance to other youth. Normal adult programs do not work with young people. Specific youth-directed programs have to be provided.

One of the biggest problems with treating teenagers is that they are present-oriented, that is they have problems recognizing consequences that are not immediate. The idea that a three month flirtation with cocaine will necessitate a lifetime of recovery is beyond their scope. They also seek instant gratification, much more than even adult addicts, and expect rewards from treatment immediately. Youth programs which include reward incentives for accomplishing different phases of treatment result in better long-term outcomes. Part of the reward structure is that they get included in a group that they can feel a part of.

OLDER AMERICANS

Because many older Americans view addiction as a character flaw rather than a disease, they are less likely to seek help for any problematic use of alcohol or other drugs. In addition, signs of addiction are often misinterpreted as part of the aging process or reaction to prescription medications that are common among the elderly. Also, because of less physical resiliency in those over 55, problematic use of alcohol or other drugs occurs at lower dosages than with younger people. The House Select Committee on Aging has reported that about 70% of hospitalized elderly persons show evidence of alcohol-related problems (although they might be in the hospital for some other condition). About 2.5 million older adults are addicted to alcohol, drugs, or both.

At present, there are few treatment programs aimed specifically at older Americans but as the percentage of older Americans grows and as the baby boomers begin to retire, the need will grow. As with other special groups, older Americans with a substance abuse problem seem to do better in groups with others their own age although mixed groups will also work.

Of nine centers set up by NIDA to study addiction, one has been designated specifically to investigate this problem in older Americans. It is located at the University of Florida in Gainesville.

ETHNIC GROUPS

Recognition of cultural variances between groups provides better treatment outcomes. Studies continue to verify that treatment specifically targeted to different ethnic groups promotes continued abstinence better than general treatment programs. Cultural competency and culturally consistent treatment are now key components of successful programming. It is imperative to note that culture includes a diverse constellation of vital elements: customs, values, rituals, norms, religious beliefs, and ideals. You can't just base a culture upon the color of the skin or general area of the world. Thus, the more specific the program is, the more effective it will be.

African American

The following ideas as to the differences in the treatment/intervention needs of inner-city, African American substance abusers are the result of years of experience working with the African American community in San Francisco by members of the Haight-Ashbury Detox Clinic and the Black Extended Family Program at Glide Memorial Church.

Higher Pain Threshold. Historically, African Americans have developed a high pain threshold to help them survive in a harsh and painful environment. Unfortunately, this greater tolerance for suffering

delays a cry for help, leading to more severe addiction and other life problems before entering treatment.

One solution to lowering the pain threshold and getting addicts to treatment sooner is educating the African American community to the true impact of drugs.

- In some urban areas, an alarmingly high incidence of African American babies are born drug affected.

- African American teenagers have a greater chance of dying from "crack"-related crimes than they do from being hit by a car.

- There are more African American men in their 20s who are in jail from drug-related offenses than are in college.

- Since African American women are using "crack" at a greater rate than other drugs except alcohol, the family structure is dissolving at an alarming rate.

- Many neighborhoods with a high African American population have an alarmingly high infant mortality rate due to drug use by pregnant women who abuse or are addicted to substances like "crack" and heroin.

Drugs as an Economic Resource. Few economic windfalls are available to inner-city African American communities. Reducing drug dealing here means a loss of income to many families. This is in contrast to the European American community where drug/alcohol abuse usually drains the finances of families.

The true economics of the process need to be taught. For example, once the dealer becomes a user, the economic drains start. Other members of the community are devastated and become dysfunctional; crime is brought to their own backyard.

"Most African Americans come into recovery by way of the criminal justice system,

very late in the whole process of addiction, and we are compelled to come to programs like Glide or Haight-Ashbury by the courts. So you have a whole different attitude from a person who has hit rock bottom and has decided they've got to seek help. The kids are more concerned about just finishing their term and finishing whatever sentence they have and getting out. They don't want to deal with counselors. They don't want to deal with advice. So what you've got is a chance, at that point, to try to hook them into some kind of system that allows them to get back into the society with a greater chance of success." Youth drug counselor

Crime Leads to Chemical Dependency. Most often, crime is the first entry into the chemical dependency subculture rather than drug use itself as with the European American community. Often, in the African American community the pattern is to make sales first and then sample the wares.

Strong Sense of Boundaries. Intervention is viewed as an inappropriate imposition or violation of one's space. There is resistance from within the community to approaching someone with a chemical dependency problem because that would violate the person's boundaries or turf but not approaching someone also perpetuates denial.

These problems are the most difficult to address. They need a major attitudinal change, i.e., is it better to respect one's turf or to attempt interventions and try to do something about the problem?

Chemical Dependency: Primary or Secondary Problem. Chemical dependency is most often viewed in the African American community as a secondary problem and not a primary one. Minority

communities often cite underemployment, poor housing, and lack of social/recreational resources as the primary problems instead of chemical dependency. This perpetuates denial and prevents many addicts from getting into treatment early. Drug users must understand that no other issues can be tackled successfully without tackling recovery first. The community needs to accept chemical dependency as a primary problem.

"Recovery is a lifetime process. That's a very difficult thing for African Americans to focus on. We're sprinters. We're real good at the 50-yard dash and the 100-yard dash, and we have a feeling that, 'Okay, it's a drug problem. Once I stop using and I put it behind me, I can forget it and go about my business.' But no. Coming up with systems and reinforcing as we do during the day and during the week that recovery is a lifetime process, you have to think more in terms of being a marathoner."
Rafiq Bilal, former director, Black Extended Family Program

Conspiracy Theory. The belief that "the rapid spread of 'crack' (and AIDS) into the African American community is deliberate genocide" is very widely held in the African American community. Given the history of slavery, segregation, and de facto segregation, it is understandable. Whether or not the conspiracy theory is true, addiction is a disease that must be treated in the individual as well as in society as a whole.

Revelations. In the African American community, organized spirituality has been found to be a key to promoting recovery. Treatment programs based in church settings have been shown to be more effective.

"The African American community is very spiritually oriented whether from involve-

ment with the church or from historical as-
sociations. Most interesting is a recovery
pattern of consecutive periods of clean
time/relapse, clean time/relapse, until a
revelation or 'snapping' occurs which results
in a continuous, sustained recovery effort.
This is different from the more classic, 'ex-
panding periods of sobriety, leading towards
more sustained, long-term recovery.'"
Rafiq Bilal, former director, Black Extended Family
Program

The Black Extended Family Program
under the guidance of Reverend Cecil
Williams uses the concept and emotional
force of the extended family to help keep
people in treatment and give them an alternative to the lonely life of the addict.
This concept reestablishes the family, spirituality, and self-worth, qualities that have
been weakened by drug use.

Hispanic

With Hispanics, it is important to understand the cultural diversity and the differences between groups as well as the similarities.

The most common similarities are

- Spanish language;
- Catholic background;
- Indian or African traits;
- Iberian heritage;
- strong family structure.

The differences are

- number of years or generations they
  have lived in the United States;
- country of origin; the three most
  prevalent being Mexico, Puerto Rico,
  and Cuba;
- level of education;
- economic status: are they Mexican mi-
  grant workers who immigrate to sur-

vive poverty and help their family back
home, are they upper-class Mexicans or
Costa Ricans looking to protect their
wealth, are they middle- and upper-
class Cubans who fled Castro a generation ago and have become a driving
force in the Florida economy, or are
they lower- middle- and upper-class
Puerto Ricans (American citizens) who
have moved to the East Coast to find a
better life for their families?

After addressing any emergency physical or mental health needs, the first thing a
treatment facility has to determine is the
level of acculturation of any Hispanic
clients coming in for treatment. For example, how well do they speak English, are
they newly arrived immigrants, how integrated are they in the predominantly Anglo
society, are they first, second or third generation Hispanics who have stayed aware of
their cultural heritage and kept contact
with relatives and friends at home, or are
they caught between two cultures without
a solid home base?

In New York, the rapid influx of Puerto
Ricans in the 1950s, '60s, and '70s often
caused a fragmentation of the extended
family system, a polarization between generations, a loss of many aspects of the
Puerto Rican culture, and an identity crisis.
These stressors, along with language differences, were found responsible (in a New
York State survey) for increases in substance abuse. With Cuban Americans,
however, the rapid integration into
American society has resulted in a level of
drug use about half that of the Mexican
American and Puerto Rican communities.

What this means in terms of treatment
is that programs have to be flexible, have a
diverse staff that has a preponderance of
Spanish-speaking and/or bilingual and bicultural counselors and administrators, and
be willing to treat the whole family since the
family is so important in Hispanic cultures.
Because Hispanic American families have

excellent networking systems, these systems can be used extensively in the treatment process. In addition, the treatment facility should be aware of the roles that each member in the family plays. This is in contrast to many Anglo families where the roles of each member can be quite variable.

The core aspects of Hispanic cultures are *dignidad, respeto, y carino*—dignity, respect, and love. Even the concept of urine testing can be a touchy subject because the request for a urine test implies a lack of trust. Another aspect is the strong role spirituality plays in Hispanic culture. In addition to a Catholic heritage, many Hispanic cultures have nonorthodox religious beliefs, such as Spiritism, Santeria, Brujeria, and Curanderism. Pentecostal and Jehovah's Witness churches are also strong in Hispanic communities.

"Some of the recent Mexican immigrants I've worked with who have an alcohol problem didn't start drinking heavily until they came to this country at the age of 25 or 30. At home, they had to care for their family and had little money. Here, they are separated from their families and have more money and so the use of alcohol and other drugs escalates. The other thing I've found is that even if an Hispanic client speaks perfect English, the fact that I'm bilingual and bicultural increases participation in treatment."

Hispanic specialist drug counselor from Washington state

Asian American

With Asian Americans, as with Hispanics, there is a wide variety of cultures.

The differences include

- a variety of distinct and separate ethnic groups, like Japanese, Filipino, Cambodian, Indian, and Samoan;

- a variety of languages, such as Korean, Chinese, Tagalog, and hundreds more;

- a variety of religions, from Buddhism and Hinduism to Animism, Islam, and Christianity;

- a variety of strong cultural characteristics based on thousands of years of history;

- a great variety of cultures even within immigrants from the same country, e.g., Cantonese, Shanghaiese, and Taiwanese;

- different levels of acculturation depending on the number of generations they have been in the United States. For example, many Chinese Americans and Japanese Americans stretch back four or five generations while the newer immigrants, such as Laotians, Viet Namese, Koreans, and Thai, go back only one or two generations.

The similarities are

- they have a strong regard for family;

- they generally have a high respect for education;

- they are less demonstrative or open in their communication about personal issues;

- they are more reserved about expressing accomplishments because they feel this would be a form of arrogant boasting;

- they are reluctant to discuss health issues or death because they superstitiously believe that it would make those situations occur.

These and other cultural and social values and traits affect treatment outcome.

Asian Americans respond more to credentialed professionals than to peer counselors and prefer individual counseling to group counseling. They rely more on their own responsibility to handle their addiction rather than a higher power or external control. They also feel that if they were to

*Educational material and promotion
of a clinic's programs have to be
directed at specific communities.*

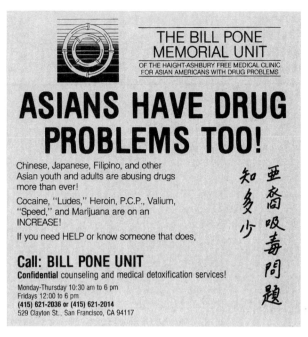

THE BILL PONE
MEMORIAL UNIT
OF THE HAIGHT-ASHBURY FREE MEDICAL CLINIC
FOR ASIAN AMERICANS WITH DRUG PROBLEMS

ASIANS HAVE DRUG PROBLEMS TOO!

Chinese, Japanese, Filipino, and other
Asian youth and adults are abusing drugs
more than ever!

Cocaine, "Ludes," Heroin, P.C.P., Valium,
"Speed," and Marijuana are on an
INCREASE!

If you need HELP or know someone that does,

Call: BILL PONE UNIT

Confidential counseling and medical detoxification services!

Monday-Thursday 10:30 am to 6 pm
Fridays 12:00 to 6 pm
(415) 621-2036 or (415) 621-2014
529 Clayton St., San Francisco, CA 94117

亞裔吸毒問題
知多少

complain about their issues, they would be imposing on others. They feel that individual honor and saving face are important issues and so they are therefore less responsive and will avoid confrontation. They prefer alternative ways of being able to express their feelings, like creative or expressive arts therapy. They require a strong incorporation of family therapy. Finally, they have strongly developed gender roles, so separate male and female groups are more effective than mixed groups.

For Asian Americans, entry into treatment usually occurs late since an admission of addiction is an admission of loss of control. Another problem is that addicts live for the addiction and for themselves rather than for the family and the community as they have been taught. Finally, the sense of family shame often keeps the family enabling and rescuing the addict again and again. On the other hand, their strong sense of family makes for greater compliance with protocols once treatment, which incorporates family therapy, has been started.

Available Programs. Because of the wide variety of Asian American cultures, the historical importance and availability of certain drugs and the wide geographic distribution in cities and states of various groups, treatment personnel must do surveys of their neighborhoods to make treatment relevant. For example, the utilization of treatment services by Asian Americans in San Francisco was extremely low in the 1980s. This was misinterpreted to mean that Asian Americans had fewer drug problems than other ethnic groups.

Community reports however found as high an incidence of drug abuse in the Asian community as in other ethnic groups, the difference being that the Asian American's drugs of choice were sedatives, particularly street Quaaludes® and Soma® (sedating muscle relaxant) which weren't focused on in most treatment programs. When the Haight-Ashbury Detox Clinic developed a specific Asian American program incorporating family therapy, treatment of sedative abuse, and personnel who were bicultural and bilingual, it resulted in a dramatic increase of Asian Americans coming into treatment at a level consistent with their overall population in the city.

Programs for Asian Americans must involve the family in any treatment or the chances of success are greatly lowered. In addition, cultural connections must be recognized and utilized to make the treatment relevant.

Native American

Native American groups have a wide variety of cultural traditions. For example, the five tribes of eastern Oklahoma who are literate, complex, and successful, have low rates of alcoholism. This is in comparison to some western mountain tribes who, in one study, were found to have a rate of alcoholism seven times the national average. In addition, drugs with an historical context, such as tobacco and peyote, are used more often in ceremonies than as recreational drugs, so the introduction of different drugs, particularly alcohol and inhalants, with no cultural tradition of restricted use, has caused numerous problems.

Bicultural and bilingual treatment personnel greatly increase the chances of successful treatment. Many tribes incorporate cultural traditions in healing, including talking circles, purification ceremonies, sweat lodges, meditative practices, shamanistic ceremonies, and even community "sings."

Detoxification centers, halfway houses, outpatient programs, and hospital units have been funded by the Indian Health Service and certain state and county governments. However, over 60% of Native Americans live away from traditional communities in multi-ethnic urban areas, so treatment centers in those locales should have the same diversity of bilingual and bicultural personnel for Native Americans as they do for other ethnic and cultural groups.

Talking circles have been used for hundreds of years in various Native American tribes as a way to solve problems and heal members of the tribe. The process is similar to peer groups, though instead of round robin talking with no interruptions there is cross talk and questions. The sessions usually last for two or three hours, though they can be much longer.

"On reservations, you get locked into a community where you don't grow and there is a minimum of interaction with other groups. There is virtually no middle class. You have a group whose members are highly religious who do not drink at all, you have a few who work for the Bureau of Indian Affairs or in limited industry and drink sparingly, and you have another group that lives to drink and drinks to live. There's not enough work, nothing to do, and often nothing to look forward to for many in this group. You're just another Indian and you're not to be trusted. You have to want to be more than just another drunken Indian.

We have to be proud of who we are before we can reach recovery. In the Native American community, the family is very tight. Everyone is your cousin or aunt or uncle. A sense of pride in your people is part of the core of spirituality that helps us survive. As part of this, we've always looked to elders for guidance. The elders would talk to you about your drinking (a form of intervention) to get you to make changes in your life. The elders have a variety of approaches. They might even do a tough love approach and tell alcoholics to leave the reservation, finish their drinking, and come back when they are sober, or they might tell them to get honest with themselves and make a sobri-

ety pledge to the medicine man or in a pipe ceremony.

We have a variety of tribes that I deal with here in Montana, such as Sioux, Northern Cheyenne, Blackfoot, and Crow. Each one has its own traditions. Unfortunately, a number of clinic directors on reservations who are brought in from the outside have trouble understanding the traditions, so they rely more on standard psychosocial therapy which is not as effective and breeds distrust. Adding to this is the fact that, for many Native Americans, hitting bottom is not as big a trigger for self-referral into treatment as it is in the Anglo community. Often, they are not aware of what bottom is. It takes intervention or court mandate to make changes. On the other hand, once they get recovery, they are much less likely to let go. I tell them that alcoholism is like the raven that has stolen your shadow. If your shadow is gone, your spirituality is gone. Be proud of who you are."

Bob Clarkson, Native American drug and alcohol counselor

Great Spirit, grant me the serenity of a dove to accept the things I cannot change, the courage of an eagle to change the things I can, and the wisdom of an owl to know the difference.

(Native American version of the Serenity Prayer used in Alcoholics Anonymous)

OTHERS

There are numerous groupings of Americans who require targeted treatment. Whether they are substance abusers who have physical disabilities, gays or lesbians, homeless, mentally challenged, elderly, or a dozen other groupings, the key seems to be involvement with peer groups who have experienced the life style, the problems, the prejudice, the homophobia, the shunning, the joys, the problems with self-esteem or relationships and can speak and help based on personal experience.

The common point that needs to be recognized is that addiction is addiction. To imagine that problems with addictive behavior would disappear if only some other conditions or problems were taken care of is a sure path to continued addictive behavior. On the other hand, the other problems, such as racism and mental instability, have to be addressed and treated at the same time because many of the roots of compulsive use lie in a subconscious effort to avoid or cope with the pain experienced in these conditions or life styles.

For example, Americans with disabilities represent a much neglected group of chemically dependent people. Despite passage of the Americans With Disabilities Act, most programs remain inaccessible to many with mobility impairment, visual impairment, and hearing impairment. That fact, plus other ways in which we deal with disabled persons in this country, promotes the concept of learned helplessness and dependency on others and on drugs. People with physical handicaps can develop a dependency which promotes greater denial in the recovery process.

TREATMENT OBSTACLES

Denial and lack of financial or treatment resources have always comprised the biggest obstacles to addiction treatment. But, as the treatment of addictive disease continues to evolve, other significant obstacles are being identified which require intervention for successful treatment outcomes.

DEVELOPMENT ARREST

The use of psychoactive drugs can delay users' emotional development and keep them from learning how to deal with life's problems. In terms of treatment, the counselors or other professionals have to be aware of the level of development in the individual. They have to be aware of how much of what they or others are teaching is being understood by the client. If a client is not fully detoxified or is not given time to start functioning normally, even the most sophisticated treatment can fall on deaf ears. More extensive assessment is one way to overcome these problems.

FOLLOW-THROUGH
(monitoring)

Nothing is more indicative of poor treatment outcome than early program dropout or lack of compliance to the treatment protocol. Ironically, client confidentiality, which is so vital to the addiction treatment process, has contributed to the problem of poor treatment compliance. Clients who have not or will not release information about their treatment progress can be noncompliant to protocols without the awareness of families, employers, or others until more destruction has resulted from their resumed addiction.

Professional licensing boards (medical, nursing, legal) now mandate release of confidentiality as a condition of retaining a license when addicts who are professionals are delivered to treatment after their addiction has been discovered. This practice, though assuring better program compliance, created another obstacle for the treatment professional. How could a therapist engage addicts into deep and sensitive issues about their addiction without being viewed as an extension of the licensing board, the family, or law enforcement? To address this obstacle, some licensing boards and employee assistance programs now employ a program monitor who oversees the progress of an addict in treatment to assure compliance to program protocols.

CONFLICTING GOALS

An individual addict's treatment goal may conflict with a program's goal. Some addicts may enter treatment merely to be able to better manage their abuse of drugs or to qualify for certain social benefits. Most treatment programs insist on an immediate commitment from their clients to a drug-free life style. This difference between goals leads to a poor treatment outcome.

Program goals may conflict with society's goals for treating addicts. Programs naturally focus on the care of their clients, using interventions which they hope will lead their clients to the best possible life outcome. Society is more interested in supporting programs which decrease the social costs of addiction (e.g. crime, health costs, accidents, and violence).

The problems of conflicting goals are best managed by development of clear program objectives and goals and better assessment and matching of clients to programs. Although these concepts seem straightforward and easy to practice, only now is investment in these two areas beginning to occur.

TREATMENT RESOURCES

The biggest obstacle continues to be lack of treatment resources. On a national basis, individuals who apply for treatment are put on a waiting list of 2 weeks to 3 months or longer before they can get into treatment. Studies have shown that for every 100 people put on waiting list, 66% will never make it into treatment. Over the past 30 years, the Haight-Ashbury Detox Clinic has found that of those put on their waiting list, 80% never access treatment. What happens to those potential clients is a matter of deep concern. Many die from drugs or from suicide while waiting for treatment. Most become more heavily involved in drugs and a high proportion end up in the criminal justice system. Since treatment has been shown to be very effective, it is a national tragedy that we continue to have long protracted waiting periods for clients wanting to access treatment.

CHAPTER SUMMARY

Introduction

1. The most prevalent mental disorder is addiction. Annually, it causes over 1/2 million deaths and intense social disruption.

Treatment Effectiveness

2. Treatment is effective. It has a 50% success rate.

3. Each dollar spent on treatment saves at least $7 to $20 in costs related to unchecked addiction.

4. Prison costs up to $40,000 per inmate a year compared to $2,000 to $4,000 for outpatient treatment or methadone maintenance.

5. Almost 2/3 of arrestees test positive for illicit psychoactive drugs, particularly cocaine and marijuana.

Broad Range of Techniques

6. Treatment options include inpatient and outpatient facilities, expensive hospitals, halfway houses, free 12-step groups, drug substitution therapies, and dozens more.

7. It is important to match the treatment program to the client's personality, problems, and background.

Beginning Treatment

8. Breaking through denial is the crucial first step to begin treatment.

9. Denial can be overcome by the addict hitting bottom or through a direct intervention (e.g., legal system, family, workplace supervisor, physician).

10. The elements of a formal intervention are love, a facilitator, intervention statements, anticipated defenses and outcomes, the intervention itself, and contingency plans.

Treatment Goals

11. The two key treatment goals are motivation towards abstinence and creating a drug-free life style. The supporting goals have to do with actually creating that better life style.

Selection of a Program

12. Diagnosis is crucial in directing the client to the best treatment program.

13. There are many diagnostic tests that are used, the most extensive being the 180-item Addiction Severity Index (ASI) test.

14. The principal programs are hospital detoxification programs, social-model detoxification programs, therapeutic communities, halfway houses, sober-living or transitional-living programs, partial hospitalization and day hospitals, and harm reduction programs.

Treatment Continuum

15. Treatment starts with detoxification and escalates through initial abstinence, long-term abstinence, and recovery.

DETOXIFICATION

16. Drugs can be cleared from the system through abstinence, medication therapy, and psychosocial therapy.

17. Detoxification medications include clonidine, phenobarbital, methadone, antipsychotics, and others.

INITIAL ABSTINENCE

18. This phase is supported through anticraving medications (e.g., naltrexone, bromocryptine, and nicotine replacements), individual counseling, and group therapy.

19. Environmental triggers cause relapse. Cue extinction or desensitization is one way to avoid relapse.

LONG-TERM ABSTINENCE

20. Addicts must accept that treatment for addiction is a lifelong process and that chemical dependency extends to a variety of substances not just the drug of choice.

21. Long-term abstinence uses individual and group therapy and 12-step groups to prolong abstinence.

RECOVERY

22. Recovery entails restructuring one's life not just staying abstinent.

23. Follow-up is important not just to satisfy government funding agencies but to know which programs work.

24. Follow-up helps tailor programs to match the client and identify clients who need to be treated again for a relapse.

Individual Versus Group Therapy

25. Individual therapy, conducted by a trained counselor, helps the recovering client address specific issues.

26. Group therapy can be facilitated, peer, 12-step, educational, topic-specific, or targeted.

27. Various 12-step groups, such as Alcoholics Anonymous, Narcotics Anonymous, and Overeaters Anonymous, use sponsors, spirituality, and the power of people telling their own stories to teach a clean and sober life style.

Treatment and the Family

28. Addiction affects the whole family, so good treatment should involve the whole family.

29. Groups such as Al-Anon, Nar-Anon and ACoA help support and educate the family and friends of alcoholics and addicts.

30. Codependency and enabling, whereby family members support the addict in his or her addiction, must be addressed in treatment.

31. Adults who were raised in addictive households carry many of their problems into adulthood and must face those problems in treatment.

Drug-Specific Treatment

32. Most people coming in for treatment are polydrug abusers even though they have a drug of choice.

33. Stimulant detoxification often initially presents treatment professionals with symptoms of psychosis and paranoia.

34. Anticraving medications and therapy help overcome anergia, euthymia, anhedonia, and craving.

35. Because smoking addiction involves nicotine craving, nicotine replacement therapies help taper tobacco craving.

36. Heroin and other opioid treatments usually need medications for withdrawal during detoxification.

37. Methadone maintenance is a harm reduction therapy that replaces a controlled opioid for an illicit, problem-causing street opioid.

38. Alcohol or sedative-hypnotic withdrawal can be life-threatening unless assisted with medical therapy which includes antiseizure medication like phenobarbital.

39. Talk-downs with emotional support and time for the drug to leave the body are the usual treatments for bad trips due to LSD or other psychedelics. Antipsychotic or antianxiety medications are also used when needed.

Target Populations

40. Treatment must be tailored to specific groups based on gender, sexual orientation, age, ethnic group, job, and even economic status.

41. Treatment for men should be different than for women. Men often blame external forces and women often blame themselves for their addiction.

42. Treatment for different ethnic groups requires bilingual and/or bicultural counselors, culture-specific treatment protocols, and acceptance of addiction as a disease.

43. African American, Hispanic American, Asian American, and Native American treatment often requires strong family involvement and accessing the spiritual roots of each community.

Treatment Obstacles

44. The major obstacles to effective treatment are developmental arrest, lack of cognition, conflicting goals, poor follow through, and lack of facilities.

Mental/Emotional Health and Drugs

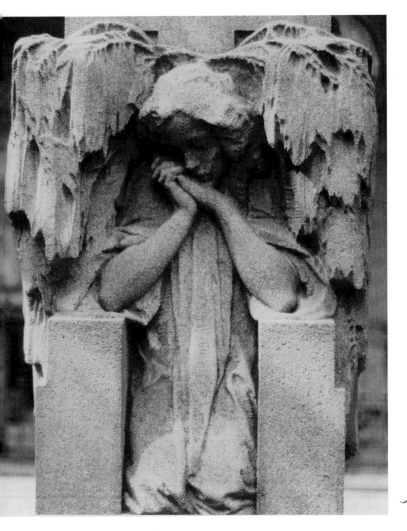

MENTAL HEALTH AND DRUGS

- **Brain Chemistry:** The neurotransmitters and other brain mechanisms involved in mental and emotional problems are the same ones affected by psychoactive drugs.

- **Epidemiology:** There is a high incidence of mental imbalances among drug users and many people with mental/emotional problems use drugs, often to self-medicate themselves.

- **Determining Factors:** Heredity, environment, and psychoactive drugs affect mental health in much the same way they affect drug use and addiction.

DUAL DIAGNOSIS OR THE MENTALLY ILL CHEMICAL ABUSER (MICA)

- **Definition:** The number of individuals suffering from both a substance abuse problem and a mental illness is growing. The decrease in inpatient mental facilities has magnified this problem.

- **Patterns of Dual Diagnosis:** A mental illness can be preexisting, potential, or drug induced (temporary or permanent). Drug use can aggravate mental illnesses or hide them.

- **Making the Diagnosis:** Because the direct effects as well as the withdrawal effects of drugs can mimic mental illnesses, initial diagnoses have to be tentative.

- **Mental Health (MH) Versus Chemical Dependency (CD):** The previous distrust between these two communities is giving way to cooperation and recognition of the relationship between drug use and mental illness.

- **Psychiatric Disorders:** Major depression, schizophrenia, bipolar disorder (manic-depression), along with anxiety disorders including personality disorders, are major psychiatric problems linked with drug use.

- **Treatment:** Drug abuse and mental illness have to be treated simultaneously or treatment will not be effective. Treatment can include individual therapy, group therapy, self-help groups, psychiatric medications, and a variety of facilities from outpatient to live-in.

- **Psychiatric Medications:** Antidepressants, antipsychotics, bipolar disorder medications, and antianxiety drugs are the principal drugs used to control mental illnesses.

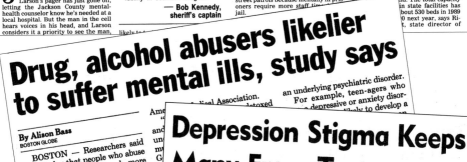

Jail's mentally ill inmates increase

By TOM HILL
of the Mail Tribune

John Larson has only a few minutes to visit with the man in solitary confinement.

Larson's pager has just gone off, letting the Jackson County mental-health counselor know he's needed at a local hospital. But the man in the cell hears voices in his head, and Larson considers it a priority to see the man, likely to...

"The Jackson County Jail is now the largest mental health facility in southern Oregon."
— Bob Kennedy, sheriff's captain

"The Jackson County Jail is now the largest mental health facility in southern Oregon," Sheriff's Capt. Bob Kennedy says.

He says the problem has the potential to take one or more deputies off street patrols because mentally ill prisoners require more staff... jail.

prisoners at a time, Kennedy says. Today, such prisoners consistently make up 20 percent of the jail's population — about 40 prisoners, he says.

Officials say cutbacks in state beds for mental patients is one of the main... nd. The total capacity in state facilities has bout 530 beds in 1989 0 next year, says Ri..., state director of

Drug, alcohol abusers likelier to suffer mental ills, study says

By Alison Bass
BOSTON GLOBE

BOSTON — Researchers said Wednesday that people who abuse alcohol or drugs are much more likely than nonabusers to suffer from pre-existing mental disorders, such as manic-depression, anxiety and schizophrenia.

...ical Association.
...toxed

an underlying psychiatric disorder. For example, teen-agers who ...depressive or anxiety disor-...ikely to develop a

Depression Stigma Keeps Many From Treatment

Sufferers urged not to blame themselves

By Clarence Johnson
Chronicle Staff Writer

Although millions of Americans have suffered from depression, most are reluctant to seek treatment, primarily because the disease is widely perceived to be a personal flaw rather than a health problem, according to two surveys released yesterday.

and dangerous moods of melancholy, the survey said.

In San Francisco, more than four out of 10 adults reported that they have suffered from depression during the Christmas season. However, 44 percent said they know little or nothing about the

---

MENTAL HEALTH AND DRUGS

BRAIN CHEMISTRY

"I didn't think that I was a mentally ill person. I thought, 'Well, I'm a drug addict and I'm an alcoholic and if I don't drink and I don't use, then it should just be a simple matter of just changing my entire life and I felt a little bit overwhelmed."
35-year-old man with major depression

The interconnections between mental/emotional health, drug use, and drug addiction are so pervasive that understanding these links gives us valuable insights into the functioning of the human mind at all levels. The reason for the links is that the neurotransmitters affected by psychoactive drugs are the same ones that are unbalanced by mental illness. Many people with mental problems are drawn to psychoactive drugs in an effort to rebalance their brain chemistry and control their agitation, depression, or other problems. The opposite is also true. For some people who abuse drugs, their chemistry becomes unbalanced enough to activate a preexisting mental illness, induce a new one, or mimic the symptoms of another.

"I wound up preferring the heroin because I felt relaxed when I would snort it. I felt like I didn't have any troubles. I felt like I had some peace of mind and the drugs that were up, like 'speed' and cocaine, made me feel really anxious."
Recovering drug abuser with major depression

This connection between mental health and drug use can be seen in the similarity between the symptoms of psychiatric disorders and either the direct effects of psychoactive drugs or the withdrawal effects. For example:

- cocaine or amphetamine intoxication mimics mania, anxiety, or paranoid psychosis;

- excessive use of downers, such as heroin, alcohol, or prescription sedative-hypnotics (e.g., Xanax®), mimic the depressed mood, lack of interest in surroundings, and excessive sleep characteristic of a major depression;

- psychedelic drugs, such as mescaline and LSD, mimic the delusional hallucinations associated with a major psychosis;

- cocaine and amphetamine withdrawals resemble a major depression;
- the direct effects of the stronger stimulants, coupled with the exhaustion of withdrawal, mimic a bipolar illness that includes manic delusions and then depression.

Beyond the more severe classifiable mental illnesses, there is also a connection between lesser emotional and mental health problems and drug use. These problems include anxiety, personality disorders, posttraumatic stress syndrome, obsessive-compulsive disorders, and even attention deficit/hyperactivity disorder.

Whenever drug use is involved, some emotional or mental imbalance is often present. Conversely, when a mental or emotional problem is involved, drug use is more likely.

EPIDEMIOLOGY

In a study by the *National Institute of Mental Health*, 37% of alcohol abusers and 53% of other substance abusers had, in addition to their drug problem, at least one serious mental illness, such as schizophrenia, major depression, or bipolar illness (manic-depression). Certain drugs increase the likelihood of mental illness. Three-fourths of cocaine abusers had a diagnosable mental disorder as did half of all compulsive marijuana users. Many were self-medicating their psychiatric disorders with street drugs.

"I believe I had depression all along, even before I started using, and so through alcohol, marijuana, and even heroin, I was treating that depression."   *Dual diagnosis client*

Conversely, 29% of all mentally ill people had a problem with either alcohol or other drugs. The overlap is even greater with certain mental disorders. Sixty-one percent of people with manic-depressive illness and 47% of people with schizophrenia also had a problem with substance abuse. Finally, in prisons, the prevalence of a psychiatric illness with an addictive disorder was a remarkable 81%.

DETERMINING FACTORS

The three main factors that affect the central nervous system's balance and therefore a human being's susceptibility to mental illness and/or addiction are heredity, environment, and psychoactive drugs.

HEREDITY AND MENTAL BALANCE

"Biology gives a newborn infant a couple of key things. It gives the biologically driven human being aspirations. Every human baby, at the time of birth, has built into their genetic program the aspirations of our species—to be touched, and held, and hold others, and to love, and to laugh with others but not to be laughed at. Not every human newborn has the genetic potential to realize that dream."
Bert Pepper, M.D., psychiatrist

How does heredity affect our mental health? Research has already shown a close link between heredity and schizophrenia, manic-depression, depression, and even anxiety. For example, the risk of a child developing schizophrenia is somewhere be-

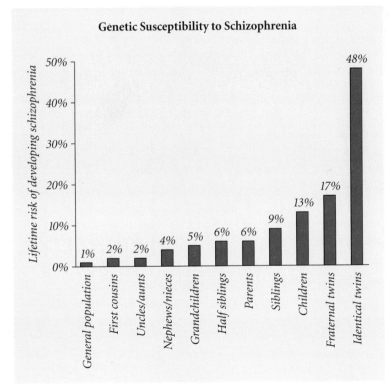

Figure 10-1 •
The risk of developing schizophrenia if a genetic relation has the disease varies with the number of shared genes. Second-degree relatives, such as nieces, only share 25% of one's genes, a parent shares 50% of the genes, and an identical twin shares 100% of the genes.
Adapted from I.I. Gottesman, *Schizophrenia Genesis* (New York: W.H. Freeman and Co., 1991)

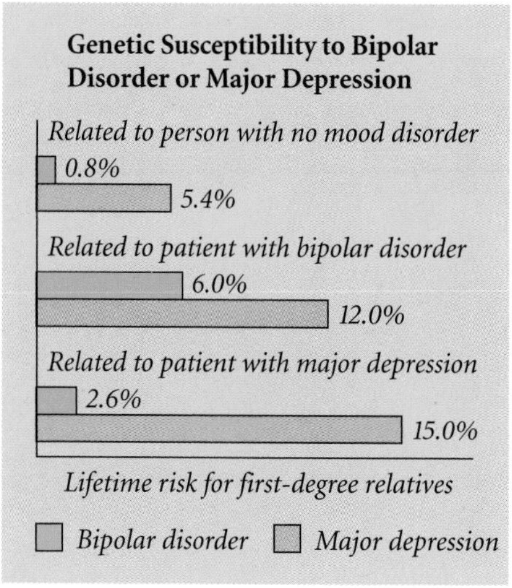

Genetic Susceptibility to Bipolar Disorder or Major Depression

Related to person with no mood disorder
0.8%
5.4%

Related to patient with bipolar disorder
6.0%
12.0%

Related to patient with major depression
2.6%
15.0%

Lifetime risk for first-degree relatives

☐ Bipolar disorder   ☐ Major depression

Figure 10-2 •

Risk of developing depression or bipolar disorder if a 1st-degree relative (parent, sibling, child) has the disease.

Adapted from Goodwin and Jamison, *Manic Depressive Illness.* (New York: W. H. Freeman and Co. 1990)

tween 0.5% to 1% if the child has no close relatives with schizophrenia. On the other hand, if the child has a close relative who has schizophrenia, the risk jumps, on average, to about 15%.

"My great uncle's got schizophrenia and my nephew's got schizophrenia. He's got it really bad because he can't control his fits. I didn't think about that growing up, only when I started hearing the voices. Then I thought, 'Hmm, just like my nephew.'"
28-year-old man with schizophrenia

Some individuals are born with an unstable brain chemistry that gives them a susceptibility to certain mental illnesses. If the inherited unstable brain chemistry is further stressed by a hostile environment or psychoactive drug use, then these people have an even higher likelihood of develop-

ing mental illness. If there is a very high genetic susceptibility, it may not take as severe an environmental stress to trigger a mental illness. If there's a low genetic susceptibility, it will take a much stronger environmental or chemical stress to trigger the illness. Even if there is a high susceptibility with strong environmental stresses, mental illness may still not develop. In fact, the statistics show that even if there is a close relative with major depression, five out of six of those people will not develop that illness.

"In my family, my mom, my aunt, and my grandmother were diagnosed as manic depressive. It runs in the family. It didn't have anything to do with drugs. It was just a lack of something in the brain."
16-year-old boy in treatment for bipolar illness

In addition, genetic links for other compulsive disorders, such as obesity, compulsive gambling, and even attention deficit disorder, have been found in twin surveys. Identical twins raised by two different sets of foster parents often exhibit the same character traits and behaviors regardless of their different environmental development.

It is important to remember that heredity affects susceptibility to drug addiction in much the same pattern that heredity affects susceptibility to mental illness. In other words, a high genetic susceptibility does not mean that mental illness or addiction will occur, only that there is a greater chance that it will occur.

"Both my parents were alcoholics. My brother's an addict and alcoholic. It runs in the family, so I basically followed in my father's footsteps—the drinking, the running around, losing wives, kids, all that."
38-year-old recovering alcoholic with major depression

The relationship between heredity, mental illness, and psychoactive drugs can be seen by examining the connection among the neurotransmitter dopamine, the drug cocaine, and schizophrenia. Heredity affects the formation of dopamine receptor sites and the ability of the brain to produce dopamine. Schizophrenia seems to be caused in part by the brain having too much dopamine. Cocaine stimulates the release of dopamine and long-term use of cocaine can induce a schizophrenic-like psychosis. With both the real psychosis and the drug-induced psychosis, excess dopamine seems to be a key element.

ENVIRONMENT AND MENTAL BALANCE

"My parents had a troubled marriage and they'd fight and argue and my mother would be beaten. I think maybe some of the rage and some of the anger manifested itself into my schizophrenia or just triggered it."
28-year-old man in treatment for schizophrenia

The neurochemistry of persons subject to extreme anxiety can be disrupted and unbalanced to the point that their reactions to normal situations are different than most people's. Such persons may react to stressful situations by running away, falling apart, becoming extremely angry, or using psychoactive drugs. The stressors they respond to don't have to be dramatic. They can merely be normal family expectations. For such individuals, a mother saying, "It's eleven o'clock, I wish you'd get out of bed," can result in extreme anger which further disrupts their balance, their thought processes, and therefore their behavior.

"After my schizophrenia became really prominent, I noticed that little things, like on-the-job stress, would get to me and I'd move on because it would trigger all sorts of problems." 28-year-old client in treatment

Well over 50% of the young adults who are psychotic and have a problem with drugs experienced at least one form of abuse when they were children and the rate is much greater for women than for men. In addition, over 75% of women addicts have suffered incest, molestation, or physical abuse as a child or adult.

"My dad beat my mom when he was under the influence of alcohol. He was an alcoholic. He also beat my older sister and me. When he came home, I was always running and hiding. A few years after he left the family, I was molested. I was screwed up but when I went into the service, I found that the marijuana and the heroin I abused in 'Nam kept my emotions under control." Vietnam veteran

The same environmental factors that can trigger a susceptibility to drug abuse can exaggerate or trigger mental/emotional problems.

PSYCHOACTIVE DRUGS AND MENTAL BALANCE

Along with heredity and environment, psychoactive drugs are the third factor that affects our mental balance. Drugs can deplete, increase, mimic, or otherwise disrupt the neurotransmitters in the brain. This disruption of brain chemistry can lead to drug addiction, mental illness, or both.

If any nervous system receives enough psychoactive drugs, it may eventually develop mental/emotional problems but it is the predisposed brain that is more likely to have prolonged and permanent difficulties.

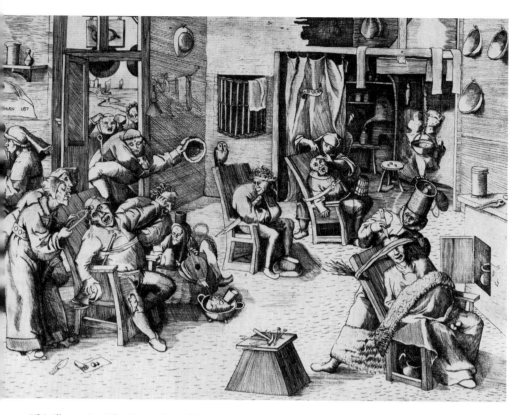

This illustration, The Extraction of the Stone of Madness *by Pieter Bruegal the Elder, a satire of ways to treat mental illness, shows that even 300 years ago, people thought that mental illness was caused by something physical inside the brain. The view of many clinicians today is that mental illness can be treated by changing the neurochemistry inside the brain through psychotropic medications.*
Courtesy of the National Library of Medicine, Bethesda

The brain that is not predisposed is the one most likely to return to its predrug functioning during abstinence.

"Apparently, through three generations of my family and our alcohol drinking or opium smoking, I inherited a tendency to manic-depression that won't awaken under just alcohol abuse. It took a more exotic drug, one that was a little bit beyond the range of a northern European family, to bring out my illness and that was marijuana."
45-year-old client with major depression

Every time a psychoactive substance enters the brain, it changes the brain's equilibrium and the brain has to adjust. When exposure to that drug has ended, the brain does not always return to its original baseline. For example, a brain predisposed to major depression can be pushed into activating that mental problem by heavy abuse of stimulant drugs. A brain predisposed towards schizophrenia can be activated by psychedelic abuse.

DUAL DIAGNOSIS OR THE MENTALLY ILL CHEMICAL ABUSER (MICA)

DEFINITION

A growing number of chemically dependent individuals are under treatment for the condition known as dual diagnosis. This is usually defined as a person having both a substance abuse problem and a diagnosable significant psychiatric problem.

The term dual diagnosis is more common in the chemical dependency treatment community. The term MICA (mentally ill chemical abuser) is preferred in the mental health treatment community. Other terms like comorbidity and "double trouble" have also been used to refer to this condition.

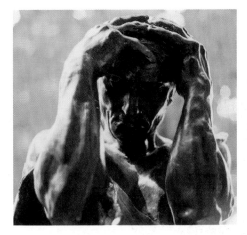

Detail of Burghers of Calais *by Auguste Rodin.*
Photo reprinted, by permission, Simone Garlaund.

"After more than 30 years of use, when I gave up the codeine and the Valium® in treatment, I started to remember the pain. You know, the first thing that flashed through my mind was my uncle's face when he was hurting me real bad when I was 10. I hadn't remembered it for 32 years."
45-year-old woman with major depression

"This previous client is a case where so much is being revealed as she gets clearer and clearer [from the drugs]. She's had major depression at different times and there may be an underlying personality disorder but there is also some posttraumatic shock syndrome in the sense that she is discovering, as she is getting clean and sober, an incest background and severe physical abuse from many persons which she was not even aware of while when she was using. She wasn't just anesthetizing her feelings. She didn't even recognize the beatings as beatings."
Haight-Ashbury Detox Clinic counselor

The psychiatric disorders most often used to define dual diagnosis when found in combination with drug abuse are

- major depression;
- schizophrenia (thought disorder);
- bipolar disorder (manic-depression).

Many treatment professionals also include other mental problems in their definition of dual diagnosis:

- anxiety disorders, e.g., panic disorder, obsessive-compulsive disorder, posttraumatic stress syndrome;
- organic disorders;
- attention deficit/hyperactivity disorder (AD/HD);

- developmental disorders;
- somatoform disorders;
- rage disorders;
- other disorders, such as sexual dysfunction and anorexia.

What this means is that a cocaine user might also be psychotic or paranoid even when not using drugs. An alcoholic might have severe depression which persists even when clean and sober.

"I have this illness, mental illness, with manic-depression and when I take the alcohol, my functioning isn't as clear-cut, not as sharp as say the average person who isn't suffering any mental problems."
52-year-old client with dual diagnosis

It is important to distinguish between having symptoms and having a major psychiatric disorder. Everyone feels blue and sad sometimes. Everyone has the capacity for grief and loneliness but this does not mean that a person is medically depressed, requiring medication or psychiatric treatment. It's really a question of severity and persistence of these symptoms.

PATTERNS OF DUAL DIAGNOSIS

Depending on which drug is used and how it is used, psychoactive substances can be related to four different patterns of dually diagnosed patients.

PREEXISTING MENTAL ILLNESS

One kind of dual diagnosis involves the person who has a clearly defined mental illness and then gets involved in drugs, for example, the teen with major depression who discovers amphetamines.

"My mom asked my little brother if he thought I'd been depressed a lot in my life, and he said I'd been depressed ever since he could remember. The 'speed' got me out of it except when I was coming down."
16-year-old boy

POTENTIAL MENTAL ILLNESS

Another kind of dual diagnosis associated with the use of psychoactive drugs occurs when there might be an underlying psychiatric problem that isn't fully developed as yet. There is no clear-cut depression nor clear-cut schizophrenia before drug use begins. There may be some unusual thought patterns but these are not significant enough to be recognized as a mental illness. When that person starts to use psychoactive drugs, the effects of those substances activate or accelerate the development of the underlying mental disturbance.

"I think it was about six years ago when I had a suspicion of being a manic-depressive but I was so drunk and I really didn't know what was wrong with me. And when I quit using drugs, I just felt horrible, even worse than I had before, like I was dying."
38-year-old client

PERMANENT DRUG-INDUCED MENTAL ILLNESS

The third kind of dual diagnosis happens when there isn't a preexisting problem but when, as a result of years of use or some extreme reaction to the drug, the user develops a chronic psychiatric problem. The toxic effects of the drug permanently imbalance the brain chemistry.

"My initial flip out was in 1986 after snorting 'crank' for six weeks straight, about half

a gram a day. Three weeks later, I had my first manic episode. Later they put me on Haldol® and then lithium. I have three diagnoses: amphetamine psychosis, psychotic-depressive, and manic-depressive."
28-year-old male client

TEMPORARY DRUG-INDUCED MENTAL ILLNESS

There is a fourth condition that is not really dual diagnosis which occurs when the drug itself or withdrawal from the drug causes a transient depression, temporary psychosis, or other apparent mental illness. The imbalance in the brain chemistry with this type of diagnosis is usually temporary and with abstinence, the mental illness will disappear within a few months to a year. This is not true dual diagnosis but only a temporary condition resulting from the toxic emotional effects of the drug.

"This 'speed' run's only been 13 days but I get these sores and I get paranoid and real crazy. After I come down, it'll be weird. It will take weeks to get back into shape. And all that other crap will disappear."
43-year-old heavy methamphetamine IV addict

MAKING THE DIAGNOSIS

ASSESSMENT

When people see a relative or friend acting oddly and having trouble coping with everyday life over a prolonged period, they don't know whether they should ascribe it to relationship problems, troubles at home, drug use, or mental illness. Substance abuse and mental health professionals have the same problem. Thus, when as-

sessing mental illness in a substance abuser, a general rule used by both mental health and substance abuse treatment professionals is that the initial diagnosis should be tentative, or as one psychiatrist said, "The diagnosis should be written in disappearing ink because as the drug clears, the symptoms will change."

"The doctor told me that a person who drank 25 years like me would probably take a year to clear. That was one reason that I never figured out that I was manic-depressive. I didn't notice it. I figured I was depressed because I was drunk all the time."
35-year-old man

The prevalence of dual diagnosis depends on when the diagnosis is made. Since many mental symptoms are a temporary result of drug toxicity or drug withdrawal, an early diagnosis may merely be drug toxicity rather than dual diagnosis. Thus the prudent chemical dependency clinician treats all dangerous symptoms but delays making a psychiatric diagnosis until the drug user has had time to get sober and out of a state of drug intoxication or drug withdrawal.

Other factors that may influence the diagnosis include

- the expertise of the clinician doing the diagnosis;
- the definition of psychiatric disorder that is used;
- the perspective of the assessment team, whether from the mental health or the chemical dependency treatment community;
- the population studied, i.e., the prevalence of dual diagnosis in a homeless drug-abusing population is greater than that seen in a group of school teachers.

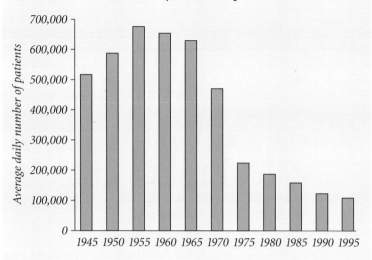

Figure 10-3 •
The psychiatric hospital census has gone down while the overall number of people diagnosed with mental illnesses has gone up.

Reasons for Increased Diagnoses

There are several possible reasons why the numbers of dually diagnosed clients on the streets seem dramatically higher in the 1990s than during the '60s and '70s. These include

- the diminishing number of inpatient mental health facilities due to decreasing mental health budgets;

- a reliance on prescribed medications, such as antidepressants or antipsychotics, so more clients are treated on an outpatient basis;

- an increased reliance, in general, on outpatient mental health facilities.

All these reasons have forced an increasing number of people with psychiatric disorders to deal with their problems on an outpatient basis or on their own. Being detached from hospital supervision, clients are more likely to exhibit poor control of their prescribed medication, thus aggravating their mental problems and making them more likely to turn to street drugs for help. Many people with mental disorders self-medicate with alcohol, heroin, amphetamines, or dozens of other drugs in an attempt to control their symptoms. As a result, the incidence of dual diagnosis among compulsive drugs users and particularly among the homeless remains extremely high.

"I had used heroin to control my depression sort of as a mood stabilizer and so withdrawing from it caused an even worse depression. When I came out of the sort of fog from the first five days of not having it, I felt better but the pink cloud feeling vanished quite quickly and was replaced with the depression that I was used to."
Patient in a halfway house with major depression

The growth of licensed professionals working in the field of chemical dependency treatment has resulted in a greater recognition and documentation of dual diagnosis. Increased abuse of cocaine and amphetamines has also increased the problem of dual diagnosis. A larger number of substance abusers means that more of them will also be dually diagnosed. Also, since stimulants are more toxic to brain chemistry than most substances, those with fragile brain chemistry are more likely to be pushed over the edge into chronic neurochemical imbalance and mental illness.

Finally, managed care and diagnosis-related group (DRG) payment for treatment services usually provide more financial incentives for the treatment of multiple medical and psychiatric problems than for just addiction treatment. This can pressure some clinicians to overdiagnose mentally ill chemical abusers (MICA).

UNDERSTANDING THE DUALLY DIAGNOSED PERSON

Understanding and adapting to the treatment complexities of the client with both a mental health problem and a drug problem are challenges for both drug treatment and mental health professionals.

"When I went into the hospital, I would tell them I had a problem, that I was on Valium® and codeine. The first thing they would then give me was a shot of Valium®. I told them that Valium® addiction was one of my problems. They still gave it to me."
40-year-old dually diagnosed woman

In the past, inability to treat a person who manifested both a drug and a mental problem, combined with an outright refusal to develop treatment strategies for the dually diagnosed client, resulted in inappropriate and potentially dangerous interactions with clients. They were often shuffled aimlessly back and forth between mental health and chemical dependency

systems without receiving adequate treatment. Even though there's been an increase in facilities that address the dually diagnosed client, inappropriate care is all too often still the rule rather than the exception. Budget considerations and lack of expertise have much to do with this problem.

Substance abuse treatment facilities do not usually want these patients because they see them as too disorganized and too disruptive, or in many cases, too inattentive to participate in group therapy which is frequently employed as the core element of treatment. Psychiatric treatment centers also avoid these patients because they're perceived as chemically dependent, disruptive, manipulative, and always relapsing into active substance abuse which interferes with medications used to treat mental illnesses.

MENTAL HEALTH (MH) VERSUS CHEMICAL DEPENDENCY (CD)

The following list contains 11 differences that have existed between the mental health treatment community and the chemical dependency treatment community. While certain differences continue, these two communities are moving toward a closer working relationship. An increasing number of facilities employ both mental health and chemical dependency staff. They offer on-site treatment for the dually diagnosed client or at least provide a cross-referral team approach to a separate mental health treatment provider.

1. Mental health (MH) used to say, "Control the underlying psychiatric problem and then the drug abuse will disappear." Chemical dependency (CD) used to say, "Get the patient

clean and sober and the mental health problems will resolve themselves." While these statements might have been true in many cases, both disciplines are coming to recognize that perhaps 1/3 to 1/2 of their clients are legitimately dually diagnosed and require concurrent treatment of both the addiction and the underlying mental problems.

2. In the MH system, limited recovery from one's problems is more readily acceptable than in CD programs where most professionals believe that lifetime abstinence from all abused drugs, including alcohol and marijuana, along with a supporting program of recovery, is necessary to ongoing recovery.

3. Male dual diagnosis clients are more reluctant to seek help from the MH system than from CD treatment programs. This is probably a result of the involuntary treatment aspects and the stigma of mental illness. Clients and their families hope that the problem is addiction from which they believe they can more fully recover than they can from mental illness. With women, the opposite is often the case. They experience more stigma about being an addict and will admit to an emotional or mental problem more readily than an addiction problem.

"I tell members of my family that I'm in a halfway house for drug addiction as opposed to mental health because it seems with drug addiction, I can get better but with mental health, people see it as a chronic, long-term problem."
19-year-old dually diagnosed male client with major depression

4. MH relies more on medication to help the client function, whereas CD programs tend to be divided between promoting a drug-free philosophy and substituting what they may consider a less damaging drug, such as methadone, in a maintenance program. One of the alternatives to methadone is the opioid antagonist naltrexone. It blocks the action of heroin and other opioids in the brain without producing psychoactive effects, thus providing a potentially viable alternative to drug maintenance. Medically oriented programs, as opposed to drug-free CD programs, will employ drugs to help clients initially detoxify before getting them into a long-term drug-free philosophy.

"I refused to take any psychiatric medication for a long time. I thought you had to be really crazy to take it and I thought that this was a big conflict which would limit my recovery. If I take medication, I'm a drug addict. But I'm glad I'm taking it now. I'm able to sleep and think better."
35-year-old client with major depression

5. MH uses case management, shepherding the client from one service to another, whereas CD programs have traditionally emphasized self-reliance because they do not want to enable clients nor make clients transfer their dependence to the program. In spite of that, case management and an HMO approach to treatment are being adapted in some CD treatment programs. Cooperation may prove successful with each care provider using services available from the other care provider. An addict can be referred to a psychiatrist while a client with depression and an addiction can be encouraged to go to 12-step groups to learn to live without drugs.

6. MH has a supportive philosophy, whereas many CD programs will use confrontation techniques. A major conflict occurs when a patient is not responding to substance abuse treatment and has a severe psychiatric disorder or is HIV infected. One can't use the same threshold of bad behavior to terminate that patient from treatment as one would with a single diagnosis patient. In dual diagnosis programs, CD may put up with more drug-using behavior when a patient also has a psychiatric disorder or HIV infection. It is difficult to medically discharge patients being treated for mental illness or HIV when they relapse into drug addiction.

7. Both the MH system and the CD system have problems with sharing information because of confidentiality laws and regulations. In general however MH shares information with allied fields more readily than CD.

8. In MH, most of the treatment team is composed of professionals: social workers, psychiatrists, psychologists, and licensed counselors. In CD programs, recovering addicts and professionals often work together. (In 1940 in the United States, there were just 9,000 psychiatrists, social workers, and psychologists. Now there are more than 100,000 psychologists, 60,000 psychiatrists, and probably 150,000 social workers, not to mention those in allied mental health professions.) The dual diagnosis clinics are likely to have staff from both disciplines.

9. MH relies heavily on scientific diagnosis and prognosis of an illness and is more process oriented. CD programs rely more heavily on the spiritual side of recovery and are more outcome oriented than process oriented. (Process oriented refers to a set of procedures which are implemented at specific times during the course of treatment to achieve positive benefits for the patient.) Cooperation is evident in recent years as MH has come to more actively utilize spiritual 12-step programs, whereas CD has come to accept the neurochemical and psychiatric roots of addiction.

"All I can tell someone is, 'I have a problem. I don't know which way you're going to deal with it or tackle it but I have a problem and I can't function, and I need help.'"
Dual diagnosis patient with major depression

10. MH pays a lot of attention to the idea of preventing the client from getting worse. In the past, CD programs, taking their cue from early 12-step fellowship beliefs, had more of a tendency to allow people to hit bottom in order to break through the denial of addiction. Most CD programs now see that approach as outmoded and dangerous. They rely more on intervention to break through denial and on diagnosis-driven treatment, using such criteria as those developed by the American Society of Addiction Medicine. The new clinics take both philosophies into account and recognize that both problems have to be treated. In particular, chemical dependency recognizes that relapse is a part of recovery and many centers allow more slips and relapses than they did in the past.

11. In MH, patient education and training are nonstructured and more individualized. In CD programs, they are more standardized, concentrating on information about the drugs themselves, the progression of addiction, and the 12-step process. Presently,

materials from both disciplines are used with the dually diagnosed client since both conditions need to be treated.

While the situation may be improving from the perspective of the MH treatment community, dual diagnosis has represented an almost insurmountable challenge to the clinical expertise of the staff of CD programs, especially to their assessment skills and even their underlying concept of recovery or sobriety. It can be difficult to differentiate an underlying psychiatric illness from a drug-induced mental illness. Often a diagnosis of mental illness is made too early in the treatment or assessment process, resulting in patients being referred to mental health programs which, most often, then reject these individuals because of their drug abuse problems.

CD programs often lack or resist developing the expertise needed to diagnose and treat mental health problems. Fiscal and other limited resource problems prevent the expansion of their services to meet the needs of dually diagnosed clients, creating a tendency to establish mental health problems as exclusionary criteria for treatment admission or continued treatment in many CD programs. Even CD programs with expertise in this area sometimes mistake psychoactive drug reaction symptoms for proof that there is an underlying psychiatric diagnosis.

RECOMMENDATIONS

The dually diagnosed patient must be treated for both disorders and is best treated in a single program when appropriate resources are available. Where programs equipped to handle dual diagnosis cases are not available, CD programs need to establish relationships with MH service providers and vice versa, so that they can work together in providing the client with their combined treatment expertise. Each needs to recognize that mental health and substance abuse treatment are both long-term propositions and therefore they need to establish both short-term and long-range services to address the problems of dual diagnosis.

OTHER DIAGNOSES

Triple Diagnosis

Triple diagnosis is the presence of AIDS or HIV disease in the dually diagnosed client. Persons with AIDS, an AIDS-related condition, an HIV-positive blood test, or persons who are a partner of someone with AIDS require additional treatment expertise and specific services to effectively address their chemical dependency.

As the AIDS epidemic continues to progress out of mainly gay and intravenous drug-using populations and into the cocaine- and other drug-using heterosexual populations, triple diagnosis will strain health department resources and further complicate treatment.

Multiple Diagnoses

As the chemical dependency treatment community becomes more aware of other simultaneous disorders which complicate the treatment of addiction, it must be must willing to accept new challenges such as

- multiple drug (polydrug) addiction;
- chronic pain in the chemically dependent individual;
- other medical disorders, such as epilepsy, cancer, heart and kidney disease, diabetes, sickle cell anemia, and even sexual dysfunction.

In addition, a variety of medical disabilities, such as hearing impairment and mobility impairment, and social concerns, such as cultural attitudes toward chemical dependency and mental health treatment and language barriers, may also provide impediments to successful treatment.

These problems require the development of future drug programs that are holistic, use several modalities, and are multidisciplinary in order to meet the challenge of the evolving complicated clinical needs of the chemically dependent patient.

The following sections will examine the different kinds of psychiatric disorders; discuss the relationship between heredity, environment, and psychoactive drugs as related to treatment of mental illness and drug addiction; then examine the various treatments available for the mentally ill substance-abusing patient, particularly the use of psychotropic medications in therapy.

PSYCHIATRIC DISORDERS

Although there are hundreds of mental illnesses as classified by the mental health community, we will describe the principal ones that are most often associated with dual diagnosis.

PRINCIPAL DUAL DIAGNOSIS DISORDERS

Schizophrenia

Schizophrenia is a thought disorder believed to be mostly inherited. It is characterized by

- hallucinations (false visual, auditory, or tactile sensations and perceptions);
- delusions (false beliefs);

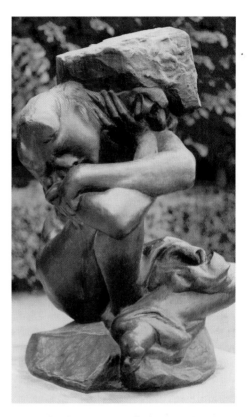

Caryatides *by Auguste Rodin.*
Photo reprinted, by permission, Simone Garlaund.

- an inappropriate affect (an illogical emotional response to any situation);
- autistic symptoms (a pronounced detachment from reality);
- ambivalence (difficulty in making even the simplest decisions);
- poor association (difficulty in connecting thoughts and ideas);
- poor job performance;
- strained social relations;
- an impaired ability to care for oneself.

The signs have to be present for at least six months for the diagnosis to be made.

"I was hearing voices and the voices wouldn't go away and they followed me wherever I went. I got into creating scenarios as to who they were and what they were doing." 28-year-old man with schizophrenia

Schizophrenia usually strikes individuals in their late teens to early adulthood and can be with them for life although occasionally, there's spontaneous remission. Schizophrenia is extremely destructive to those with the illness and to the friends and families around them.

When diagnosing schizophrenia, clinicians try to determine what drugs are being used by the patient. If they don't, they may end up with a false or incomplete diagnosis. Clinicians can accomplish this assessment by taking a thorough medical history or by using urinalysis. Unfortunately, a large percentage of drug or alcohol problems is missed.

Several abused drugs mimic schizophrenia and psychosis, producing symptoms which can be easily misdiagnosed. Cocaine and amphetamines, especially when used to excess, will cause a toxic psychosis that is almost indistinguishable from a true paranoid psychosis. Steroids can also cause a psychosis. Drug-induced paranoia can be indistinguishable from true paranoia. Most drugs, but particularly the stimulant MDMA ("ecstasy"), related stimulant/hallucinogens, and even marijuana, can cause paranoia.

Psychedelics, such as LSD, peyote, and psilocybin, and PCP disassociate users from their surroundings, so all arounder abuse can also be mistaken for a thought disorder. Also, withdrawal from downers can be mistaken for a thought disorder because of extreme agitation. Many of the psychiatric symptoms should disappear as the body's drug levels subside upon treatment and detoxification.

Major Depression

A major depression is likely to be experienced by 1 in 20 Americans during their lifetimes. It is characterized by

- depressed mood;
- diminished interest and diminished pleasure in most activities;
- disturbances of sleep patterns and appetite;
- decreased ability to concentrate;
- feelings of worthlessness;
- suicidal thoughts.

All of these symptoms may persist without any life situation to provoke them. For example, a patient with major depression may win a lot of money in a lottery and respond to it by being melancholy or depressed.

For the diagnosis to be made accurately, these feelings have to occur every day, most of the day, for at least two weeks running. Organic causes, such as an illness or drug abuse, should rule out a diagnosis of major depression as should natural reactions to the death of a loved one, separation, or a strained relationship.

"The depression just came when it wanted to come. I just sat there and thought about something and I got depressed. The anger came because every male that has ever been in my life has beaten me or used me, you know, mentally and physically—not sexually thank goodness." Severely depressed 17-year-old female

The withdrawal symptoms which occur with most stimulant addictions (cocaine or amphetamine) and the comedown or resolution phase of a psychedelic (LSD, "ecstasy") result in temporary drug-induced depression, which is almost indistinguishable from that of major depression.

Bipolar Affective Disorder (formerly called manic-depression)

A bipolar disorder is characterized by alternating periods of depression, normalcy, and mania. The depression phase is described above. The depression is as severe as any depression seen in psychiatry. If untreated, many bipolar patients frequently attempt suicide. The mania, on the other hand, is characterized by

- a persistently elevated, expansive, and irritated mood;
- inflated self-esteem or grandiosity;
- decreased need for sleep;
- increased pressure to keep talking;
- flight of ideas;
- distractibility;
- increase in goal-directed activity or psychomotor agitation;
- excessive involvement in pleasurable activities that have a high potential for painful consequences (e.g., drug abuse, gambling, or inappropriate sexual advances).

These mood disturbances are severe enough to cause marked impairment in job, social activities, and relationships.

"The manic feeling is a real feeling of elation and euphoria. There's that grinding angry sort of—I don't really get angry and violent. Well, I did in jail but I don't really want to hurt anybody or anything. And as far as being depressed goes, I can really say I've only been depressed about three times, once to the point of being suicidal."
30-year-old man with a bipolar affective disorder

Bipolar affective disorder usually begins in a person's 20s and affects men and women equally. Many researchers believe this disease is genetic.

Toxic effects of stimulants or psychedelic abuse will often resemble a bipolar disorder. Users experience swings from mania to depression depending upon the phase of the drug's action, the surroundings, and their own subconscious feelings and beliefs.

OTHER PSYCHIATRIC DISORDERS

Anxiety Disorders

Anxiety disorders are the most common psychiatric disturbances seen in medical offices. They are

1. Panic disorder with and without agoraphobia (fear of open spaces)

   "I'd be waiting for my prescription at a drugstore and someone would just look at me and all of a sudden, my whole body just went inside itself and I started shaking. My heart was racing. I couldn't say anything. I crossed my arms in front of me and I was just in total panic. I couldn't move. All I did was shake inside like I was terrified. And my mind kept saying there's nothing to be scared of but I couldn't control it. I had no idea what really triggered it. My husband would come up and hold me and sit there and say, 'Breathe.' And after a couple of minutes, I would be all right and I would use one of my pills for anxiety, Lorazepam®, a benzodiazepine. I think that my use of cocaine over a period of

several years messed up my neuro-chemistry, particularly my adrenaline system. Then I was always afraid of being someplace where I would have an attack and not be able to get help."
42-year-old woman with a panic disorder

2. Agoraphobia without history of panic disorder—a generalized fear of open spaces

3. Social phobia—fear of being seen by others as acting in a humiliating or embarrassing way, such as eating in public

4. Simple phobia—irrational fear of a specific thing or place

5. Obsessive-compulsive disorder (OCD) —uncontrollable intrusive thoughts and irresistible often distressing actions, such as cutting one's hair or repeated hand washing

"I had a number of obsessions. The obvious one right now is my hair. I cut my hair obsessively in a crewcut, constantly, by my own hand. The thought would just come into my mind. It was something I didn't really have control over. I would smoke marijuana almost as compulsively as I cut my hair."
Client with an obsessive-compulsive disorder

6. Posttraumatic stress disorder—persistent reexperiencing of the full memory of a stressful event outside usual human experience, such as combat, molestation, or a car crash. It is usually triggered by an environmental stimulus, e.g., a car backfires and the combat veteran's mind relives the stress and memory of combat. This disorder can last a lifetime and be very disabling.

"I broke down after about six months over in Vietnam and I was in charge of

a gun crew. And when I broke down from seeing the deaths and all the abuse over there, some people's lives were lost. I'm responsible and it hurts. When I was medically evacuated back to the States, I immediately jumped into alcohol and heroin."*
42-year-old Vietnam veteran with posttraumatic stress syndrome

7. Generalized anxiety disorder—unrealistic worry about several life situations that lasts for six months or more

8. Other anxiety disorders

Sometimes it is extremely difficult to differentiate the anxiety disorders. Many are defined more by symptoms than by specific names. Some of the more common symptoms in anxiety disorders are shortness of breath, muscle tension, restlessness, stomach irritation, sweating, palpitations, restlessness, hypervigilance, difficulty concentrating, and excessive worry. Often, anxiety and depression are mixed together. Some physicians think that many anxiety disorders are really an outgrowth of depression.

Toxic effects of stimulant drugs and withdrawal from opioids, sedatives, and alcohol (downers) also cause symptoms similar to those described in anxiety disorders and can be easily misdiagnosed as such.

Organic Mental Disorders

Organic mental disorders are problems of brain dysfunction brought on by physical changes in the brain caused by aging, miscellaneous diseases, injury to the brain, or psychoactive drug toxicities. Alzheimer's disease is one example of an organic mental disorder. People suffer unusually rapid death of brain cells, resulting in memory loss, confusion, and loss of emotions, so they gradually lose the ability to care for themselves. Mental confusion from heavy marijuana use in an elderly patient can mimic symptoms of this disorder.

Developmental Disorders

Developmental disorders include mental retardation, eating disorders, gender identity disorders, attention deficit disorders, autism, speech disorders, and disruptive behavior disorders. Heavy and frequent use of psychedelics, like LSD or PCP, can be mistaken for developmental disorders.

Somatoform Disorders

Somatoform disorders have physical symptoms without a known or discoverable physical cause and are likely to be psychologically caused, e.g., hypochondria (abnormal anxiety over one's health accompanied by imaginary symptoms of illness). Cocaine, amphetamine, and stimulant psychoses can create a delusion that the user's skin is infested with bugs when no infection exists.

The Passive-Aggressive, Antisocial, and Borderline Personality Disorders

Personality disorders are characterized by inflexible behavioral patterns that lead to substantial distress or functional impairment. Most of these personalities act out, that is, exhibit behavioral patterns that have an angry hostile tone, that violate social conventions, and that result in negative consequences. Anger is intrinsic to all three of these personality disorders, as are chronic feelings of unhappiness and alienation from others, conflicts with authority, and family discord. These disorders frequently coexist with substance abuse and are particularly hard to treat because of relapse to drug use or disruption in treatment.

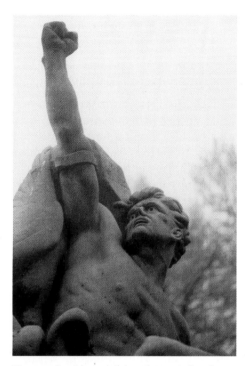

Photo reprinted, by permission, Simone Garlaund.

TREATMENT

The close association of unbalanced brain chemistry with the distorting effects of heredity, environment, and psychoactive drugs suggests that treatment of mental illness and/or addiction should be directed towards rebalancing the brain chemistry.

REBALANCING BRAIN CHEMISTRY

Heredity and Treatment

As yet, we cannot alter a person's genetic code. We can't change a person with alcoholic marker genes that signal a susceptibility to alcoholism, drug addiction, or other addictive behavior. We can't alter a teenager with a mother and grandmother who have schizophrenia. We can only alert some people that they are more at risk for a certain mental illness, drug addiction, or other compulsive behavior.

Environment and Treatment

If we can't correct heredity, we can suggest a change in the environment itself. Also, through external treatment, we can attempt to correct some of the damage done by the environment.

If people change where and how they live, they can avoid those stressors and environmental cues which keep them in a state of turmoil, continually unbalance their neurochemistry, and make them more likely to abuse drugs, thereby intensifying their mental illness. For example, to help restore healthy ways of living, people can leave an abusive relationship, avoid their drug-using associates, get enough sleep, avoid situations that make them angry, seek out new friends in self-help groups to avoid isolation, and make sure they get good nutrition.

Hard as it might be, changing one's external environment is much easier than changing one's brain chemistry through manipulation of thoughts, feelings, or emotions.

Psychotherapy

"Look into the depths of your own soul and learn first to know yourself, then you will understand why this illness was bound to come upon you and perhaps you will thenceforth avoid falling ill."
Sigmund Freud, 1924

Psychoanalysis and psychotherapy, which were originated by Sigmund Freud in the late 1800s, are ways of helping the dually diagnosed patient. They help clients explore their past to enable them to neutralize or minimize the emotional and neurochemical imbalance caused by heredity or the traumas and stresses of childhood, e.g., remembering sexual abuse that happened when they were a young child.

Individual or group therapy can be effective but, by necessity, it has to be a long-term undertaking (even a lifetime project) to be truly effective in changing individuals or at least in minimizing the damage they do to themselves.

"I go to Emotions Anonymous. I go there and it helps because I became a drug addict by not being able to deal with my emotions and my feelings." 25-year-old client

Psychoactive Drugs and Treatment

Finally, psychoactive drugs themselves can be used to treat mental illness. This form of treatment is attempted by both psychiatrists and by patients themselves who may self-medicate their condition with the use of abusable drugs. Of course there are dangers in self-medication. The uncontrolled use of street drugs, such as cocaine or some prescription medications like Ritalin®, can distort one's neurochemistry and thereby magnify or trigger mental problems.

"I took both alcohol and lithium for my manic-depression. The difference is that one is faster working. The alcohol works quickly, the lithium takes time to get there. But the alcohol caused other problems in my life in addition to my depression. I think I'll stick to the lithium." 50-year-old woman

There is an ever expanding group of drugs called psychotropic medications (e.g., antidepressants, antipsychotics or neuroleptics, and antianxiety drugs) that are prescribed by physicians to try to counteract neurochemical imbalance caused by mental illness or addiction. These drugs can help the dually diagnosed client to lead

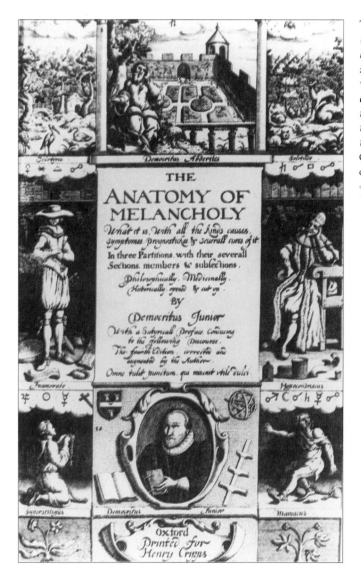

The Anatomy of Melancholy (1660) by Robert Burton is a book about depression which shows that some civilizations were aware of mental illness and wrote about ways to treat it. This book even examines the benefits of confessing grief to a friend.

Courtesy of the National Library of Medicine, Bethesda

a less destructive life. (We will examine the various psychotropic medications in detail later.)

The following Table 10-1 is a review of many of the relationships between brain chemistry, drug addiction, and mental illness. Column 1 lists the neurotransmitters (the brain's messengers), column 2 describes the natural regulatory function of the neurotransmitters, column 3 lists the street drugs that strongly affect those neurotransmitters, column 4 describes the mental illnesses associated with the disrupted neurotransmitters, and column 5 lists drugs used to correct the disruptions.

When studying the table, notice how many different neurotransmitters are affected by a single street drug, especially cocaine or alcohol. Also notice the physical and mental traits that are affected by a neurotransmitter and how a street drug affects those functions.

TABLE 10–1 THE RELATIONSHIP BETWEEN NEUROTRANSMITTERS, THEIR FUNCTIONS, STREET DRUGS, MENTAL ILLNESS, AND PSYCHOTROPIC MEDICATIONS

Neurotransmitter	Some Major Functions	Street Drugs Which Disrupt the Neurotransmitter	Associated Mental Illnesses	Medications Used to Rebalance Neurotransmitter
Serotonin	Mood stability; appetite, sleep control, sexual activity aggression, self-esteem	Alcohol, nicotine, amphetamine, cocaine, PCP, LSD, MDMA ("ecstasy")	Anxiety, depression, bipolar disorder, obsessive-compulsive disorder	BuSpar®, tricyclic antidepressant, lithium, MAO inhibitors, Prozac®, Zoloft®, tryptophan, Ritanserin®, Anafranil®, Paxil®
Dopamine	Muscle tone/control, motor behavior, energy, reward mechanism, attention span, pleasure, emotional stability	Cocaine, nicotine, PCP, amphetamine, caffeine, LSD, marijuana, alcohol, opioids	Schizophrenia, Parkinson's disease	Lithium, MAO inhibitors, phenothiazine antipsychotics, thiazine antipsychotics, tyrosine, taurine
Norepinephrine and epinephrine	Energy, motivation, eating, attention span, pleasure, heart rate, blood pressure, dilation of bronchi, assertiveness, alertness, confidence	Cocaine, nicotine, amphetamine, caffeine, marijuana	Depression, manic-depression, anxiety, narcolepsy, sleep problems, attention deficit/hyperactivity disorder	Tricyclic antidepressants, lithium, MAO inhibitors, phenothiazine, antipsychotics, prescription amphetamines, Ritalin®, clonidine, barbiturates, benzodiazepines, beta blockers (Propranolol®), tyrosine, d,1 phenylalanine
Endorphin enkephalin	Pain control, reward mechanism, stress control (physical and emotional)	Heroin, other opioids, PCP, alcohol, marijuana, anabolic steroids	Schizophrenia, depression	Methadone, LAAM, Trexan®, buprenorphine, d,1 phenyla-lalanine

TABLE 10-1   (Continued)

Neurotransmitter	Some Major Functions	Street Drugs Which Disrupt the Neurotransmitter	Associated Mental Illnesses	Medications Used to Rebalance Neurotransmitter
GABA (gamma amino butyric acid)	Inhibitor of many neuro-transmitters, muscle relax-ant, control of aggression, arousal	Alcohol, marijuana, barbiturates, PCP, benzodiazepines	Anxiety and sleep disorders	Benzodiazepines, glutamine
Acetylcholine	Memory, learning, muscular reflexes, aggression, alertness, blood pressure, heart rate, sexual behavior, mental acuity, sleep, muscle control	Marijuana, nicotine, alcohol, PCP, cocaine, amphetamine, LSD	Alzheimer's disease, schizophrenia, tremors	Phenothiazine antipsychotics, Artane®, Cogentin®, lecithin, choline
Cortisone, corticotrophin	Immune system, healing, stress	Heroin, anabolic steroids, cocaine	Schizophrenia, depression, insomnia, anxiety	Corticosteroids (Prednisone®, cortisone), ACTH
Histamine	Regulator of emotional behavior, sleep, inflammation of tissues, stomach acid, secretion, allergic response	Antihistamines, opioids	Depressive illness	Antihistamines, tricyclic antidepressants

Starting Treatment

With many dually diagnosed clients it is hard to know where to start treatment: the mental illness, the addiction, or both simultaneously right from the beginning.

"I start where the pain is. One patient, for example, couldn't talk about his marijuana use without talking about how depressed and suicidal he was. We addressed the pain, the pain being his massive depression, and then we enabled him, by doing that, to back off his marijuana use. In the case of another patient, she was in such a tormented state in terms of anxiety, panic, fear, and depression behind her use of benzodiazepines and codeine that we had to start detoxing immediately and we had to explain to her that we would be looking at the depression and the anxiety and probably medicating them as we detoxed her off her primary drugs of abuse."
Haight-Ashbury Detox Clinic counselor

A suicidal situation obviously needs to be attended to regardless of the cause. Similarly, if patients are dangerous—homicidal or aggressive in some dangerous fashion—they have to be managed, often in a psychiatric facility. When these presentations are less malignant and less dangerous to self or others, then the treatment facility generally says, "What does it take to manage them?" And the first rule of thumb is that the patient has to be somewhat cooperative and manageable, so detoxification is usually the first step.

Impaired Cognition

Unfortunately, many clinicians involved in treatment believe that once dually diagnosed individuals put down the booze or drugs, they should be able to engage in treatment but that's not always the case. Reviewing screening exams on neurocognitive function at a veteran's hospital, researchers found that approximately 50% of the patients were mildly to severely impaired.

For the treatment provider, what this means is the patient can repeat things but the information and therapy don't sink in. It takes from two weeks to six months after detoxification for reasoning, memory, and thinking to come back to a point where the dually diagnosed individual can begin to engage in treatment. Treatment has to be tailored to the person's ability to process the information that the doctor and staff are providing.

Developmental Arrest

Drug abuse and mental illness often result in a pause in emotional development. Take the case of a young man in his late teens or early 20s who's full grown and intelligent but has been using drugs since the age of 11 or 12 and has also had emotional and mental problems. This type of patient comes to treatment with all kinds of difficulties. One of the worst problems is that he's suffered developmental arrest at age 11 or 12, the point where most people begin to work through issues and stresses in their lives. Most people mature through all the struggles and go on to become adults but those who use drugs, who have avoided difficult emotions, and have not gone through that process of maturation will still experience the emotions that they avoided five or six years ago.

"It's all those issues as a child that I seemed to take into my adulthood and they come out. I'd get my buttons pressed. Someone gets me a little pissed off. You know, I really thought when I came into recovery I would-

n't be angry anymore. Well, it took me almost three years in treatment to realize
that anger is a legitimate feeling. It's how I
deal with it today and how I used to deal
with it. That's what I'm learning about."
30-year-old dually diagnosed client

What happens is that many dually diagnosed clients have the character traits
that are normal in children but abnormal
in adults, thus making treatment extremely
difficult. Dr. Bert Pepper, a psychiatrist who
treats young dually diagnosed clients, lists
11 of these characteristics.

1. They have a low frustration tolerance.
2. They can't work persistently for a goal
   without constant encouragement and
   guidance, partially because of their low
   tolerance for frustration.
3. They lie to avoid punishment.
4. They have mixed feelings about independence and dependence and then,
   feeling hostile about dependency, they
   test limits.
5. They test limits constantly because
   they haven't learned them yet or have
   rejected them.
6. Their feelings are expressed as behaviors. They cry, run away, and hit rather
   than talk, reason, explain, or apologize.
7. They have a shallow labile affect which
   means a shallowness of mood. Give
   kids a toy, they laugh, take it away, they
   cry.
8. They have a fear of being rejected. Extreme rejection sensitivity can even be
   expressed as paranoid schizophrenia.
9. Some live in the present only but most
   of the older teens or young adults live
   in the past. Most dually diagnosed
   clients have no hope for the future,
   possibly because they remember the
   past too well or have troubles thinking.
10. Denial is a common characteristic in
    young children. One form is a refusal
    to deal with unpleasant but necessary
    duties. Another form is an unwilling-
    ness to stop something that's pleasur-
    able, like kids playing roughhouse un-
    til one gets hurt badly.
11. They have the feeling that "Either
    you're for me or against me," a black
    and white approach to every judgment
    in life, with no modulation or moder-
    ation.

These characteristics are also very common in those being treated solely for
chemical dependency.

What these characteristics suggest is
that any treatment program has to be
highly structured. What the client needs to
do is learn all those behaviors, ideas, and
emotions that were not learned in youth or
adolescence because of the drugs, the mental illness, or the turmoil of growing up.

These difficulties are all chronic or even
lifelong problems which cannot be treated
with short-term therapy. These are problems of living, of living sober, and of living
with the symptoms of the mental illness.
The best treatment is inpatient care because it requires a great deal of monitoring
and continuity over a fairly long period of
time. Unfortunately, resources (financial
and professional) for long-term inpatient
care do not usually exist.

PSYCHIATRIC MEDICATIONS

PSYCHOPHARMACOLOGY

The field of medicine that specializes in
the use of medications to help correct or
help control mental illnesses is called psychopharmacology. The scope of this branch

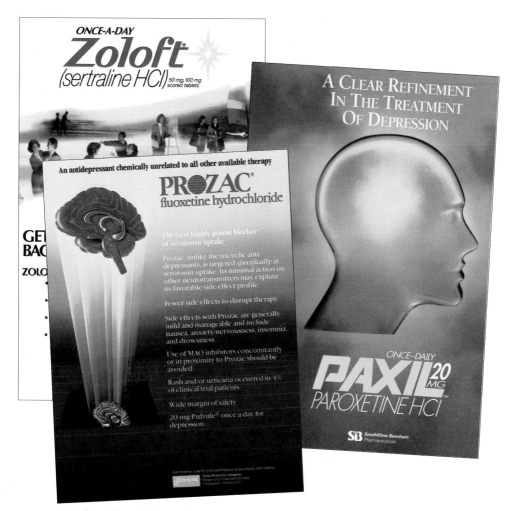

These three ads for antidepressants are for serotonin reuptake inhibitors. Newer ones are being constantly developed.

of medicine has grown rapidly in the last 10 years, producing hundreds of new medications and a new approach to mental illness.

Quite often, the dual diagnosis patient does need medication for the psychiatric disorder: tricyclic antidepressants for endogenous depression, lithium for a bipolar disorder (e.g., manic-depression), and antipsychotic (neuroleptic) medication for a thought disorder. These medications have

to be handled carefully because the individual has difficulty dealing with drugs. The clinician has to make sure the medication used for the psychiatric problem does not aggravate or complicate the substance abuse problem.

Medications are used on a short-term, medium-term, or even lifetime basis to try to rebalance the brain chemistry that has become unbalanced either through hereditary anomalies, environmental stress, and/or the use of psychoactive drugs. These medications are used in conjunction with individual or group therapy and with life style changes.

One of the biggest debates in treatment centers is about the level of medication that should be used. Some clinicians look at psychotropic medications as a last resort. Others feel that they should be the first step in treatment. However, there is no question that judicious use of medications has freed many people suffering from mental illness from a life of misery.

PHARMACOLOGY

The various psychiatric medications currently in use affect the manner in which neurotransmitters work in different ways.

- They (e.g., phenothiazines) can increase or inhibit the release of neurotransmitters and even block the receptor sites.

- They can block the reuptake of neurotransmitters by the sending neuron, thus increasing the amount of neurotransmitters available in the synaptic gap (Prozac® and Zoloft® work this way on serotonin).

- They (Nardil® and MAO inhibitors) can speed up or inhibit the metabolism of neurotransmitters , thereby enhancing the action of adrenaline or dopamine.

- They can enhance the effect of existing neurotransmitters (benzodiazepines, such as Valium®, increase the effects of GABA).

Besides manipulating brain chemistry, some drugs act directly to control symptoms. Drugs such as beta blockers (Propranolol®) calm the sympathetic nervous system which controls heart rate, blood pressure, and other functions which can go out of control in a panic attack or drug withdrawal state. They also calm the brain.

One problem with psychotropic medications is that it's very hard to design a drug that will only work on a certain neurotransmitter in a certain way. There are always side effects and since every patient and every illness are different, constant monitoring of each patient's reaction to the drug and the dosage is an absolute necessity. A careful explanation of the drug and a specific plan of use are necessary.

"The medication that we are talking about giving you in this treatment program is really designed to correct some of the damage that you did to your body and to your mind with the drugs or damage that had been happening as a result of some emotional or psychological problem. It does not mean you're sick, it does not mean you're defective, and it does not mean you're weak. It just means that your biochemistry has somehow gotten out of balance and the medications that we're recommending, especially the antidepressant medications, are to rebalance those chemicals and bring you to a point where you can fully and effectively function and then begin to work on your other problems."

Stanley Yantis, M.D., psychiatrist to a client with dual diagnosis

PSYCHIATRIC MEDICATIONS VERSUS STREET DRUGS

One of the advantages of physician prescribed medications over street drugs is that generally, except for benzodiazepines and stimulants, they are not addicting. But sometimes, prescribing psychiatric medications for clients can cause problems for dually diagnosed clients because they are often taught to stay away from all drugs during recovery.

When using street drugs, patients feel a great deal of control over which drugs they ingest, inject, or otherwise self-administer. The same patients when receiving medication from a doctor say that they are not in control any more of what is being given them. Thus they are more apt to rely on street drugs rather than on psychiatric medications for relief of their emotional problems.

"Before I came to the clinic, I thought that using antidepressants was taboo. I wanted to use street drugs but not any of these clinical ones. There's a stigma to it. I used marijuana to deal with my depression and I could take it when I felt I needed it, not a pill that I had to take every so often as prescribed by my psychiatrist."
35-year-old client with depression and a problem with marijuana

This next section which classifies and discusses the specific drugs is rather technical and may best be used as a reference source.

CLASSIFICATION OF PSYCHIATRIC MEDICATIONS

Some of the major groups of psychotropic medications are tricyclic antidepressants, MAO inhibitors, serotonin reuptake inhibitors, antipsychotics (neuroleptics), anxiolytics (antianxiety drugs), lithium, beta blockers, and sleeping pills.

We will discuss the drugs under the heading of the mental illness that they are generally used to treat (see Table 10-2). There is some overlap, for example, when a drug used for depression, such as Prozac®,

is also used to treat obsessive-compulsive disorder or when an antidepressant is also used for bipolar disorder.

DRUGS TO TREAT DEPRESSION

Many in the psychiatric field feel that depression causes and in turn is caused by an abnormality of the neurotransmitters norepinephrine (adrenaline) and serotonin, plus a few other neurotransmitters. Antidepressants are meant to increase the amount of serotonin or norepinephrine available to the brain to correct this imbalance.

Tricyclic Antidepressants

Tricyclic antidepressants, such as imipramine (Tofranil®) and desipramine (Norpramine®), are thought to block reabsorption of these neurotransmitters by the sending neuron and so increase the activity of those biochemicals. This blocking effect in turn forces the synthesis of more receptor sites for these neurochemicals. The delay in the creation of new receptor sites may account for the lag time in effecting a change in the patient's mood. It usually takes two to six weeks for a patient to respond to the drug.

The tricyclics are very effective on patients with chronic symptoms of depression. People without depression do not get a lift from tricyclic antidepressants as they do with a stimulant. In fact, most of these medications actually cause drowsiness.

"The antidepressants did not get me high as far as what I could feel. It wasn't like feeling drunk or stoned. You don't get that sensation. The high I got is more like a lift, a mood lift. It's the difference between being lethargic and sad or active and happy."
35-year-old man with depression and a marijuana problem

The tricyclic antidepressants, available mainly as pills, can be dangerous if too many are taken, so it is important to monitor patient compliance with prescribed dosage and to get constant feedback from the patient as to the effects and side effects. Major side effects are dry mouth, blurred vision, inhibited urination, hypotension, and sleepiness.

"I went off antidepressants and after a month, six weeks, I began getting depressed again but I had to be convinced that I was depressed again. And they said, 'You really should go back on medication,' and I didn't want to admit that I didn't want to be on medication. I wanted to exist without it."
35-year-old patient with major depression

These drugs are also dangerous to the heart, especially if they are taken with stimulants, depressants, or alcohol. Patients must abstain from abusing drugs while being treated with tricyclic antidepressants.

Monamine Oxidase Inhibitors

MAO inhibitors, such as phenelzine (Nardil®), tranylcypromine (Parnate®), and isocarboxazid (Marplan®), are also used to treat depression. These very strong drugs work by blocking an enzyme which metabolizes neurotransmitters including norepinephrine and serotonin. This, in essence, raises the level of these neurotransmitters. Unfortunately, MAO inhibitors have several potentially dangerous side effects, so care and close monitoring are necessary in their use. They do give fairly quick relief from a major depression and panic disorder but the user has to be on a special diet and remain aware of the possibility of high blood pressure, headaches, and several other side effects. Combined use of MAO inhibitors with abused stimulants, depressants, and alcohol can be fatal.

Newer Antidepressants

The newer antidepressants, such as Prozac®, Deseryl®, Paxil®, Zoloft®, Welbutrin®, and Xanax®, work through a variety of mechanisms.

Prozac®(fluoxetine). The most popular of the new antidepressants, Prozac® has received a large amount of publicity both pro and con since its release in 1988. It seems quite effective in the treatment of depression with fewer side effects than tricyclic antidepressants or the MAO inhibitors. It is also used to treat obsessive-compulsive disorders and panic disorder.

Prozac® is classified as a serotonin reuptake inhibitor because it increases the amount of serotonin available to the nervous system. The amount needed to be effective varies widely from patient to patient and has to be adjusted. It generally takes two to four weeks for the full effect to be felt. The side effects are usually insomnia, nausea, diarrhea, headache, and nervousness. Most of the side effects are mild and will go away in a few weeks.

Paroxetine (Paxil®) and sertraline (Zoloft®) also work to block serotonin uptake and have similar side effects as Prozac®.

Xanax®. Alprazolam (Xanax®) a benzodiazepine sedative-hypnotic, though not labeled as a treatment for depression, has been used clinically by several doctors to control mild depression and anxiety but if the patient also has a drug problem, benzodiazepines are only recommended for detoxification or immediate relief.

Stimulants

In the past, amphetamine or amphetamine congeners, such as Dexedrine®,

TABLE 10–2 MEDICATIONS USED TO HANDLE PSYCHIATRIC PROBLEMS

MAJOR DEPRESSION

Tricyclic antidepressants: imipramine (Tofranil®, Janimine®), desipramine (Norpramin®, Pertofrane®), amitriptyline, (Elavil®, Endep®), nortriptyline (Pamelor®), doxepin (Sinequan®, Adapin®), trimipramine (Surmontil®), protriptyline (Vivactil®), maprotiline (Ludiomil®)

Monoamine oxidase (MAO) inhibitors: phenelzine (Nardil®), tranylcypromine (Parnate®), isocarboxazid (Marplan®), pargyline (Eutonyl®), selegiline

New antidepressants: fluoxetine (Prozac®), trazodone (Desyrel®), amoxapine (Asendin®), alprazolam (Xanax®), bupropion (Welbutrin®), sertraline (Zoloft®), Ritanserin®, paroxetine (Paxil®)

Stimulants used as antidepressants: amphetamines, (Dexedrine®, Biphetamine®, Desoxyn®), methylphenidate (Ritalin®), pemoline (Cylert®)

BIPOLAR AFFECTIVE DISORDER (manic-depression)

Lithium: (Eskalith®, Lithobid®)

Others: carbamazepine (Tegretol®), valproic acid (Depakene®), clonazepam (Klonopin®)

SCHIZOPHRENIA

Phenothiazines: trifluoperazine (Stelazine®), fluphenazine (Proloxin®, Permitil®), perphenazine (Trilafon®), chlorpromazine (Thorazine®), thioridazine (Mellaril®), mesoridazine (Serentil®)

Others: halperidol (Haldol®), thiothixene (Navane®), loxapine (Loxitane®), molindone (Moban®, Lidone®), clozapine (Clozaril®), pimozide (Orap®)

GENERALIZED ANXIETY DISORDER

Benzodiazepines:
Short acting (2–4 hour duration of action): alprazolam (Xanax®), oxazepam (Serax®), lorazepam (Ativan®), triazolam (Halcion®), temazepam (Restoril®)
Long acting (6–24 hour duration of action): diazepam (Valium®), chlordiazepoxide (Librium®), clorazepate (Tranxene®), clonazepam (Klonopin®), prazepam (Centrax®), halazepam (Paxipam®)

Nonbenzodiazepines: buspirone (BuSpar®)

OBSESSIVE-COMPULSIVE DISORDER (OCD)

Clomipramine (Anafranil®), sertraline (Zoloft®), fluoxetine (Prozac®)

PANIC DISORDER

First-line drugs (medications which should be tried first to control panic): imipramine (Tofranil®), desipramine (Norpramin® or Pertofrane®), alprazolam (Xanax®)

Second-line drugs: phenelzine (Nardil®), tranycypromine (Parnate®), clonazepam (Klonopin®)

Beta blockers: propranolol (Inderal®), atenolol (Tenormin®)

TABLE 10–2 (Continued)

SOCIAL PHOBIA
Beta blockers: propranolol (Inderal®), atenolol (Tenormin®)
MAO inhibitors: phenelzine (Nardil®)

POSTTRAUMATIC STRESS SYNDROME
First-line drugs: benzodiazepines and sedatives in treatment of generalized anxiety disorder
Second-line drugs: antipsychotics as in the treatment of schizophrenia

SLEEPING DISORDER
Sleeping pills: flurazepam (Dalmane®), triazolam (Halcion®), temazepam (Restoril®)

Biphetamine®, Desoxyn®, Ritalin®, and Cylert®, were used to treat depression. They work by increasing the amount of norepinephrine and epinephrine in the central nervous system. They were mood elevators when used in moderation but the problem was that since tolerance develops rapidly, and the mood lift proved to be too alluring, misuse and addiction developed fairly rapidly with the drugs. The overuse led to various physical and mental problems, such as agitation, aggression, paranoia, and psychosis. Ritalin® is occasionally prescribed for elderly patients with depression and for young patients with attention deficit disorder. But for a dually diagnosed client, these drugs should be used with utmost caution.

Drugs Used to Treat Bipolar Disorder (manic-depression)

Antidepressants, such as the tricyclics or, recently, Welbutrin® or Prozac®, are initially used to treat severe depression in the bipolar patient and antipsychotics, such as Thorazine® or Haldol®, are initially used to treat the severe manic phase. However, the main drug used for the treatment of bipolar illnesses over the last 30 years is lithium.

Lithium. Lithium is started concurrently with an antidepressant or an antipsychotic. Lithium is a long-term medication taken for years, even a lifetime. Clinicians are careful when making the diagnosis since the patient might be in the manic phase which resembles schizophrenia or the depressive phase which resembles unipolar depression. Misdiagnosis can be dangerous since long-term treatment of these other conditions is quite different.

Lithium doesn't really prevent a person from having moods. The patients still have high and low swings. What it does is dampen them. Because the high swings aren't as high and the depressions aren't as low, lithium helps the bipolar patient function. About 80% of bipolar patients respond to lithium. Symptoms begin to change within 10 to 15 days after starting the drug.

"The way manic-depression works, at least for me, is the medicine can control about 20% of it. The other 80% is me. I have to learn how to control my moods with my mind because the medication is only a small part." 40-year-old with bipolar disorder

Others

Tegretol® (carbamazepine) is used in patients who do not respond to lithium alone. It seems to help patients who have more rapid "cycling" of their highs and lows. Depakene® (valproic acid) is used if the bipolar patient fails to respond to lithium and Tegretol®. Its use with the bipolar patient is still limited to cases resistant to other medications.

Drugs Used to Treat Schizophrenia (antipsychotics or neuroleptics)

In the early 1950s, a new class of drugs, phenothiazines, was found to be effective in controlling the symptoms of schizophrenia. Some of the drugs, such as Thorazine®, Mellaril® Proloxin®, and Compazine®, were initially referred to as major tranquilizers. More recently, nonphenothiazines, like Haldol®, Loxitane®, and Moban®, have been developed. They act like phenothiazines and have similar side effects.

Researchers found that one of the major causes of schizophrenia is an excess of dopamine, a condition that is usually inherited. Most of the antipsychotic medications work by blocking the dopamine receptors in the brain, thereby inhibiting the effects of the excess dopamine. Generally, antipsychotic drugs do work but they do not cure schizophrenia. They can also cause serious side effects. The various side effects differentiate the drugs.

The main side effects of antipsychotics usually have to do with the decrease in dopamine in the system. From Table 10-1 (p. 440), you can see that dopamine controls muscle tone and motor behavior. By decreasing the dopamine, symptoms such as ticks, jumpiness, and the inability to sit still are common. Parkinsonian syndrome (mainly a tremor but also loss of facial expression and slowed movements), akathisia

(agitation, jumpiness exhibited by 75% of patients), akinesia (temporary loss of movement and apathy), and even the more serious tardive dyskenesia (involuntary movements of the jaws, head, neck, trunk and extremities) are the most common complications when using these medications. Often, drugs such as Cogentin®, Artane®, or Kemadrin®, or even Benadryl® are prescribed to block side effects.

Patients on antipsychotics can seem drugged but for people suffering from schizophrenia who are agitated or violent, the sedative effect is very useful. These drugs are dangerous when used as a sleeping pill by patients who do not have schizophrenia or are not violent and agitated. The drugs can actually cause symptoms of mental illness in patients who are not schizophrenic. They also have severe side effects.

Antipsychotic drugs in general are also classified as high potency (Haldol®, Stelazine®, Prolixin®, Trilafon®, Navane®) and low potency (Thorazine®, Mellaril®, Loxitrane®, Moban®).

In an emergency situation, patients are generally started on a high-potency antipsychotic. They are given several weeks to obtain a full response. If there is no response, either the dose can be raised or another drug tried. Most clinicians prefer to use low doses of these medications. The low-potency antipsychotics are used when patients also have problems sleeping. Manic patients are candidates for low-potency antipsychotic use.

Since antipsychotics are so potent, attempts are made to stop or decrease the dose of these medications as soon as possible, i.e., when the symptoms subside. This philosophy is particularly important in treating elderly patients.

Recently, atypical antipsychotic drugs have been tested. Clozaril® (clozapine) is effective in the 30% of patients who do not respond to standard antipsychotic drug therapy. Unfortunately, weekly blood tests are necessary to monitor the side effects of Clozaril®, making use very expensive.

Patients who have been dually diagnosed with schizophrenia often self-medicate with heroin and other opioids to control their symptoms. Alcohol, other sedative-hypnotics, and even marijuana or inhalants are used as well. Since all of these street drugs have dangerous toxic effects when combined with antipsychotic drugs, patients are exhorted to cease using them while under psychiatric treatment.

Drugs Used for Anxiety Disorders

For generalized anxiety disorder, as well as some of the other anxiety disorders, the benzodiazepines are widely used. The most commonly used are Xanax®, Valium®, Librium®, and Tranxene®. Developed in the early 1960s, the benzodiazepines were considered safe substitutes for barbiturates and the meprobamates (Miltown®, Equanil®). They act very quickly, particularly Valium®. The calming effects are apparent within 30 minutes. Some of the benzodiazepines are long acting (Valium®, Librium®, Tranxene®, Klonopin®, Centrax®) and some are short acting (Halcion®, Ativan®, Restoril®). The main problem with these drugs is that they are habit forming, even at clinical dosages, and do have withdrawal symptoms, so they are almost always avoided with the dually diagnosed patient for whom they can retrigger drug abuse. If the drug must be used, dosages are kept as low as possible and the patient is monitored for addiction or relapse.

Buspirone (BuSpar®) is the only other drug labeled for generalized anxiety disorder. It is a serotonin modulator and will block the transmission of excess serotonin which is considered to be one of the causes of the symptoms of many forms of anxiety.

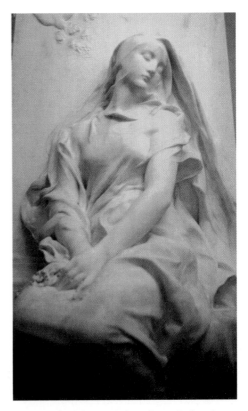

Photo reprinted, by permission, Simone Garlaund.

It also mimics serotonin, so it can also substitute for low levels of serotonin, a feature used by some doctors to treat depression. It takes several weeks to work and is not nearly as initially dramatic as the benzodiazepines, so many patients are reluctant to use it. Its advantage, however, is that side effects are minimal and it is definitely not habit forming.

Drugs for Obsessive-Compulsive Disorder (OCD)

For the obsessive-compulsive disorder, almost every type of psychotropic medication has been used in the past, usually with relatively poor results. Anafranil® (clomipramine) has recently been used with reasonable results. It is a serotonin reuptake inhibitor like Zoloft® and Prozac®.

Drugs for Panic Disorder

Several drugs are used to control panic disorder (as opposed to panic attacks). Panic attacks occur in someone who has panic disorder, in those on a bad LSD trip, in someone having an extreme reaction to a stimulant, in a heart patient experiencing rapid heart beating (tachycardia), and in reactions to various medications. Panic disorder consists of multiple panic attacks accompanied by fear and anxiety about having more panic attacks. Situations where a panic attack might occur are also to be avoided. It is sometimes difficult to distinguish between a panic attack and a panic disorder.

Beta blockers calm the symptoms of a panic attack, such as rapid heart rates, hypertension, and difficulty breathing, because they block excess muscular activity in the vascular system and lungs. Beta blockers also have a calming effect on the brain, which is helpful in treating panic disorders. It takes about one hour for the medicine to work, so many people with a panic disorder or social phobia will take a dose one hour before entering a stressful situation.

CHAPTER SUMMARY

MENTAL HEALTH AND DRUGS

Brain Chemistry

1. The neurotransmitters that are involved in mental illness are the same ones involved in drug abuse and addiction.

2. The direct effects of many psychoactive drugs, as well as the withdrawal effects, mimic various mental illnesses.

Epidemiology

3. About 37% of alcohol abusers and 53% of drug abusers also have a serious mental illness.

4. Up to 81% of those in prison with a drug problem also have a mental illness.

Determining Factors

5. Heredity, environment, and psychoactive drugs affect one's susceptibility to mental illness in much the same way they affect susceptibility to drug abuse.

6. The risk of developing a mental illness depends on heredity. The risk of people developing schizophrenia if they have a close relative with schizophrenia jumps from 1% to 15%, for major depression it jumps from 5% to 15%, and for a bipolar illness, it jumps from 1% to 12%.

7. Environment can increase susceptibility to mental illness. Physical abuse in childhood is very common (50% to 75%) in those who are psychotic.

8. Psychoactive drugs can alter neurochemistry and aggravate preexisting mental illnesses, trigger latent ones, or create new ones.

DUAL DIAGNOSIS OR THE MENTALLY ILL CHEMICAL ABUSER (MICA)

Definition

9. Dual diagnosis is defined as a condition in which a person has both a substance abuse problem and a diagnosable significant psychiatric problem.

10. The three main psychiatric disorders used to define dual diagnosis are schizophrenia (a thought disorder), major depression (a mood disorder), and bipolar disorder (manic-depression).

11. Other mental illnesses used by some to define dual diagnosis include anxiety disorders, such as panic disorder, phobia, obsessive-compulsive disorder, posttraumatic stress syndrome, organic disorders, developmental disorders, somatoform disorders, attention deficit/hyperactivity disorder and other personality disorders.

Patterns of Dual Diagnosis

12. The four different patterns of dual diagnosis are a preexisting mental illness that is aggravated by drug use, a potential mental illness that is triggered by drug use, a permanent mental illness induced by drug use, and a temporary mental illness that is induced by drug use.

Making the Diagnosis

13. A psychiatric diagnosis should always be conditional since abusable drugs can directly or indirectly mimic some mental illnesses.

14. The number of dually diagnosed patients has increased due to better diagnosis techniques, shrinking numbers of inpatient mental health facilities, greater numbers of drug abusers, and a reliance on psychiatric medications.

Mental Health (MH) Versus Chemical Dependency (CD)

15. Four main differences between the mental health (MH) treatment community and the chemical dependency (CD) treatment community are the following:

   a. MH says control the psychiatric problem and the drug abuse will disappear. CD says get the patient clean and sober and the mental health problem will disappear;

   b. in MH, limited recovery is more acceptable, whereas in CD, most believe that lifetime abstinence is possible;

   c. MH often uses psychiatric drugs to treat the dual diagnosis patient, whereas CD promotes a drug-free philosophy;

   d. MH has a supportive philosophy, whereas CD uses a confrontive philosophy.

16. Health professionals need to combine the two philosophies of treatment to develop programs that treat both mental illness and addiction.

17. Triple diagnosis is usually the coexistence of a mental health problem, a drug addiction, and an HIV diagnosis.

Psychiatric Disorders

18. Schizophrenia, a thought disorder, is characterized by hallucinations, delusions, an inappropriate affect, poor association, and an impaired ability to care for oneself.

19. Major depression is characterized by a depressed mood, diminished interest and pleasure in most activities, sleep and appetite disturbances, feelings of worthlessness, and suicidal thoughts.

20. A bipolar affective disorder involves manic phases alternating with depressive phases.

21. Anxiety disorders include panic disorder, obsessive-compulsive disorder, posttraumatic stress disorder, and a generalized anxiety disorder.

22. Other mental illness include an organic mental disorder (e.g., Alzheimer's disease), developmental disorders (e.g., attention deficit/hyperactivity disorder), somatoform disorders (e.g., hypochondria), and various personality disorders.

Treatment

23. Treatment for dual diagnosis can be done with psychotherapy, counseling, the group process, and/or with psychiatric medications.

24. Usually both the addiction and the mental problem need to be treated simultaneously.

25. Impaired cognition and developmental arrest make treatment of dual diagnosis difficult. Many people coming in for treatment are much younger emotionally than they are physically.

Psychiatric Medications

26. The major classes of psychiatric drugs are antidepressants, MAO inhibitors, antipsychotics, antianxiety drugs, lithium, and beta blockers.

27. Psychiatric medications manipulate brain chemistry and relieve symptoms of mental illness. They can also cause undesirable side effects.

28. Many with mental illnesses try to self-medicate with street drugs or alcohol.

29. Drugs used to treat depression are tricyclic antidepressants, MAO inhibitors, amphetamines, and newer antidepressants, such as Prozac® and Zoloft®.

30. Some of the drugs used to treat schizophrenia are the phenothiazines, such as chlorpromazine (Thorazine®), halperidol (Haldol®), clozapine (Clozaril®).

31. The main drug used to treat a bipolar disorder is lithium.

32. The principal drugs used to treat anxiety are the benzodiazepines, such as Valium® and Xanax®, and the nonbenzodiazepine, BuSpar® (buspirone).

REVIEW QUESTIONS

CHAPTER 1
HISTORY AND CLASSIFICATION

History of Psychoactive Drugs

1. What are four natural ways (such as meditation) that people since ancient times have changed their perception of reality without using drugs?
2. What natural sources did all psychoactive drugs come from in prehistoric times?
3. Name two ancient civilizations, a psychoactive drug they each used, and how the drug was put into people's bodies.
4. Describe three reasons opium was used in ancient civilizations.
5. What are three reasons that psychedelic plants, such as henbane and belladonna, were used in the Middle Ages?
6. What are three psychoactive drugs that Islamic cultures used instead of alcohol?
7. Ergot poisoning was caused by mold on what substance?
8. Which chemical process increased the concentration of alcoholic beverages in the Middle Ages?
9. In which area of the world were peyote and psilocybin mushrooms first used? On which continent were coca leaves first used?
10. Name two psychoactive substances that were introduced from one part of the world to another. Indicate which country or region of the world exported it and which country or region of the world adopted it.
11. Name two reasons tobacco became popular in Europe in the 1600s.
12. In Europe and the Middle East, which two popular cure-alls used opium?
13. Which country was plagued by the Gin Epidemic in the eighteenth century?

14. Name two of the first inhalants used in America and Europe.
15. Which two countries fought the Opium Wars?
16. Which three drugs had their potency increased by new refinement or delivery methods in the nineteenth century? Indicate the natural form of the drug and the refined form.
17. Name two organizations in the nineteenth century involved in limiting the use of alcohol.
18. List three factors that drastically increased cigarette sales at the end of the nineteenth and beginning of the twentieth centuries.
19. Name one of the major U.S. laws enacted at the beginning of the twentieth century to limit the use of psychoactive drugs.
20. What were two reasons that the Eighteenth Amendment banning the sale of alcohol in the United States was repealed?
21. Which organization was started in the 1930s to help people with a drinking problem?
22. In which year was the growing and sale of marijuana banned by the Marijuana Tax Act?
23. Give an example of the upper-downer cycle in the use of psychoactive drugs in America by naming two consecutive decades (or periods of time) and the kinds of drugs that were used.
24. Which method of drug use fueled the cocaine epidemic of the mid-1980s?
25. Name three psychoactive drugs that are used in "rave" clubs in the 1990s.
26. What is the main difference in the marijuana of the 1990s compared to the marijuana of the 1960s and 1970s?
27. Which two psychoactive drugs are causing the most premature deaths in the 1990s?

Classification of Psychoactive Drugs

28. Give a medical use, a religious use, and an emotional use for alcohol.
29. Cite examples of a chemical name, a trade name, and a street name for two psychoactive drugs.
30. Name the three major classes of psychoactive drugs.
31. Name three classes of other psychoactive drugs.
32. Name three stimulants.
33. Name three depressants.
34. Name three psychedelics.
35. Name two inhalants.

CHAPTER 2
HEREDITY, ENVIRONMENT, PSYCHOACTIVE DRUGS

How Psychoactive Drugs Affect Us

1. Name five ways that drugs can enter the body.
2. Which is the fastest method of use for drugs to reach the central nervous system and affect the brain? Which is the slowest?
3. Describe precisely the route that a swallowed drug would take to get to the brain.
4. Name the three parts of the nervous system.
5. What are three functions of the old brain?
6. What are three functions of the new brain?
7. Does drug craving reside in the old brain or the new brain?
8. What are the four parts of a nerve cell?
9. Describe precisely the way that a signal will cross the synaptic gap.
10. In which structures are neurotransmitters stored in the nerve cell?
11. Describe how stimulant drugs affect the movement of neurotransmitters.
12. Describe how opioids affect the movement of neurotransmitters.
13. Name three different neurotransmitters.
14. What biological process makes a drug user take greater quantities of psychoactive drugs to receive the same effect?
15. Name three different kinds of tolerance.
16. Describe one physiological change that occurs with the prolonged use of a psychoactive drug, such as alcohol, due to tissue dependence.
17. List three effects of heroin and their subsequent withdrawal effects.

18. Which two organs are most responsible for ridding the body of drugs?
19. Name four factors which determine how fast a psychoactive drug is metabolized by the body.

From Experimentation to Addiction

20. Name seven reasons why a person might use a psychoactive drug.
21. Describe two desirable effects of alcohol and two undesirable effects.
22. What are three factors that determine the level at which a person is using a psychoactive drug?
23. Name the six levels of drug use.
24. What is the main hallmark of drug abuse?
25. List four characteristics of addiction.
26. What are three current theories of addiction?
27. List four physical features which can be passed on through heredity.
28. Name two susceptibilities which can be passed on through heredity.
29. What does the presence of an alcoholism-associated gene signify in regards to alcoholism?
30. Name the major environmental factor that can affect someone's brain chemistry.
31. Name three neighborhood environmental factors that can increase one's susceptibility to drug abuse.
32. How can people with no hereditary or environmental risk factors become addicts?
33. Besides heredity, environment, and the use of psychoactive drugs, which factor can also increase one's susceptibility to abuse drugs?
34. According to the compulsion curve, what moves a person from low susceptibility to high susceptibility?
35. Will a person who has become addicted to a psychoactive drug return to his or her original susceptibility level if drug use ceases?

CHAPTER 3
UPPERS

1. Name five stimulants and list them from strongest to weakest.
2. List four plants whose leaves, nuts, or fruit are used as stimulants.
3. Which neurotransmitter is most responsible for the stimulation caused by uppers?
4. What are three major effects of stimulants?

5. How does stimulation of the reward/pleasure center cause stimulant users to lose their appetite?
6. What is the major problem caused by the release of energy chemicals due to extended use of stimulants?
7. What effects do cocaine and amphetamines have on blood pressure and heart rate?
8. What are the three most common ways to put cocaine into the body? Which is the fastest route to the brain?
9. What are three major differences between cocaine and amphetamines?
10. What usually causes death with an amphetamine or cocaine overdose?
11. What are two other names for smokable cocaine?
12. What properties of smokable cocaine enable it to be smoked?
13. What are two economic reasons for the spread of smokable cocaine?
14. What were amphetamines originally prescribed for?
15. Which properties of amphetamines contribute to its abuse compared to cocaine?
16. What are four symptoms of prolonged amphetamine use?
17. Why does an amphetamine "crash" occur?
18. Name three ways amphetamines can be put into the body.
19. Why does the methamphetamine known as "ice" cause more intense mental effects than amphetamines which are eaten or snorted?
20. What are the two main uses of amphetamine congeners?
21. What does AD/HD stand for?
22. Do the amphetamine congeners have an addiction liability?
23. What are three possible ingredients in lookalikes or over-the-counter stimulants?
24. Which body system is most affected by lookalikes or over-the-counter stimulants?
25. In which part of the world is the use of khat widespread?
26. Name three plant stimulants that are popular in the Middle East.
27. Which has the most caffeine: a six-ounce cup of coffee, six ounces of chocolate, or a six-ounce cup of tea?
28. What are three symptoms of caffeine withdrawal?
29. Name two routes through which nicotine is absorbed by the body.
30. In which part of the world did tobacco smoking originate?
31. Is nicotine more likely to cause heart problems or cancer?
32. Is the tar which is found in tobacco smoke more likely to cause heart problems or cancer?
33. What is the main reason that tobacco is so addictive?
34. What are three other reasons that cigarette smoking is so addictive?
35. What are some of the symptoms of nicotine withdrawal?

CHAPTER 4
DOWNERS: OPIATES/OPIOIDS AND SEDATIVE-HYPNOTICS

1. What are the three main groups of downers (depressants)?
2. List four other groups of downers.

Opiates/Opioids

3. What is the difference between opiates and opioids?
4. Name three opiates and three opioids.
5. What processes, discoveries, or inventions have increased the addiction liability of opiates and opioids?
6. Which method of using opioids gets the drugs to the brain the fastest?
7. What is the main medical use of opioids?
8. What are two other medical uses of opioids?
9. Which neurotransmitter transmits pain and which one blocks pain?
10. Which neurotransmitter ultimately activates the reward/pleasure center of the brain?
11. List four withdrawal effects of heroin.
12. What effect does heroin have on the eyes of a user?
13. Name three methods of using heroin.
14. Which areas of the world are the largest producers and exporters of heroin?
15. What is the main type of heroin supplied by Mexico to the United States?
16. What is the main use of codeine?
17. What is the range of purity of street heroin?
18. What are two dangerous problems with using heroin intravenously?
19. Name the ingredients in two different kinds of "speedballs."
20. Name four of the lesser known opioids.

21. Which opioid lasts longer in the body, heroin or methadone?

Sedative-Hypnotics

22. What are the two main classes of sedative-hypnotics?
23. What are three uses of sedative-hypnotics?
24. Which major class of sedative-hypnotics is more likely to cause an overdose?
25. Are sedative-hypnotics more similar to opioids or alcohol in terms of effects?
26. Name two barbiturates.
27. What are two overdose effects of barbiturates?
28. Name the most common drugs found in patients in a hospital emergency room.
29. Name three different benzodiazepines.
30. Which is the main organ for metabolizing Valium®?
31. Which is the main neurotransmitter affected by benzodiazepines?
32. Name two sedative-hypnotics which are not benzodiazepines or barbiturates.
33. What are two ways addicts can get prescription sedative-hypnotics or prescription opioids?
34. What is the biggest danger with drug synergism when using two depressant drugs?
35. Name the process in which a user builds a tolerance to heroin and uses Darvon® to relieve the withdrawal.

CHAPTER 5
DOWNERS: ALCOHOL

1. Describe how alcohol might have been discovered.
2. Which legal psychoactive drug causes the most deaths?
3. What are two other technical names for grain alcohol?
4. Beer fermentation uses which plants? Which plants are used for fermenting wine?
5. What is the approximate percentage of alcohol in beer? Wine? Vodka?
6. What are four factors that speed the rate of absorption of alcohol by the body?
7. What are four factors that slow the rate of absorption of alcohol by the body?
8. What are the final two products of alcohol metabolism which are excreted from the body?

9. Is alcohol metabolized at a variable or continuous rate?
10. What does BAC stand for?
11. Name four groups of people who should avoid even low-level use of alcohol.
12. What are two health benefits of low-dose use of alcohol?
13. Describe two major psychological effects of low-dose use of alcohol.
14. Which is the main inhibitory neurotransmitter affected by alcohol?
15. What is the legal BAC intoxication level in most states?
16. What are three dangerous effects of high-dose use of alcohol?
17. What three factors help determine whether a person will become an alcoholic?
18. The liver's ability to process greater and greater amounts of alcohol contributes to which two physiological phenomena that can eventually lead to alcoholism?
19. After frequent high-dose use, which is more dangerous: alcohol withdrawal or heroin withdrawal?
20. Describe the major effect of cirrhosis of the liver for alcoholics.
21. What are three dangerous effects of long-term high-dose use of alcohol?
22. Which drug is usually most dangerous in combination with alcohol: a benzodiazepine or cocaine?
23. Besides direct health effects, describe three ways that alcohol can cause death.
24. Which is most often a major psychological effect of long-term use of alcohol: anxiety, mania, or depression?
25. What do FAS and FAE stand for?
26. Describe two symptoms of FAS.
27. Name three reasons why the use of alcohol can cause violence.
28. Name three diseases caused by excessive use of alcohol.
29. Name two countries that have a higher per capita consumption rate of alcohol than the United States.
30. What percentage of Americans over 12 years of age have at least one drink of an alcoholic beverage each month: 25%, 50%, or 75%?
31. What percentage of all hospital admissions were due to direct or indirect medical complications from alcohol: 5–10%, 25–30%, or 55–60%?

32. Do negative health consequences from drinking develop faster with women or men?
33. Is heavy drinking least prevalent in the Caucasian, African American, or Hispanic community?
34. What are the six levels of alcohol use?
35. What does MAST stand for?

CHAPTER 6
ALL AROUNDERS

1. Name three psychedelics used more than 500 years ago.
2. List four other psychedelics in addition to the three named in question one.
3. Which are the two best known indole psychedelics?
4. What are two factors, other than the direct effects of the psychedelic itself, that help determine what effect a psychedelic will have?
5. What is a common physical effect of many psychedelics, particularly low-dose LSD?
6. Which phenomenon is "a mistaken idea that is not swayed by reason": a hallucination, a delusion, or an illusion?
7. What is synesthesia?
8. What are two street names for LSD?
9. Does LSD have its greatest effect in the cerebellum, the midbrain, or the brain stem?
10. How many micrograms are considered a full psychedelic dose of LSD?
11. Name two ways LSD can be taken into the body.
12. What is a usual physical effect of psychedelic mushrooms when ingested?
13. What is the active ingredient in most psychedelic mushrooms?
14. What is the active ingredient in peyote?
15. Is the use of peyote more likely to cause delusions, illusions, or hallucinations?
16. What are two slang names for MDMA?
17. Is MDMA more a stimulant or a psychedelic?
18. Name four drugs, besides MDMA, which are used at "rave" clubs.
19. Name an active ingredient in a nightshade plant, such as belladonna.
20. Are anticholinergic psychedelics more likely to cause illusions or hallucinations?
21. What used to be a medical use of PCP?
22. Name three ways that PCP can be put in the body.
23. Describe three effects of PCP.
24. What is a medical use for ketamine?

25. What are three ways cannabis plants can be used?
26. Which is the most widely used psychoactive drug in the United States?
27. What is the name of the neurotransmitter that mimics THC?
28. Name two species of marijuana plant.
29. What is the purpose of the sinsemilla-growing technique?
30. Describe two short-term physical effects of smoking marijuana.
31. Describe two short-term mental effects of smoking marijuana.
32. What are four reasons that people will smoke marijuana?
33. Which is more dangerous to the mucous membranes of the respiratory system: smoking marijuana, smoking cigarettes, or smoking cigarettes and marijuana?
34. Describe three withdrawal effects that occur upon cessation of long-term marijuana smoking.
35. What does the phrase "the mirror that magnifies" mean in relation to smoking marijuana?

CHAPTER 7
OTHER DRUGS, OTHER ADDICTIONS

Other Drugs

1. What are the three major classes of inhalants?
2. Name three different volatile solvents which are used for their psychedelic effects.
3. Name a volatile nitrite.
4. What are three different effects of volatile nitrites?
5. List two methods of using inhalants.
6. What are three warning signs to help one recognize stimulant abuse in another person?
7. What is a long-term dangerous effect of solvent inhalant abuse?
8. What are two reasons for the increase in the use of drugs in sports?
9. Name two different therapeutic drugs used in sports.
10. What are two desired effects of anabolic-androgenic steroids?
11. What are two undesired side effects of anabolic-androgenic steroids?
12. Is cocaine or an amphetamine more likely to be used to enhance performance at an athletic event?

13. What are two other nonsteroidal drugs used to enhance performance?
14. What is the psychedelic ingredient in Raid® or Lysol®?
15. What are three advertised effects of "smart drugs" and "smart drinks?"

Other Addictions

16. What four types of compulsive behaviors have many of the same symptoms as drug abuse and addiction?
17. Give two reasons that people engage in compulsive behaviors.
18. Name two nondrug compulsive behaviors that have been proven to have a strong hereditary component.
19. What kind of studies show the strong linkage between heredity and compulsive behaviors or addiction?
20. What does the presence of a marker gene such as the DRD$_2$ A$_1$ allele gene signify?
21. Is there more than one marker gene for compulsive behavior?
22. Name three different types of gambling or games of chance which are legal in states other than Nevada and New Jersey.
23. Approximately what percentage of Americans are compulsive gamblers: 1-3%, 11-13%, or 21-23%?
24. Why do many governments support gambling?
25. List four symptoms of compulsive gambling.
26. Alcoholism is common in 10% to 30%, 30% to 50%, or 50% to 70% of all compulsive gamblers?
27. What does GA stand for to a heavy bettor?
28. Name the three main eating disorders.
29. What are two symptoms of bulimia?
30. Which eating disorder could be described as a weight phobia?
31. In compulsive overeaters, what usually triggers the desire to eat instead of food hunger?
32. List three ways to change the habit of compulsive overeating.
33. What are the two most common compulsive sexual behaviors?
34. Name three symptoms of cyberaddiction.
35. Since all compulsive behaviors, including addiction, have similar roots, can they be treated in a similar fashion? Why or why not?

CHAPTER 8
DRUG USE AND PREVENTION: FROM CRADLE TO GRAVE

1. Describe a likely way that an infant, a 16-year-old boy, and a grandmother would have a problem with "crack" cocaine.

Prevention

2. What are three goals of prevention?
3. What are three methods used to achieve the goals of prevention?
4. What are four prevention tactics that have been tried over the years?
5. Name the three components of the public health models of drug abuse prevention.
6. What are four government agencies that are involved with supply reduction in the United States?
7. Under demand reduction, who is the target audience for secondary prevention?
8. Describe three methods of harm reduction?
9. What is one of the biggest barriers to effective prevention programs?

From Cradle to Grave

10. Which psychoactive drug has the earliest first use by adolescents?
11. Name one of the three psychoactive drugs that has the latest age of first use.
12. Which barrier protects the fetus from most substances except nutrients and psychoactive drugs?
13. Describe precisely two ways in which a fetus could be exposed to the HIV virus.
14. What is a specific fetal effect of cocaine? Heroin? Alcohol?
15. Which prevention program can keep a fetus from being drug exposed?
16. Which are the three most commonly used psychoactive drugs in high schools and colleges in the United States?
17. Name five factors that increase a teenager's risk for drug abuse.
18. Name the four factors that predict a child's resiliency to drug abuse as described by Stephen Glenn and Richard Jessor.
19. What percentage of college students binge drink: 44%, 66%, or 88%?
20. Describe three symptoms of secondhand drinking.

21. What are two methods that colleges use to reduce problem drinking on campus?
22. Which are the three facets of sexual behavior that are impacted by psychoactive drugs?
23. Which physical effect of alcohol decreases sexual performance?
24. What are two effects of psychoactive drug use that can lead to high-risk sexual practices?
25. Which is the most common sexually transmitted disease?
26. Name three diseases caused by contaminated needles used by drug abusers.
27. Drug abuse costs American business $30, $70, or $140 billion per year?
28. Name three ways that drug abuse can cost a business money.
29. What does EAP stand for and what kinds of problems does it handle?
30. What are the two most common uses of drug testing?
31. How long after use does it take before a drug (besides alcohol) is first detectable through urine testing?
32. Which drug remains detectable in the urine for the longest period of time?
33. Which drug is excreted from the body at a defined continuous rate?
34. Name three reasons that drugs and alcohol have more of an effect on the elderly.
35. What are two factors that prevent people from recognizing drug abuse in the elderly?
36. Why doesn't one prevention program work for all people?

CHAPTER 9
TREATMENT

1. What is the most prevalent mind disorder in the United States?
2. About how much does each dollar spent for drug abuse treatment save society?
3. What is the most effective duration of drug treatment?
4. Drug abuse treatment reduces recidivism (repeat offenses)in prisoners by 10% to 20%, 30% to 50%, or 60% to 80%?
5. Name two different treatment options.
6. Name four target populations for drug abuse treatment.
7. Who else besides an addict exhibits signs of denial of a drug abuse problem?
8. What are three methods for breaking through denial?

9. Name two of the four parts of an intervention statement.
10. One of the goals of drug abuse treatment is moving the client towards abstinence. What is the other goal?
11. What are two supporting goals of treatment?
12. Name five different treatment programs and specify whether they are inpatient or outpatient.
13. What are two of the factors concerning the drug abuser that should be known when an intervention group selects a treatment program?
14. What is the most commonly used test for addiction?
15. About how many people are treated in drug programs each year in the United States?
16. What are the four steps in the treatment continuum?
17. Name two drugs that can be used to help detoxify a drug abuser.
18. Name two different types of psychosocial therapy.
19. During initial abstinence, what factor is most likely to trigger relapse?
20. During long-term abstinence, what is the crucial idea that an addict must accept?
21. Name two natural highs that could help an addict stay abstinent during recovery.
22. What are three ways to measure success in a treatment program?
23. What are two different kinds of individual therapy?
24. Overall, is individual counseling or group therapy more effective in drug treatment?
25. Name three types of drug treatment groups.
26. Name four groups based on the 12-step process.
27. What are steps 1 and 2 in the 12 steps of Alcoholics Anonymous?
28. What are two self-help groups for the families of addicts?
29. Name three approaches to treating the family of an addict or alcoholic.
30. What are three dysfunctional behaviors manifested by the relatives or addicts or alcoholics?
31. What does ACoA stand for?
32. Polydrug abuse is the most common reason people go into treatment. True or false.
33. What is the most common psychiatric presentment for someone at the end of a long stimulant run?

34. What is a common drug therapy for tobacco addiction?
35. What is the usual treatment for a "bad trip" due to LSD?
36. Withdrawal after long-term high-dose use from which two drugs can cause life-threatening symptoms?
37. What is the major difference in men and women's attitudes as to the cause of addiction?
38. What two changes could a treatment center make to be culturally specific?
39. Which two institutions' involvement in African American drug treatment have been proven effective?
40. Name four obstacles to effective drug treatment.

CHAPTER 10
MENTAL/EMOTIONAL HEALTH AND DRUGS

Mental Health and Drugs

1. Give two examples of how the direct effects of a psychoactive drug can mimic a mental illness. Name the drug and the illness.
2. Give two examples of how the withdrawal effects of a psychoactive drug can mimic a mental illness. Name the drug and the illness.
3. In U.S. prisons, what is the prevalence of a psychiatric disorder if the prisoner has a substance abuse problem: 40%, 60%, or 80%?
4. The abuser of which substance is more likely to have a psychiatric problem: alcohol, heroin, or cocaine?
5. If someone has a close-order relative with schizophrenia, what is the likelihood, on average, that that person will also develop schizophrenia: 2%, 5%, 15% or 30%?
6. Which other mental illnesses have a strong hereditary component?
7. What is a very strong predisposing environmental factor that can make a person more susceptible to mental illness?
8. Name two ways that psychoactive drugs can determine whether a person has a mental illness.

Dual Diagnosis or the Mentally Ill Chemical Abuser (MICA)

9. Define dual diagnosis.
10. Name the three mental illnesses that are most often used to define dual diagnosis.
11. Name three other mental illnesses that are also found in dually diagnosed clients.
12. Name four ways that the use of psychoactive drugs can produce a dually diagnosed individual.
13. Why should the initial diagnosis of dual diagnosis be written in disappearing ink?
14. Name four factors that might account for the increase in dually diagnosed clients.
15. Name three differences between the mental health (MH) treatment community and the chemical dependency (CD) treatment community.
16. Which community is more likely to let a client hit bottom before starting treatment: MH or CD?
17. Define triple diagnosis.
18. List two symptoms of schizophrenia.
19. List two symptoms of major depression.
20. List two symptoms of bipolar-affective disorder.
21. Name four types of anxiety disorders.
22. What is psychopharmacology?
23. Describe three ways that a dually diagnosed individual can reduce environmental stress that might trigger his or her mental illness.
24. What are three approaches used to treat mental illness?
25. Name three different classes of drugs used to treat depression.
26. What is the main drug used to treat manic-depression?
27. Name two drugs used to treat anxiety.
28. Which neurotransmitter is most involved in schizophrenia and the cocaine high?
29. What are two differences between street psychoactive drugs and psychiatric medications?

BIBLIOGRAPHY

In the preparation of this book we have conducted hundreds of interviews with health care professionals, drug abusers, former drug abusers, research scientists, and criminal justice professionals. We have also consulted hundreds of books, pamphlets, magazine articles, and studies. The following list includes those we found most valuable. (Several hundred newspaper articles are not included.)

GENERAL DRUG INFORMATION USED IN ALL CHAPTERS

Abadinsky, Howard. *Drug Abuse: An Introduction.* Chicago, IL: Nelson-Hall, 1989.

American Society of Addiction Medicine. *Syllabus for the Review Course in Addiction Medicine.* Washington, DC: American Society of Addiction Medicine, 1990.

Fleming, Michael F. and Kristen Lawton Barry. *Addictive Disorders.* St. Louis, MO: Mosby-Year Book, Inc., 1992.

Forest, Gary G. and Robert H. Gordon. *Substance Abuse, Homicide, and Violent Behavior.* New York: Gardner Press, 1990.

Friedman, Lawrence S., et. al. eds. *Source Book of Substance Abuse and Addiction.* Baltimore, MD: Williams & Wilkins, 1996.

Goldstein, Avram. *Addiction: From Biology to Drug Policy.* New York: W.H. Freeman and Company, 1994.

Goode, Erich. *Drugs in American Society.* 4th ed. New York: McGraw-Hill, Inc., 1993.

Institute for Substance Abuse Research. *Drugs of Abuse Digest.* 9th ed. Vero Beach, FL, 1993.

Jaffe, Jerome H. *Encyclopedia of Drugs and Alcohol.* 4 vols. New York: Macmillan Library Reference USA, 1995.

Jones, Lee, and Victoria Kimbrough. *Great Ideas.* New York: Cambridge University Press, 1987.

Julien, Robert M. *A Primer of Drug Action: A Concise, Nontechnical Guide to the Actions, Uses, and Side Effects of Psychoactive Drugs.* 7th ed. New York: W. H. Freeman and Company, 1995.

Leccese, Arthur P. *Drugs and Society: Behavioral Medicines and Abusable Drugs.* Englewood Cliffs, NJ: Prentice Hall, 1991.

Liska, Ken. *Drugs and the Human Body with Implications for Society.* 4th ed. New York: Macmillan Publishing Company, 1990.

Longenecker, Gesina L. *How Drugs Work: Drug Abuse and the Human Body.* Emeryville, CA: Ziff-Davis Press, 1994.

Lowinson, Joyce H., Pedro Ruiz, and Robert Millman. *Substance Abuse: A Comprehensive Textbook.* 2d ed. Baltimore, MD: Williams & Wilkins, 1992.

Marnell, Tim. ed. *Drug Identification Bible.* 2d ed. Denver, CO: Drug Identification Bible®, 1995.

Miller, Norman S. *Comprehensive Handbook of Drug and Alcohol Addiction.* New York: Marcel Dekker, Inc., 1991.

O'Brian, Robert, Sidney Cohen., et. al. *The Encyclopedia of Drug Abuse.* 2d ed. New York: Facts on File, 1992.

Physicians' Desk Reference. Montvale, NJ: Medical Economics Data Production, 1995.

Pinger, Robert R., Wayne A. Payne, Dale B. Hahn, and Ellen J. Hahn. *Drugs: Issues for Today* 2d ed. St. Louis, MO: Mosby-Year Book, Inc., 1995.

Ray, Oakley and Charles Ksir. *Drugs, Society & Human Behavior.* 7th ed. St. Louis, MO: Mosby-Year Book, Inc., 1995.

Silverman, Harold M. *The Pill Book: The Illustrated Guide to the Most-Prescribed Drugs in the United States.* 7th ed. New York: Bantam Books, 1996.

Stafford, Peter. *Psychedelics Encyclopedia.* 3d expanded ed. Berkeley, CA: Ronin Publishing, Inc., 1992.

U.S. Department of Health and Human Services, National Institutes of Health. *National Survey Results on Drug Use from The Monitoring the Future Study, 1975-1995.* GPO, 1996.

——. *National Survey Results on Drug Use from The Monitoring The Future Study, 1975-1995. Vol. I. Secondary School Students.* GPO, 1996.

——. *National Survey Results on Drug Use from The Monitoring The Future Study, 1975-1995. Vol. II. College Students and Young Adults.* Washington, DC: GPO, 1996.

——. *Women and Drugs: A New Era for Research.* NIDA Research Monograph 65. Rockville, MD: GPO, 1986.

Venturelli, Peter J. *Drug Use in America: Social, Cultural, and Political Perspectives.* Boston: Jones and Bartlett Publishers, 1994.

Weil, Andrew and Winifred Rosen. *From Chocolate to Morphine: Everything You Need To Know About Mind-Altering Drugs.* 2d ed. Boston/New York: Houghton Mifflin Company, 1993.

The White House. *The National Drug Control Strategy: 1996.* GPO. 1996.

Zerkin, Leif and Jeffery H. Novey, eds *Journal of Psychoactive Drugs, 1967-1996.* Available through Haight-Ashbury Publications, 409 Clayton Street, San Francisco, CA 94117.

OTHER PUBLICATIONS, BOOKS, AND ARTICLES USED IN SPECIFIC CHAPTERS

Chapter 1—Psychoactive Drugs: History and Classification

Armstrong, David and Elizabeth Metzger Armstrong. *The Great American Medicine Show: Being an Illustrated History of Hucksters, Healers, Health Evangelists, and Heroes from Plymouth Rock to the Present.* New York: Prentice Hall, 1991.

Beeching, Jack. *The Chinese Opium Wars.* New York: Harcourt Brace Jocanovich. 1975.

Brecher, Edward M. and the Editors of Consumer Reports. *Licit and Illicit Drugs.* Boston: Little, Brown and Company, 1972.

Cowan, David L. and William H. Helfand. *Pharmacy: An Illustrated History.* New York: Harry N. Abrams, Inc., 1990.

Lyons, Albert S. and R. Joseph Petrucelli, II. *Medicine: An Illustrated History.* New York: Harry N. Abrams, Inc., 1978.

McKenna, Terence. *Food of the Gods: The Search for the Original Tree of Knowledge.* New York: Bantam Books, 1992.

Musto, David F. *Alcohol in American History.* New York: Scientific American Magazine, 1996.

——. *The American Disease: Origins of Narcotic Control.* New York: Oxford University Press, 1987.

——. *Opium, Cocaine and Marijuana in American. History.* New York: Scientific American, July 1991.

Schivelbusch, Wolfgang. *Tastes of Paradise: A Social History of Spices, Stimulants, and Intoxicants.* New York: Pantheon Books, 1980.

Seymour, Richard G. and David E. Smith. *Still Free After All These Years, 1967-1987.* San Francisco: Partisan Press, 1986.

Silver, Gary and Michael Aldrich. *The Dope Chronicles: 1850-1950.* San Francisco: Harper and Row Publishers, 1979.

Starks, Michael. *Cocaine Fiends and Reefer Madness: An Illustrated History of Drugs in the Movies.* New York: Cornwall Books, 1982.

U.S. Congress. House. *Perspectives on the History of Psychoactive Substance Use.* Research Issues 24. DHEW Publication no. (ADM) 79-810. Rockville, MD. GPO, 1979.

Chapter 2—Heredity, Environment, Psychoactive Drugs

ABC's of the Human Mind. Pleasantville, NY: Reader's Digest, 1990.

Barondes, Samuel H. *Molecules and Mental Illness.* New York: Scientific American Library, 1993.

Blum, Kenneth, John G. Cull, Eric R. Braverman, and David E. Comings. "Reward Deficiency Syndrome." *American Scientist Magazine* 84 (March-April 1996):132-145.

Blum, Kenneth and James E. Payne. *Alcohol and the Addictive Brain.* New York: The Free Press, 1991.

Chafetz, Michael D. *Nutrition and Neurotransmitters: The Nutrient Bases of Behavior.* Englewood Cliffs, NJ: Prentice Hall, 1990.

Cohen, Sydney. *The Chemical Mind: The Neurochemistry of Addictive Disorders,* Minneapolis, MN: CompCare® Publishers, 1988.

Glants, Meyer and Roy Pickens. *Vulnerability to Drug Abuse.* Washington, DC: American Psychological Association, 1992.

Harvey, Richard A. and Pamela C. Champe. *Pharmacology*. Philadelphia, PA: J.B. Lippincott Company, 1992.

Kandel, Eric R., James H. Schwartz, and Thomas M. Jessel. *Principles of Neural Science*. 3d ed. New York: Elsevier, 1991.

Krause, Carol. *How Healthy Is Your Family Tree?* New York: Fireside, 1995.

Lullmann, Heinz, Klaus Mohr, Albrecht Ziegler, and Detlef Bieger. *Color Atlas of Pharmacology*. New York: Thieme Medical Publishers, 1993.

Miller, David and Kenneth Blum. *Overload: Attention Deficit Disorder and the Addictive Brain*. Kansas City, MO: Andrews and McMeel, 1996.

Mind and Brain. New York: W. H. Freeman and Company, 1993.

Restak, Richard M., M.D. *Receptors*. New York: Bantam Books, 1994.

Seeburger, Francis F. *Addiction and Responsibility: An Inquiry into the Addictive Mind*. New York: The Crossroad Publishing Company, 1993.

Seymour, Richard B. and David E. Smith. *Drugfree: A Unique, Positive Approach to Staying Off Alcohol and Other Drugs*. New York: Harrington, 1987. Available through Haight-Ashbury Publications, 409 Clayton St., San Francisco, CA 94117.

——. *The Guide to Psychoactive Drugs*. New York: Harrington, 1987. Also available through Haight-Ashbury Publications.

Snyder, Solomon H. *Drugs and the Brain*. New York: Scientific American Library, 1986.

Chapter 3—Uppers

American Medical Association, Department of Substance Abuse. *Balancing the Response to Prescription Drug Abuse*. Chicago, IL: American Medical Association, 1990.

The Coke Book. New York: Berkeley Books, 1984.

Gold, Mark S. *800-COCAINE*. Toronto: Bantam Books, 1984.

Grinspoon, Lester and James B. Bakalar. *Cocaine: A Drug and Its Social Evolution*. New York: Basic Books, Inc., 1985.

Heimann, Robert K. *Tobacco & Americans*. New York: McGraw-Hill Book Company, Inc. 1960.

Lee, David. *Cocaine: Consumer's Handbook*. Berkeley, CA: And/Or Press, 1976.

Smith, David E. and Donald R. Wesson. *Treating Cocaine Dependency*. Center City, MN: Hazelden Foundation, 1988.

U.S. Congress. House. Committee on Energy and Commerce. Subcommittee on Health and the Environment. *Advertising of Tobacco Products*. 99th Cong., 2d sess., 1986. Serial 99-167.

——. Committee on Labor and Human Resources. *Tobacco Product Education and Health Protection Act of 1990*. 101st Cong., 2d sess., 1990. S 1883. pts. 1 and 2.

——. *Hearings on Tobacco Advertising*. 100th Cong., 1st sess., 1987. Serial 100-20.

——. Subcommittee on Oversight and Investigations. *Cigarette Advertising and the HHS Anti-Smoking Campaign*. 97th Cong., 1st sess., 1981. Serial 97-66.

——. Subcommittee on Transportation and Hazardous Materials. *Tobacco Issues*. 101st Cong., 1st sess., 1989. pts. 1 and 2. Serial 101-85 and 101-126.

——. Subcommittee on Transportation, Tourism, and Hazardous Materials. *Cigarettes: Advertising, Testing, and Liability*. 100th Cong., 2d sess., 1988. Serial 100-217.

——. *Tobacco Product Education and Health Protection Act of 1991*. S.1088. 102d Cong., 1st sess., 1991.

U.S. Department of Health and Human Services. Substance Abuse and Mental Health Services Administration. Center for Substance Abuse Treatment. *Assessment and Treatment of Cocaine-Abusing Methadone-Maintained Patients*. Rockville, MD: DHHS Publication no. (SMA) 94-3003, 1994.

White, Peter T. *Coca*. Washington, DC: National Geographic Magazine, Vol. 175, no.1, Jan 1989.

Chapter 4—Downers: Opiates/Opioids and Sedative-Hypnotics

Browning, Frank and the Editors of Ramparts. *Smack!* New York: Harrow Books, 1972.

Colvin, Rod. *Prescription Drug Abuse: The Hidden Epidemic: A Guide for Coping and Understanding*. Omaha, NE: Addicus Books, Inc., 1995.

Smith, David E., Donald R. Wesson, and Donald J. Tusel. *Treating Opiate Dependency*. Center City, MN: Hazelden. 1989.

U.S. Department of Health and Human Services. Substance Abuse and Mental Health Services Administration. Center for Substance Abuse Treatment. *Treatment of Opiate Addiction With Methadone*. Rockville, MD: DHHS Publication no. (SMA) 94-2061, 1995.

——. *LAAM in the Treatment of Opiate Addiction*. Rockville, MD: DHHS Publication no. (SMA) 95-3052, 1994.

——. *Membranes and Barriers: Targeted Drug Delivery*. Rockville, MD: NIH Publication no. 95-3889, 1995.

——. National Institutes of Health. *Opioid Peptides: Medicinal Chemistry*. Research Monograph no. 69. DHHS Publication no. (ADM)87-1454. Rockville, MD, 1987.

——. *Progress in Opioid Research*. Research Monograph no. 75. DHHS Publication no. (ADM)87-1507. Rockville, MD, 1987.

Zackon, Fred M. *Heroin: The Street Narcotic*. New York: Chelsea House, 1992.

Chapter 5—Downers: Alcohol

Basini, Richard A. *How to Cut Down Your Social Drinking*. New York: G. P. Putnam's Sons, 1985.

Gorski, Terence T. *The Staying Sober Workbook*. rev. ed. Independence, MO: Herald House/Independence Press, 1992.

Hester, Reid K. and William R. Miller, eds. *Handbook of Alcoholism Treatment Approaches: Effective Alternatives*. Boston: Allyn and Bacon, 1989.

Kinney, Jean, and Swen Leaton. *Loosening the Grip: A Handbook of Alcohol Information*. 5th ed. St. Louis, MO: Mosby-Year Book, Inc., 1995.

Matthews, Jim. *Beer, Booze, and Books: A Sober Look at Higher Education*. Peterborouogh, NH: Viaticum Press, 1995.

O'Brien, Robert and Morris Chafetz. *The Encyclopedia of Alcoholism*, 2d ed. New York: Facts on File, 1991.

Pernanen, Kai. *Alcohol in Human Violence*. New York: The Guilford Press, 1991.

Schlaadt, Richard G. *Alcohol Use & Abuse*. Guilford, CT: The Dushkin Publishing Group, Inc., 1992.

U.S. Congress. House. Subcommittee on Telecommunications, Consumer Protection, and Finance. *Beer and Wine Advertising: Impact of Electronic Media*. 99th Cong., 1st sess., 1985. Serial 99-16.

——. Select Committee on Children, Youth, and Families. *Confronting the Impact of Alcohol Labeling and Marketing on Native American Health and Culture*. 102d Cong., 2d sess., 1992.

U.S. Congress. Senate. Committee on Commerce, Science, and Transportation. Subcommittee on Consumer Affairs. *Alcohol Beverage Advertising Act*. S.664. 102d Cong., 2d sess., 1992.

——. *The Sensible Advertising and Family Education Act*. S.674. 103d Cong., 1st sess., 1993.

U.S. Department of Health and Human Services. National Institutes of Health.

U.S. Department of Health and Human Services. National Institutes of Health. *Alcohol and Health: From the Secretary of Health and Human Services, September 1993*. Eighth Special Report to the U. S. Congress.

——. *Alcohol and Interpersonal Violence: Fostering Multidisciplinary Perspectives*. Research Monograph no. 24. NIH Publication no. 93-3496. Rockville, MD, 1993.

Vaillant, George E. *The Natural History of Alcoholism Revisited*. Cambridge, MA: Harvard U.P., 1995.

Chapter 6—All Arounders

Furst, Peter T. *Hallucinogens and Culture*. San Francisco, CA: Chandler & Sharp Publishers, Inc., 1976.

Herer, Jack. *The Emperor Wears No Clothes: Hemp and the Marijuana Conspiracy*. Van Nuys, CA: Queen of Clubs Publishing, 1991.

High Times Magazine. New York: Transhigh Corp., 1967 to present.

Keys, John D. *Chinese Herbs*. Rutland, VT: Charles E. Tuttle Co., Inc., 1976.

Lyttle, Thomas, editor. *Psychedelics*. New York: Barricade Books Inc., 1994.

McKenna, Terence. *Food of the Gods: The Search for the Original Tree of Knowledge, A Radical History of Plants, Drugs, and Human Evolution*. New York: Bantam Books, 1992.

Milkman, Harvey and Stanley Sunderwirth. *Craving for Ecstasy*. Lexington, MA: Lexington Books, 1987.

Ott, Jonathan. *Hallucinogenic Plants of North America*. Berkeley, CA: Wingbow Press, 1976.

Richardson, Jim. *Sinsemilla*. Berkeley, CA: And/Or Press, 1976.

Schultes, Richard Evans and Albert Hoffman. *The Botany and Chemistry of Hallucinogens*. Springfield, IL: Charles C. Thomas, 1980.

——*Plants of the Gods*. Rochester, VT: Healing Arts Press, 1992.

Smith, Michael Valentine. *Psychedelic Chemistry*. Port Townsend, WA: Loompanics Unlimited, 1981.

Von Bibra, Baron Ernst. *Plant Intoxicants.* Rochester, VT: Healing Arts Press, (1855; reprint, 1995).

Chapter 7—Other Drugs, Other Addictions

Arnheim, Daniel D. and William E. Prentice. *Principles of Athletic Training.* 8th ed. St. Louis, MO: Mosby-Year Book, Inc., 1993.

Banks, Robert, Jr., editor. *Substance Abuse in Sport: The Realities.* Dubuque, IA: The United States Sports Academy/Kendall/Hunt Publishing Co., 1990.

Bilodeau, Lorrainne. *The Anger Workbook.* Minneapolis, MN: CompCare® Publishers, 1992.

Carnes, Patrick. *Out of the Shadows: Understanding Sexual Addiction.* 2d ed. Minneapolis, MN: CompCare® Publishers, 1992.

Dean, Ward and John Morgenthaler. *Smart Drugs & Nutrients.* Santa Cruz, CA: B & J Publications, 1990.

Estes, Ken and Mike Brubaker. *Deadly Odds: Recovery From Compulsive Gambling.* New York: Fireside/Parkside, 1994.

Heinemann, Allen W. *Substance Abuse & Physical Disability.* New York: The Hayworth Press, 1993.

Meeks, Linda, Philip Heit, and Randy Page. *Violence Prevention.* Blacklick, OH: Meeks Heit Publishing Company, Inc., 1995.

Miller, Merlene and David Miller. *Reversing the Weight Gain Spiral: The Groundbreaking Program for Lifelong Weight Control.* New York: Ballantine Books, 1994.

Mottram, D. R. *Drugs in Sport.* Champaign, IL: Human Kinetics Books, 1988.

Siegel, Michele, Judith Brisman, and Margot Weinshel. *Surviving An Eating Disorder: Strategies for Family and Friends.* New York: Harper and Row Publishers, 1988.

Tricker, Ray and David L. Cook. *Athletes at Risk: Drugs and Sport.* Dubuque, IA: Wm. C. Brown Publishers, 1990.

U.S. Congress. House. Hearing before the Subcommittee on Crime of the Committee on the Judiciary, House of Representatives, March 22, 1990. *Abuse of Steroids in Amateur and Professional Athletics.*

——. Office of the Inspector General. *Adolescent Steroid Use.* 1991.

U.S. Department of Health and Human Services. National Institutes of Health. *Inhalant Abuse: A Volatile Research Agenda.* NIH Publication no. 93-3475. Rockville, MD, 1992.

Wadler, Gary I. and Brian Hainline. *Drugs and the Athlete.* Philadelphia, PA: F.A. Davis Company, 1989.

Chapter 8—Drug Use and Prevention: From Cradle to Grave

Alcamo and Wistreich. *Aids and Sexually Transmitted Diseases.* Dubuque, IA: Wm. C. Brown Publishers, 1994.

Anspaugh, David J., Michael H. Hamrick, and Frank D. Rosato. *Wellness: Concepts and Applications.* St. Louis, MO: Mosby-Year Book, Inc., 1991.

Bates, Carson, and James Wigtil. *Skill-Building Activities for Alcohol and Drug Education.* Boston: Jones and Bartlett Publishers, Inc., 1994.

Brill, Naomi I. *Working with People.* 4th ed. New York: Longman, 1990.

Cottrell, Randall R. *Wellness: Stress Management.* Guilford, CT: The Dushkin Publishing Group, Inc., 1992

Dugan, Timothy F., and Robert Coles, eds. *The Child in Our Times.* New York: Brunner/Mazel, Inc., 1989.

Elias, Maurice J., and Steven E. Tobias. *Problem Solving/Decision Making.* National Education Association of the United States, 1990.

Ellis, Dave. *Becoming a Master Student.* 7th ed. Boston: Houghton Mifflin Company, 1994.

Fox, C. Lynn and Shirley E. Forbing. *Creating Drug-Free Schools and Communities: A Comprehensive Approach.* New York: Harper Collins Publishers, 1992.

Gerstein, Dean R. and Lawrence W. Green, eds. *Preventing Drug Abuse: What Do We Know?* Washington, DC: National Academy Press, 1993.

Hazelden. *Refusal Skills.* Center City, MN: Hazelden Foundation, 1993.

Holstein, Michael E., William E. Cohen and Paul J. Steinbroner. *A Matter of Balance: Personal Strategies for Alcohol and Other Drugs.* Ashland, OR: CNS Publications, Inc., 1995.

Jackson, Tom. *Activities That Teach.* Cedar City, UT: 1993.

Legalizing Drugs. San Diego, CA: Greenhaven Press, Inc., 1996.

Miller, Merlene, and Terence T. Gorski. *Lowering the Risk.* Independence, MO: Herald House/Independence Press, 1991.

National Association of Secondary School Principals. *Classrooms Under the Influence: Reaching Early Adolescent Children of Alcoholics.* Reston, VA: 1994.

National Research Council. *Preventing Drug Abuse.* Washington, DC: National Academy Press, 1993.

Presley, Cheryl A., Philip W. Meilman, and Rob Lyerla. *Use, Consequences, and Perceptions of the Campus Environment. Vol 1, Alcohol and Drugs on American College Campuses.* Carbondale, IL: The Core Institute, 1993.

——. *Alcohol and Drugs on American College Campuses: Use, Consequences, and Perceptions of the Campus Environment.* Carbondale, IL: Southern Illinois University, 1993.

U.S. Congress. Office of Technology Assessment. *Technologies for Understanding and Preventing Substance Abuse and Addiction.* n.d.

——. Committee on the Judiciary. *Hearing on Domestic Violence.* 103d Cong., 1st sess., 1993. Serial J-103-2.

U.S. Department of Education. *Alcohol and Drug Programs at Higher Education Institutions.* Higher Education Surveys Report, Survey Number 18. 1995.

U.S. Department of Health and Human Services. National Institutes of Health. *Adolescent Drug Use Prevention: Common Features of Promising Community Programs.* GAO/PEMD-92-2. Rockville, MD, 1992.

——. *Children: Getting a Head Start Against Drugs.* Teacher's Guide by Sylvia Carter and Ura Jean Oyemade. DHHS Publication no. (SMA)93-1970. 1993.

——. *Cultural Competence for Evaluators: A Guide for Alcohol and Other Drug Abuse Prevention Practitioners Working With Ethnic/Racial Communities.* DHHS Publication no. (ADM) 92-1884. 1992.

——. *Drug Abuse Prevention Research.* DHHS Publication no. (ADM) 83-1270. Rockville, MD, 1993.

——. *Etiology of Drug Abuse: Implications for Prevention.* NIDA Research Monograph 56. Rockville, MD, 1985.

——. *Evaluation and Management of Early HIV Infection.* Clinical Practice Guideline, Number 7. AHCPR Publication no. 94-0572. 1994.

——. *Experiences With Community Action Projects: New Research in the Prevention of Alcohol and Other Drug Problems.* CSAP Prevention Monograph 14. 1993.

——. *Making the Case for Prevention: A Discussion Paper on Preventing Alcohol, Tobacco, and Other Drug Problems.* 1993.

——. *Parents: Getting a Head Start Against Drugs. Activity Book and Trainer's Guide.* Authored by Sylvia Carter and Ura Jean Oyemade. DHHS Publication no. (SMA)93-1971. 1993.

——. *Preventing Tobacco Use Among Young People: A Report of the Surgeon General.* 1994.

——. Public Health Service. *Prevention Plus III: Assessing Alcohol and Other Drug Prevention Programs at the School and Community Level: A Four-Step Guide to Useful Program Assessment.* Publication no. (ADM)91-1817. Rockville, MD, 1991.

——. *Proceedings of a National Conference on Preventing Alcohol and Drug Abuse in Black Communities.* DHHS Publication no. (ADM)89-1648. 1990.

——. *Signs of Effectiveness II. Preventing Alcohol, Tobacco, and Other Drug Use: A Risk Factor/Resiliency-Based Approach.* DHHS Publication no. (SAM) 94-2098. 1994.

——. *Social Networks, Drug Abuse, and HIV Transmission.* Research Monograph 151. NIH Publication no. 95-3889, 1995.

U.S. Department of Justice. Bureau of Justice Statistics. *Drugs, Crime, and the Justice System.* 1994.

U.S. General Accounting Office. Committee on Education and Labor, House of Representatives. Report to the Chairman, Subcommittee on Select Education. *Adolescent Drug Use Prevention.* PEMD-92-2.

Weston Woods Institute. *Counseling Children of Alcoholics: Fostering Resiliency.* Weston, CT: The Media Group of Connecticut, Inc., 1994.

The White House. *Preventing Crime and Promoting Responsibility: 50 Programs That Help Communities Help Their Youth.* The President's Crime Prevention Council, 1995.

Chapter 9—Treatment

Bell, Tammy L. *Adolescent Relapse Warning Signs.* Independence, MO: Herald House/Independence Press, 1989.

CALADATA: Evaluating Recovery Services: California Alcohol and Drug Treatment Assessment Execu-

tive Summary. Sacramento, CA: California Department of Alcohol and Drug Programs Resource Center, 1994.

Carnes, Patrick. *A Gentle Path Through the Twelve Steps.* Minneapolis, MN: CompCare® Publishers, 1993.

Davis, Kenneth, Howard Klar, and Joseph T. Coyle. *Foundations of Psychiatry.* Philadelphia: W.B. Saunders, 1991.

Galanter, Marc and Herbert D. Kleber. *Textbook of Substance Abuse Treatment.* Washington, DC: The American Psychiatric Press, 1994.

Goldenberg, Irene, and Herbert Goldenberg. *My Self in Family Context.* Belmont, CA, 1991.

Gorski, Terence T. *Addictive Relationships: Why Love Goes Wrong in Recovery.* Independence, MO: Herald House/Independence Press, 1993.

Kus, Robert J., R.N., Ph.D. *Addiction and Recovery in Gay and Lesbian Persons.* New York: Harrington Park Press, 1995.

Lewis, Judith A., Robert Q. Dana, and Gregory A. Blevins. *Substance Abuse Counseling.* 2d ed. Pacific Grove, CA: Brooks/Cole Publishing Company, 1994.

Moore, Thomas. *Care of the Soul.* New York: Harper Collins Publishers, Inc., 1992.

Oregon Prevention Resource Center. *A Guide to Self-Help Groups for Alcohol and Drug Addiction.* Salem, OR, 1991.

Pita, Dianne Doyle. *Addictions Counseling.* New York: The Crossroad Publishing Company, 1994.

U.S. Department of Health and Human Services. National Institutes of Health. National Institute on Drug Abuse. *Cue Extinction: In-Service Training Curriculum.* NIH Publication no. 993-3692. Rockville, MD, 1993.

——. *Drug Abuse Among Minority Youth: Methodological Issues and Recent Research Advances.* NIDA Research Monograph 130. Rockville, MD, 1993.

——. *Youth and Drugs: Society's Mixed Messages.* OSAP Prevention Monograph 6. DHHS Publication no. (ADM) 90-1689. Rockville, MD, 1990.

U.S. Department of Justice. National Institute of Justice. *The Effectiveness of Treatment for Drug Abusers Under Criminal Justice Supervision.* 1995.

——. *Speaking Out Against Drug Legalization.* 1995.

U.S. Federal Bureau of Prisons. *Understanding Substance Abuse & Treatment.* Washington, DC, 1992.

Chapter 10—Dual Diagnosis

American Psychiatric Association. *Diagnostic and Statistical Manual of Mental Disorders.* 4th ed. DSM-IV. Washington, DC: American Psychiatric Association, 1994.

Barondes, Samuel H., M.D. *Molecules and Mental Illness.* New York: Scientific American Library, 1993.

Bourne, Edmund J. *The Anxiety & Phobia Workbook.* Oakland, CA: New Harbinger Publications, Inc., 1990.

Davis, Kenneth, Howard Klar, and Joseph T. Coyle. *Foundations of Psychiatry.* Philadelphia: Harcourt Brace Jovanovich, Inc., 1991.

Evans, Katie and J. Michael Sullivan. *Dual Diagnosis: Counseling the Mentally Ill Substance Abuser.* New York: The Guilford Press, 1990.

Keltner, Norman L. and David G. Folks. *Psychotropic Drugs.* St. Louis, MO: Mosby-Year Book, Inc., 1993.

Salloum, Ihsan M., M.D., and Dennis C. Daley. *Understanding Major Anxiety Disorders and Addiction.* Center City, MN: Hazelden Foundation, 1994.

U.S. Department of Health and Human Services. Substance Abuse and Mental Health Services Administration. Center for Substance Abuse Treatment. *Approaches in the Treatment of Adolescents with Emotional and Substance Abuse Problems.* Rockville, MD: DHHS Publication no. (SMA) 93-1744, 1993.

——. *Assessment and Treatment of Patients with Coexisting Mental Illness and Alcohol and Other Drug Abuse.* Rockville, MD: DHHS Publication no. (SMA) 95-3061, 1995.

——. *Coordination of Alcohol, Drug Abuse, and Mental Health Services.* Rockville, MD: DHHS Publication no. (SMA) 93-1742, 1993.

INDEX